Recent Advances in

Obstetrics and Gynaecology 23

Recent Advances in Obstetrics and Gynaecology 22
Edited by John Bonnar and William Dunlop

SECTION ONE: **Obstetrics**
Advances in the management of the antiphospholipid syndrome
Shehnaaz Jivraj, Rajendra S. Rai

The clinical implications of thrombophilia in pregnancy
John R. Higgins, Joanne Said

Clinical applications of fetal therapy
José L. Bartha, Peter W. Soothill

Investigation and management of the small fetus
Stephen A. Walkinshaw, Lindsay Cochrane

Management of abnormal liver function in pregnancy
Mark D. Kilby, Katherine J. Barber

Can the high Caesarean section rates be reduced?
Michael S. Robson

Maternal and neonatal morbidity following operative delivery in the second stage of labour
Deirdre J. Murphy

SECTION TWO: **Gynaecology**
The evidence-based practice of assisted reproduction
Hassan N. Sallam

Menorrhagia and bleeding disorders
Rezan A. Kadir, Demetrious L. Economides

Evidence-based surgical treatment for dysfunctional uterine bleeding
David E. Parkin, Stuart Jack

Evaluation of arterial embolisation of uterine fibroids
John Reidy, Bruce McLucas

Reducing the complications of minimal access pelvic surgery
Fiona Reid, Anthony R.B. Smith

Advances in the surgical management of vaginal prolapse
Patrick Hogston

Advances in the treatment of endometrial cancer
Rick D. Clayton, Desmond P.J. Barton

Index

ISBN 1–85315–529–2

ISSN 0143 6848

Recent Advances in

Obstetrics and Gynaecology 23

Edited by

John Bonnar MA MD (Hons) FRCOG FRCPI

Emeritus Professor of Obstetrics and Gynaecology, Trinity College,
University of Dublin; Fellow of Trinity College, Dublin;
Trinity Centre for Health Sciences, St James' Hospital, Dublin, Ireland

William Dunlop PhD FRCSEd FRCOG

Professor of Obstetrics and Gynaecology,
School of Surgical and Reproductive Sciences,
University of Newcastle upon Tyne,
Royal Victoria Hospital,
Newcastle upon Tyne, England

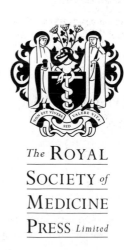

The ROYAL
SOCIETY *of*
MEDICINE
PRESS *Limited*

© 2005 Royal Society of Medicine Press Ltd

Published by the Royal Society of Medicine Press Ltd
1 Wimpole Street, London W1G 0AE, UK
Tel: +44 (0)20 7290 2921
Fax: +44 (0)20 7290 2929
Email: publishing@rsm.ac.uk
Website: www.rsmpress.co.uk

British Library Cataloguing in Publication Data
A catalogue record for this book is available from the British Library

ISBN 1-85315-605-1
ISSN 0143-6848

Distribution in Europe and Rest of World:
Marston Book Services Ltd
PO Box 269
Abingdon
Oxon OX14 4YN, UK
Tel: +44 (0)1235 465500
Fax: +44 (0)1235 465555
Email: direct.order@marston.co.uk

Distribution in the USA and Canada:
Royal Society of Medicine Press Ltd
c/o Jamco Distribution Inc
1401 Lakeway Drive
Lewisville, TX 75057, USA
Tel: +1 800 538 1287
Fax: +1 972 353 1303
Email: jamco@majors.com

Distribution in Australia and New Zealand:
Elsevier Australia
30-52 Smidmore Street
Marrikville NSW 2204, Australia
Tel: +61 2 9517 8999
Fax: +61 2 9517 2249
Email: service@elsevier.com.au

Commissioning editor - Peter Richardson
Editorial assistant - Hannah Wessely

Editorial services and typesetting by GM & BA Haddock, Midlothian, Scotland, UK
Printed and bound by Krips b.v., Meppel, The Netherlands

Contents

Section one: **OBSTETRICS**

1. Antenatal screening for Down's syndrome 1
   Stephen Ong, Martin Whittle

2. Preterm labour: prediction and treatment 15
   Honest Honest, Khalid S. Khan

3. Preterm prelabour rupture of the membranes 27
   Penny C. McParland, David J. Taylor

4. Dysfunctional labour 39
   Mark Tattersall, Siobhan Quenby

5. Domestic violence: opportunities for effective responses
   in maternity services 53
   Loraine Bacchus, Susan Bewley

6. Group B streptococcus in pregnancy 65
   Peter Brocklehurst, Sara Kenyon

7. Place of birth: evidence for best practice 77
   Otto P. Bleker, Leonie A.M. van der Hulst,
   Martine Eskes, Gouke J. Bonsel

8. Confidential Enquiries: learning lessons in maternal and
   perinatal health 101
   Mary C.M. Macintosh

9. Risk management in obstetrics   119
   James Walker

Section two: **GYNAECOLOGY**

10. Deciding on the appropriate surgery for stress incontinence   133
    Lucia M. Dolan, Paul Hilton

11. What's new in polycystic ovary syndrome?   147
    Adam H. Balen, Martin R. Glass

12. Update on endometrial ablation   159
    Michael J. Gannon, Peter O'Donovan

13. Total or subtotal hysterectomy – what is the evidence?   169
    Helga Gimbel

14. Pelvic imaging of endometriosis   183
    Gormlaith C. Hargaden, Mary Keogan

15. Surgery for advanced endometriosis   193
    Enda McVeigh, Philippe R. Koninckx

16. Emergency contraception: a global overview among
    potential users   209
    Deborah N. P. Haggai

Section Three: **GYNAECOLOGICAL ONCOLOGY**

17. Diagnosis and management of pre-invasive cervical
    glandular neoplasia   219
    Alaa A. El-Ghobashy, C. Simon Herrington

18. Recent advances in the surgical management of
    cervical cancer   231
    M. Hannemann, J. Bailey, J. Murdoch

19. Overview of ovarian cancer screening   243
    Adam N. Rosenthal, Ian Jacobs

Index   260

Contributors

Loraine Bacchus BSc MA PhD
Research Associate, Kings College London, Florence Nightingale School of Nursing and Midwifery, Women's Health Academic Unit, St Thomas's Hospital, London, UK

Jo Bailey FRCS(Ed) MRCOG
Subspecialty Trainee in Gynaecological Oncology, Directorate of Obstetrics and Gynaecology and ENT, United Bristol Healthcare NHS Trust, St Michael's Hospital, Bristol, UK

Adam H. Balen MD FRCOG
Professor of Reproductive Medicine and Surgery, The General Infirmary, Leeds, UK

Susan Bewley MB BS MA MD FRCOG
Consultant Obstetrician/Maternal Fetal Medicine, Women's Services Directorate, St Thomas's Hospital, London, UK

Otto P. Bleker MD PhD FRCOG
Professor of Obstetrics and Gynaecology, Academic Medical Center, Amsterdam, The Netherlands

Gouke J. Bonsel MD PhD
Professor of Public Health Methods, Department of Social Medicine, Academic Medical Center, Amsterdam, The Netherlands

Peter Brocklehurst MBChB FRCOG MSc (Epidemiology)
Director, National Perinatal Epidemiology Unit, University of Oxford, Oxford, UK

Lucia M. Dolan MB BCh MRCGP MRCOG
Consultant Gynaecologist and Sub-specialist in Urogynaecology, Edinburgh Royal Infirmary, Edinburgh, UK

Alaa A. El-Ghobashy MD MRCOG
Specialist Registrar in Obstetrics and Gynaecology, Bradford Royal Infirmary, Bradford, West Yorkshire, UK

Martine Eskes MD PhD
Obstetrician and Gynaecologist, Medical Advisor at the Health Care
Insurance Board (CVZ), Diemen, The Netherlands

Michael J. Gannon MB PhD FRCSI FRCOG
Consultant Obstetrician and Gynaecologist, Midland Regional Hospital,
Mullingar, Ireland

Helga Gimbel MD
Specialist Registrar, Department of Obstetrics and Gynaecology, Hillerød
County Hospital, Hillerød, Denmark

Martin R. Glass MD FRCOG
Consultant Obstetrician and Gynaecologist, The General Infirmary, Leeds, UK

Deborah N. P. Haggai MBBCh FWACS MSc Reproductive Health
Consultant/Lecturer, Department of Obstetrics and Gynaecology, Ahmadu
Bello University Teaching Hospital, Zaria, Kaduna State, Nigeria

Michael Hannemann MBBCh MRCOG PhD
Specialist Registrar, Directorate of Obstetrics and Gynaecology and ENT,
United Bristol Healthcare NHS Trust, St Michael's Hospital, Bristol, UK

Gormlaith C. Hargaden MB MRCPI FFR(RCSI)
Specialist Registrar in Radiology, Department of Radiology, St James's
Hospital, Dublin, Ireland

C. Simon Herrington MA DPhil FRCP FRCPath
Professor of Pathology, University of St Andrews, St Andrews, Fife, UK

Paul Hilton MD FRCOG
Consultant Gynaecologist, Directorate of Women's Services, Royal Victoria
Infirmary, Newcastle upon Tyne, UK

Honest Honest MBChB
Specialist Registrar in Obstetrics & Gynaecology, Birmingham Womens'
Hospital, Birmingham, UK

Ian Jacobs MD FRCOG
Professor of Gynaecological Oncology and Director, Institute of Women's
Health, University College London, Elizabeth Garrett Anderson Hospital,
London, UK

Sara Kenyon RM MA (Applied Health Studies)
Senior Research Fellow, Reproductive Sciences Section, Department of
Cancer and Molecular Studies, University of Leicester, Leicester, UK

Mary Keogan MB MRCPI FRCR
Consultant Radiologist, Department of Radiology, St James's Hospital,
Dublin, and Senior Lecturer in Radiology, Trinity College Dublin, Ireland

Khalid S. Khan MRCOG MSc
Professor of Obstetrics and Gynaecology, Birmingham Women's Hospital,
Edgbaston, Birmingham, UK

Philippe R. Koninckx MD PhD
Professor of Obstetrics and Gynaecology, Catholic University Leuven,
Belgium and Head of Division of Endoscopic Surgery. Visiting Professor and
Honorary Consultant, University of Oxford, UK

Mary C.M. Macintosh MA MRCOG MD
Medical Director, CEMACH, Chiltern Court, London, UK

Penny C. McParland PhD MRCOG
Reproductive Science Section, Department of Cancer Studies and Molecular
Medicine, University of Leicester, Leicester Royal Infirmary, Leicester, UK

Enda McVeigh MB BCh BAO MPhil MRCOG
Senior Fellow and Honorary Consultant, Nuffield Department of Obstetrics
and Gynaecology, John Radcliffe Hospital, University of Oxford, Oxford, UK

John Murdoch MD FRCOG
Consultant, Directorate of Obstetrics and Gynaecology and ENT, United
Bristol Healthcare NHS Trust, St Michael's Hospital, Bristol, UK

Peter O'Donovan MB FRCS FRCOG
Professor of Obstetrics and Gynaecology, Bradford Royal Infirmary, Bradford, UK

Stephen Ong MD MRCOG
Subspecialty Trainee in Fetal and Maternal Medicine, Department of Fetal
Medicine, Birmingham Women's Hospital, Birmingham, UK

Siobhan Quenby MD
Senior Lecturer/Honorary Consultant, School of Reproductive and
Developmental Medicine, Liverpool Women's Hospital, Liverpool, UK

Adam Rosenthal PhD MRCOG
Clinical Lecturer in Gynaecological Oncology, Institute of Women's Health,
University College London, Elizabeth Garrett Anderson Hospital, London, UK

Mark Tattersall BMBCh
Specialist Registrar, School of Reproductive and Developmental Medicine,
Liverpool Women's Hospital, Liverpool, UK

David J. Taylor MD FRCOG
Reproductive Science Section, Department of Cancer Studies and Molecular
Medicine, University of Leicester, Leicester Royal Infirmary, Leicester, UK

Leonie A.M. van der Hulst MA
Midwife and Sociologist, Department of Obstetrics and Gynaecology,
Academic Medical Center, Amsterdam, The Netherlands

James J. Walker MD FRCP(Edin) FRCPS(Glas) FRCOG
Professor of Obstetrics and Gynaecology, University of Leeds, UK and Clinical
Specialty Adviser (Obstetrics), National Patient Safety Agency, London, UK

Martin Whittle MD FRCOG FRCP(Glas)
Professor and Head of Academic Department of Obstetrics and Gynaecology,
Department of Fetal Medicine, Birmingham Women's Hospital, Birmingham, UK

Stephen Ong Martin Whittle

1

Antenatal screening for Down's syndrome

Screening for Down's syndrome was originally based on maternal age, justified by the observation that the incidence of the condition rises significantly from when the woman is 35 years of age. In the past, women aged over 35 (and certainly 37 years of age) were offered amniocentesis or chorionic villus sampling. In the 1970s, when only 5% of the population was greater than 35 years of age, this seemed a reasonable approach, although such an approach would only detect 30% all Down's affected pregnancies. Changing population demographics has meant that in parts of the UK, 15% of women are more than 35 years of age.[1] If they were all to be offered an invasive test this would result in a detection rate of 54%. However such a high intervention rate for a relatively low detection rate would be unacceptable.

Clearly, a more efficient method of screening was required and in the early 1980s it was observed that a low α-fetoprotein (AFP) level was associated with Down's syndrome.[2] AFP, which had until that time been effective in the screening for neural tube defects, became the first biochemical test to be used to screen for Down's syndrome.[3] However, it became apparent that AFP was a weak test with about a 35% detection rate for a 5% false positive rate.[4] A second analyte, human chorionic gonadotrophin (hCG), was introduced in the late 1980s (the double test). This produced a detection rate of about 58% for a 5% false positive rate, and this method of screening became the 'gold standard' for screening both in the UK and North America for some time.

The triple test, which required the use of a third analyte, oestriol, in addition to AFP and hCG, further reduced the false positive rate, although some

Stephen Ong MD MRCOG
Subspecialty Trainee in Fetal and Maternal Medicine, Department of Fetal Medicine, Birmingham Women's Hospital, Birmingham B15 2TG, UK

Martin Whittle MD FRCOG FRCP(Glas) (for correspondence)
Professor and Head of Academic Department of Obstetrics and Gynaecology, Department of Fetal Medicine, Birmingham Women's Hospital, Birmingham B15 2TG, UK. (E-mail: m.j.whittle@bham.ac.uk)

Table 1 Maternal serum screening in the second trimester: the detection rate at a fixed 5% false-positive rate

Marker	Detection rate (%)
Maternal age alone	30
Double test	58
Triple test	69
Quadruple test	76

Adapted from Wald et al.[20]

authorities disputed this fact. Nevertheless, the National Screening Committee recommended that all units should use the triple test by 2005. A further analyte, inhibin, was also recently suggested[5] and incorporated into the quadruple test. The precise value of inhibin has yet to be established.

The aim of further developments in screening was to improve detection rates whilst trying to keep intervention rates as low as possible. The efficacy of Down's screening tests can be judged by the detection rate at a fixed false-positive rate (the false-positive rate is equivalent to the screen-positive rate but is not always the same as the intervention rate).[6] Table 1 shows comparisons for current test regimens used to screen for Down's syndrome pregnancies in the second trimester at a fixed false-positive rate of 5%.

By the end of the 1990s, several issues emerged concerning screening for Down's syndrome: (i) first trimester screening became a distinct possibility; (ii) there was a general desire to continue improving detection rates and reducing intervention rates; (iii) it became obvious that the provision of information and counselling was generally lacking; and (iv) many healthcare workers began canvassing for a better infrastructure and the development of a formal national screening programme.

FIRST TRIMESTER SCREENING

There can be little doubt that many women welcome an early screening test. The motive for this is uncertain. Early reassurance is undoubtedly the most important reason but the opportunity for an early diagnosis of an affected pregnancy and its termination must also be important.

Although the debate concerning first and second trimester screening has abated somewhat, the issue is still an important one. Proponents of second trimester screening have argued that:

1. Second trimester screening is safe and well established and the woman has time to consider her choices.

2. The screening test is reasonably good.

3. The use of AFP in the second trimester also allows screening for neural tube defects.

4. The diagnostic test from second trimester screening is amniocentesis and not CVS, with its attendant implications of service availability and procedure-related loss rate.

Conversely, those favouring first trimester screening argue that:

1. Screening at this gestation allows for termination of pregnancy of an affected pregnancy at an earlier stage.

2. The test is efficient although some identified affected pregnancies would miscarry spontaneously.

3. An early normal result gives reassurance to the woman.

4. The efficiency of the first trimester result should mean that single markers of Down's syndrome in later pregnancy can be ignored.[7]

In the late 1980s and early 1990s, the improved quality of ultrasound images meant that even in early pregnancy it was possible to observe fetal abnormalities such as cystic hygroma, anencephaly and more subtle changes such as nuchal translucency (NT). NT is the fluid-filled space which appears behind the fetal neck (Fig. 1) and it was shown that increased NT was associated with Down's syndrome. NT normally measures between 1–2 mm and increases with gestation. The Fetal Medicine Foundation, led by Professor Nicolaides, specified strict criteria for obtaining a satisfactory measurement.[8]

Over the last few years, there has been much controversy concerning the detection rate of Down's syndrome using NT. In population studies, detection rates have been reported ranging from as low as 29% to as high as 91%.[9–12] However, it is interesting to note that the combined detection rate from programmes controlled by the Fetal Medicine Foundation in London is 72%.[10,11] In contrast, the combined detection rate from 6 studies outside the Fetal Medicine Foundation is only 50%.[12] There may be many reasons for the wide variation in detection rates including time available for NT measurements, under-ascertainment of Down's syndrome cases, and the use of incorrect denominator data.[12] Regardless, workers from the Fetal Medicine Foundation maintain that nuchal translucency with maternal age alone has a detection rate of 76.8% at a 4.2% false-positive rate.[8] This is at variance with the

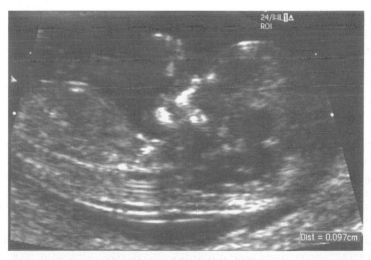

Fig. 1 Thermal image of nuchal translucency measurement.

results from the much quoted Serum, Urine and Ultrasound Screening Study (SURUSS).[13] SURUSS suggests that nuchal translucency 'has a poor performance as a screening test for Down's syndrome on its own or with maternal age alone'. Results from SURUSS estimated that NT had a 60% detection rate for a 5% false-positive rate at 10 weeks' gestation or a 69% detection rate at 12–13 weeks' gestation. Nicolaides from the Fetal Medicine Foundation has argued[8] that of the 47,053 singleton pregnancies in SURUSS, 11,025 (23.4%) women had no valid NT measurement because it was undertaken at an inappropriate gestation (n = 4228 pregnancies), the sonographer was unable to obtain a measurement (n = 3416) or that none of the images were of acceptable quality (n = 3881). He points out that achieving reliable NT measurements is dependent not only on training and adherence to standards but is also heavily dependent on the motivation of the sonographer. Nicolaides draws attention to the curious fact that, in interventional studies, successful measurements were obtained in > 99% of cases whilst in observational studies, such as SURUSS (where the sonographers recorded the measurement but did not act on the result), a successful measurement was only obtained in 78% of cases.

On balance, it is probable that in appropriately trained hands, NT would allow the detection of about 77% of Down's syndrome babies for a false-positive rate of about 4%. Second trimester results are not strictly comparable, however, because the spontaneous loss of affected pregnancies is high in the first trimester – 43% being lost by term, in contrast to 23% by term after 16 weeks.[14]

Training for first trimester screening is of particular concern. The Fetal Medicine Foundation has a successful training programme in place which sets strict criteria and continuously monitors the quality of images from trainees. Establishing a similar national programme would be challenging but not impossible. An NT service is labour intensive and requires experienced personnel who may need to be diverted from other vital radiology services (such as oncology imaging). In addition, an accurate measurement of NT mandates equipment of high quality with the capability of producing measurements in tenths of a millimetre.

Apart from improvements in ultrasound, the value of biochemical markers, such as PAPP-A and free βHCG, in the first trimester has also been established. PAPP-A is currently the single best serum marker with a 42% detection rate for a 5% false-positive rate.[15] PAPP-A is best used between 8–13 weeks' gestation and is less effective as a marker after 13 weeks.[16] In cases of Down's syndrome, PAPP-A has a concentration 2.5 times lower compared to unaffected pregnancies, with a median of 0.4 multiple of the median.[17]

Although free βHCG performs better in the second trimester as a marker, it is also useful in the first trimester. At 8–13 weeks' gestation, βHCG has a 25% detection rate for a 5% false-positive rate.[15] Free βHCG is twice as high in Down's syndrome compared to unaffected pregnancies with a median of 1.9 multiples of the median.[17]

PAPP-A, free βHCG, nuchal translucency measurement and maternal age are independent of one another. It is for this reason that the combination of these markers (combined test) provides an effective screening tool. Initial reports suggested that the combined test had an 85% detection rate for a 5%

false-positive rate.[18] Indeed, the SURUSS report would suggest that one of the benefits of including biochemistry is that it may compensate for less than perfect NT measurement.

While there may have been a difference in opinion regarding the usefulness of NT between workers from the Fetal Medicine Foundation and the SURUSS study, there seems to be less disagreement regarding the combined test. The Fetal Medicine Foundation suggests a detection rate of 87% at a 5% false-positive rate,[8] SURUSS suggests a detection rate of 85% at a 6.1% false-positive rate,[13] and the FASTER (First and Second Trimester Evaluation of Risk) trial suggests a detection rate of 85% at a 7.6% false-positive rate.[19]

IMPROVEMENT STRATEGIES

IMPROVING DETECTION RATES AND REDUCING INTERVENTION RATES

Whilst much work was being done to develop reliable methods for first trimester screening, other workers were less concerned about the gestation at which the test was performed and concentrated their efforts on improving detection rates and reducing intervention rates. The simultaneous use of markers from both the first and second trimesters constituted the integrated test. This involved first trimester nuchal translucency and PAPP-A plus a second trimester quadruple test. Mathematical modelling suggested that such a screening method would prove more efficient than screening using markers from either trimester alone.[20] The effect was larger than one would expect because first trimester screening, using nuchal translucency and PAPP-A levels, was largely independent of second trimester serum markers.[16] The utility of this approach emerged from SURUSS using modelling of the results from the first and second trimesters. The results were impressive. Fixing the false positive rate at 5%, the integrated test had a detection rate of 94% compared to the first trimester combined test of 85%. Fixing the detection rate at 85%, the integrated test has a false positive rate of 1.2% compared to the first trimester combined test of 6.1%. In real terms, this represents an 80% reduction in false positives (and hence amniocentesis performed) for the same number of Down's syndrome pregnancies detected.

In units where ultrasound facilities are not able to support the measurement of nuchal translucency, an integrated test without nuchal translucency (serum integrated test) could be used. An example of a serum integrated test is PAPP-A in the first trimester plus the quadruple test in the second trimester. This approach provides an 85% detection rate for a 2.7% false-positive rate (Table 2), materially better than any first or second trimester screening test performed alone.

The main conclusions from the SURUSS report were:

'Our results show that overall, on the basis of efficacy, safety, and cost, the integrated test is the test of choice. Adding other markers provided little benefit'.

The integrated test also received support from the FASTER trial where preliminary results suggest a detection rate of 85% at a 2.8% false-positive rate.[19] The FASTER trial also indicated that:

'Integrated screening has the lowest false positive rate at each detection rate'.

Table 2 A comparison of Down's screening tests at a fixed 85% detection rate

Tests (including maternal age)	Measurements	False-positive rate (%) for an 85% detection rate
Integrated test	NT, PAPP-A at 10 weeks; AFP, μE_3, free βHCG and inhibin A at 14–20 weeks	1.2
Serum-integrated test	PAPP-A at 10 weeks; AFP, μE_3, free βHCG and inhibin A at 14–20 weeks	2.7
Combined test	NT, free βHCG and PAPP-A at 10 weeks	6.1
Quadruple test	AFP, μE_3, free βHCG and inhibin A at 14–20 weeks	6.2
Triple test	AFP, μE_3, free βHCG at 14–20 weeks	9.3
Double test	AFP and free βHCG at 14–20 weeks	13.1
NT measurement	NT at 12–13 weeks	20.0

Adapted from Wald et al.[13]

Integrated and serum-integrated tests are now being 'field tested' but results are not yet available. To perform either the integrated or serum-integrated test, information from the first trimester is held until information from the second trimester is available and then appropriately combined. Proponents of the integrated approach are keen to stress that holding information from the first trimester is not the same as withholding information from the woman. Nicolaides is less convinced about the feasibility of the integrated test. He argues that the test assumes complete compliance by the pregnant woman in a 2-stage process that is separated by one month without receiving any information on whether the fetus looks normal, and assumes the woman will accept a second rather than first trimester diagnosis and termination.[8] Nicolaides argues that SURUSS itself highlights the immense difficulties that may be encountered. Of the 47,053 women that were recruited, 9691 (20.6%) did not attend for second trimester screening. However, if studies confirm that these screening regimens are efficient and acceptable to women, these may be the preferred tests (although the use of NT measurements, as previously mentioned, has considerable resource implications).

Apart from research organisations, government bodies have also been attempting to improve standards for Down's screening. In October 2003, guidance was issued by the National Institute for Clinical Excellence on the routine antenatal care of pregnant women. Incorporated into this was guidance on screening for Down's syndrome.[21] This was complimented by a statement from the Department of Health in November 2003 which set out 'The Model of Best Practice' to which all trusts should aspire.[22] In this document, 'benchmark timeframes' were set whereby all units should offer Down's screening with a detection rate of at least 60% with a false-positive rate of 5% or less by 2004/05. The next benchmark timeframe is April 2007. By then, all units should be offering a test which has a detection rate greater than 75% with a false-positive rate of less than 3%. These performance measures should be age-standardised and based on a cut-off of 1 in 250 at term. The following tests meet this standard:[23]

1. From 11 to 14 weeks – the combined test (NT, hCG and PAPP-A).

2. From 14 to 20 weeks – the quadruple test (hCG, AFP, μE_3, inhibin A).

3. From 11 to 14 weeks **and** 14 to 20 weeks – the integrated test (NT, PAPP-A plus hCG, AFP, μE_3, inhibin A) and the serum integrated test (PAPP-A plus hCG, AFP, μE_3, inhibin A)

The figures concerning the benchmark timeframes are, of course, average figures for the whole programme. It is important to remember that the detection rate and false-positive rate are very maternal-age sensitive. Those responsible for managing Down's syndrome screening in a relatively old population can expect to observe both a higher detection rate and higher false-positive rate than their colleagues in an identical service delivered to a younger population. However, they can both expect to have the same age-standardised rates and therefore, a single set of regional or national age standardised targets can be set.[24]

IMPROVEMENT OF PATIENT INFORMATION AND UNDERSTANDING

One of the major problems in the NHS is to provide women with comprehensible information at an appropriate time. Women who arrive for their first antenatal visit, which will rarely be before 8–10 weeks, will be bombarded with a range of information from brochures and discussions about pregnancy care. It takes a healthcare professional 6–15 min to counsel a woman about Down's screening.[23] In a recent study, 19% of women reported that prenatal screening was not fully discussed and 30% of women said that 'options after the test' were not mentioned.[25]

It seems likely that, particularly with first trimester screening for Down's syndrome, women may not be clear about what they are agreeing to. One study of a so-called 'one-stop clinic' found that 95% of women agreed to being screened.[26] This is remarkable given that screening may potentially result in an invasive procedure that could harm the pregnancy. However, 27% of women at the clinic said that they had 'never really made up their mind, but went along with what was being offered'. Furthermore, 45% of women said 'since they had been offered a screening test as part of routine care they assumed they would be having it'.[25]

In addition, an increasing problem in many large cities is the rising proportion of women for whom English is not the native language. The problem of communication when screening in the second trimester is rather less severe because women will have some time to reflect on their decision and discuss issues with their family and friends. It is obvious that the eventual diagnosis of an affected pregnancy is delayed but it seems likely that individual women will be clearer about their eventual decision.

Several initiatives have been established to improve communication. First, the National Screening Committee identified professional leads for all regions in England who subsequently established networks, comprising mainly midwives responsible for the management of Down's screening programmes in individual trusts.

Second, improved comprehensible literature has been produced at the national level. As a rule, many units produce their own literature of a quality that helps the healthcare professional explain the screening process and helps the patient understand Down's syndrome. In a recent survey, 92% of units had some form of literature available to women about Down's screening. Disappointingly, 17% of units were producing leaflets that were designed 'only' by laboratory staff and only 59% of units were currently offering literature in a language other than English.[23]

Third, the UK Government is keen to promote the use of the internet for the provision of information in health care.[27] However, in a recent survey of units providing information for Down's screening, 38% of respondents either did not have access or did not know how to access the internet,[23] let alone having access to a comprehensive web site. Although healthcare workers in general have a healthy scepticism of Government initiatives, most would recognise the potential of electronic communication. Therefore, it is important that women are encouraged to access these sources and to seek out the information they need for themselves.

DEVELOPING A NATIONAL SCREENING PROGRAMME

It is generally accepted that there is a large variation in standards and practice in the screening for Down's syndrome across the UK. To some extent this arose from the way in which Down's syndrome screening was introduced in the 1980s on the back of the AFP screening programme for open neural tube defects. This was regrettable in itself but when a second (βHCG) and a third analyte (oestriol) were shown to improve detection, implementation became even more patchy and haphazard. Implementation depended largely on local resources and enthusiasm rather than a defined policy. Not only were there technical problems but the difficulties of ensuring adequate counselling prior to women undergoing the test were not satisfactorily addressed. Indeed, this aspect was largely unfunded and often undertaken by midwives with no specific training or support. Obstetricians tended to take a back seat apart from those with an interest in prenatal diagnosis. Although the RCOG produced a working party report[28] suggesting the need for an adequate infrastructure, trained counsellors, co-ordinators, quality control and audit, the advice was largely ignored. In 1996, the UK National Screening Committee (UK NSC) was established to advise ministers on screening issues. Not surprisingly, in 1998 it found that there was inequity in the provision of services provided and variation in the type and quality of service.

Apart from the various screening methods employed by trusts, one serious deficiency concerns the availability of dating scans. Accurate dating is an essential component of the screening programme and indeed the use of ultrasound in early pregnancy reduces intervention rates by 1–2%. A recent ultrasound survey in England has shown that only 55% of units offer a first trimester dating scan.[29] In fact, nationally, about 13% of units currently offer screening for Down's syndrome without a dating scan.[23]

Since 1998, the UK NSC has made efforts to address this inequity.[30] Aside from creating the 'benchmark timeframes' that all units should aspire to, it has suggested other standards as follows:

1. A formal clinical arrangement for antenatal screening programmes. For instance, there should be a dedicated screening co-ordinator to oversee the antenatal screening programme. Each trust should also have a multidisciplinary steering committee which meets regularly and is responsible to the chief executive.

2. Those involved in Down's screening should have formal training by recognised bodies.

3. Adequate information including written information should be the norm.

4. There should be agreed ultrasound screening standards including generic standards for measuring the crown rump length and nuchal translucency. All women must have a dating scan before undergoing Down's screening.[30]

5. There should be agreed laboratory standards. These include accreditation by an appropriate body and demonstration of external audit. In addition, the laboratory must have a sufficient workload of at least 1000 Down's syndrome screen specimens per year. If a laboratory has between 1000 to 5000 specimens per annum, the laboratory must be part of a network of other screening laboratories and audit its results accordingly.

Although there remains much work to be done in achieving a screening programme that is equitable and acceptable to all, these standards do go some way to address the problems.

SOFT MARKERS

Continued improvements with ultrasound technology have allowed the identification of increasing numbers of soft markers. Soft markers are not structural abnormalities but ultrasound phenomena associated particularly with an increased risk of aneuploidy. Most fetuses with an isolated soft marker will be normal at birth. The predictive power of such markers, their value in everyday practice and their use in screening programmes remain controversial.[31] Yet many women are informed of their presence and some are offered further tests.

Over the last decade, there have been two examples in which rapid improvements in technology had overtaken the obstetrician's understanding of soft markers. These are the identification of choroid plexus cyst and renal pelvic dilatation in screening for Down's syndrome. Choroid plexus cysts are found in 1% of fetuses examined before 20 weeks. These structures may, when found in isolation, indicate an overall risk of aneuploidy of about 1 in 150.[32] But their most common association is with trisomy 18 which is almost universally fatal. Hence, the residual risk of Down's syndrome is 1 in 880. Renal pelvic dilatation was also originally thought to be fairly strongly associated with Down's syndrome,[33] supposedly giving a risk of 1 in 100. However, this association only holds when renal pelvic dilatation is found with other markers.[34]

Since then, much work has been carried out to delineate the value of soft markers. In a 6-year review of data from Oxford, Boyd and colleagues reported that ultrasound soft markers were responsible for a 12-fold increase in false-positive rate in the detection of malformations.[35] In a balanced argument, they conceded that applying the term 'false positive' in a discussion of soft markers (as opposed to structural anomalies such as a cardiac defect) may not be appropriate given that soft markers are known to be normal variants and only raise suspicion of an abnormality. Nevertheless, it is true that the moment a suspicion of abnormality is raised, there is an impact on the pregnancy whatever the outcome.[36]

Smith-Bindman and colleagues were more critical of the wide-spread use of soft markers. In a meta-analysis of 56 studies of soft markers in the second trimester, they reported that the number of women needed to be screened to detect a single case of Down's syndrome was very high,[37] being 87,413 for choroid plexus cyst, 4454 for femur length, 19,425 for echogenic bowel and 30,404 for renal pelvic dilatation. If all these women who screened positive had an invasive test, there would be a loss of 4.3, 1.2, 1.0 and 2.6 babies, respectively, for every case of Down's syndrome detected.

In general, the value of soft markers in screening for Down's syndrome remains uncertain and, as indicated above, the process is more likely to do harm than good. It is probably best to rationalise their use by employing nuchal fold thickness (the marker shown to be of greatest value), or the presence of two or more markers, as indications for possible intervention. Even this approach could be modified if there were a robust initial screening programme in place.

FUTURE DEVELOPMENTS

FETAL NASAL BONES

It was realised some time ago that the nasal bones of Down's babies are poorly formed. In 2003, Cicero et al.[38] reported that fetuses with Down's syndrome could potentially be detected in the first trimester because of the ultrasound finding of an absent nasal bone. The technique for assessing the nasal bone is challenging but its appearance is striking. An experienced sonographer would need to perform, on average, 80 supervised scans before achieving competency.[39] To date, there have been a number of studies on the subject which in total have involved 15,822 pregnancies. In these studies, an adequate image was obtained in 97.4% of cases. The nasal bone was absent in 176 of 12,652 normal fetuses (1.4%) and absent in 274 of 397 (69.0%) fetuses with Down's syndrome.[8,40]

However, other workers were less optimistic. Welsh and Malone[41] reported an ability to examine the fetal nasal bone in just 75.9% of fetuses and that the nasal bone was seen in all 9 of their Down's cases. In another study, which was retrospective and involved examining previous photographs, the nasal bone was reported to be present in all 5 cases of Down's syndrome.[42] Nicolaides maintains, however, that the reported images in both these studies are flawed as they fall short of the rigorous standards set by the Fetal Medicine Foundation.

Using data obtained by Cicero[43] (who reported a detection rate of 73% for a false-positive rate of 0.5%), the use of nasal bones together with the combined test will give a detection rate of 95% with a false-positive rate of 5% in the first trimester, or a detection rate of 95% with a 1% false-positive rate using the integrated approach.[13] Further work is required in this area, but these preliminary results do seem promising.

FETAL DUCTUS VENOSUS

Doppler ultrasound of the ductus venosus in normal pregnancy should, in theory, demonstrate a forward biphasic pulsatile flow. In fetuses with aneuploidy or a cardiac defect, there is an association with reverse flow at the time of atrial contraction. Between 59–93% of aneuploid fetuses will demonstrate an abnormal ductus venosus flow velocity. In contrast, 2–21% of normal fetuses will have an abnormal ductus venosus waveform.[44,45] Therefore, it has been suggested that assessment of ductus venosus waveforms could be used to complement existing nuchal translucency screening programmes and hopefully further improve the detection rate and reduce false-positive rates.

There are a number of reasons why this may not be appropriate. First, the ductus venosus in the first trimester is small, measuring about 2 mm.[45] A typical Doppler gate using reasonable ultrasound equipment will measure 0.5–2 mm. Placement of the gate may therefore become an issue. For instance, if the gate is placed too proximally near the umbilical sinus, the normal continuous venous flow from the umbilical vein will obscure absence of flow during an atrial contraction in the ductus venosus. Conversely, placement of the gate too distally near the inferior vena cava might lead to the incorrect conclusion that flow is reversed (reversal of flow is normal in the inferior vena cava). Second, it has not been established that the sonographic features of increased nuchal translucency and an alteration in ductus venosus waveforms are completely independent. If these variables are not independent of each other, then using them in combination to derive a risk of Down's syndrome will be statistically incorrect.[46] If, however, the technical difficulties can be overcome and the independence of ductus venosus waveforms from other sonographic parameters can be established, then we may yet see the emergence of a powerful first trimester sonographic screening tool in the form of nuchal translucency, ductus venosus and the detection of nasal bone used in combination.

Key points for clinical practice

- Screening for Down's syndrome has until relatively recently been largely technology driven.
- There has been inadequate emphasis given to vital issues such as information for women, training for staff and audit of programmes. *(continued on next page)*

Key points for clinical practice *(continued)*

- The National Screening Committee and National Institute for Clinical Excellence have defined screening standards for Down's syndrome and provided a framework for their delivery.

- Whilst the methods of screening to deliver these standards have been defined, the exact methods used in a locality will be dictated by factors including both human and equipment resource.

- New observations, such as nasal bone and ductus venosus flow, must not be introduced until properly evaluated by appropriate studies.

References

1. Wellesley D, Boyle T, Barber J, Howe DT. Retrospective audit of different antenatal screening policies for Down's syndrome in eight district general hospitals in one health region. *BMJ* 2002; **325**: 15.
2. Merkatz IR, Nitowsky HM, Macri JN, Johnson WE. An association between low maternal serum alpha-fetoprotein and fetal chromosomal abnormalities. *Am J Obstet Gynecol* 1984; **148**: 886–894.
3. Cuckle HS, Wald NJ, Lindenbaum RH. Maternal serum alpha-fetoprotein measurement: a screening test for Down syndrome. *Lancet* 1984; **1**: 926–929.
4. Wald NJ, Densem JW, Smith D, Klee GG. Four-marker serum screening for Down's syndrome. *Prenat Diagn* 1994; **14**: 707–716.
5. Wald NJ, Kennard A, Hackshaw A, McGuire A. Antenatal screening for Down's syndrome. *J Med Screen* 1997; **4**: 181–246.
6. Haddow JE, Palomaki GE. Biochemical screening for neural tube defects and Down syndrome. In: Rodeck CH, Whittle MJ. (eds) *Fetal Medicine. Basic science and clinical practice*. London: Churchill Livingstone, 1999: 373–388.
7. Ritchie K, Boynton J, Bradbury I *et al. Routine ultrasound scanning before 24 weeks of pregnancy*. Health Technology Assessment Report: NHS Quality Improvement Scotland, 2003.
8. Nicolaides KH. Nuchal translucency and other first-trimester sonographic markers of chromosomal abnormalities. *Am J Obstet Gynecol* 2004; **191**: 45–67.
9. Taipale P, Hiilesmaa V, Salonen R, Ylostalo P. Increased nuchal translucency as a marker for fetal chromosomal defects. *N Engl J Med* 1997; **337**: 1654–1658.
10. Theodoropoulos P, Lolis D, Papageorgiou C, Papaioannou S, Plachouras N, Makrydimas G. Evaluation of first-trimester screening by fetal nuchal translucency and maternal age. *Prenat Diagn* 1998; **18**: 133–137.
11. Snijders RJ, Noble P, Sebire N, Souka A, Nicolaides KH. UK multicentre project on assessment of risk of trisomy 21 by maternal age and fetal nuchal-translucency thickness at 10–14 weeks of gestation. Fetal Medicine Foundation First Trimester Screening Group. *Lancet* 1998; **352**: 343–346.
12. Malone FD, Berkowitz RL, Canick JA, D'Alton ME. First-trimester screening for aneuploidy: research or standard of care? *Am J Obstet Gynecol* 2000; **182**: 490–496.
13. Wald NJ, Rodeck C, Hackshaw AK, Walters J, Chitty L, Mackinson AM. First and second trimester antenatal screening for Down's syndrome: the results of the Serum, Urine and Ultrasound Screening Study (SURUSS). *Health Technol Assess* 2003; **7**: 1–77.
14. Morris JK, Wald NJ, Watt HC. Fetal loss in Down syndrome pregnancies. *Prenat Diagn* 1999; **19**: 142–145.
15. Haddow JE, Palomaki GE, Knight GJ, Williams J, Miller WA, Johnson A. Screening of maternal serum for fetal Down's syndrome in the first trimester. *N Engl J Med* 1998; **338**: 955–961.
16. Wald NJ, George L, Smith D, Densem JW, Petterson K. Serum screening for Down's

syndrome between 8 and 14 weeks of pregnancy. International Prenatal Screening Research Group. *Br J Obstet Gynaecol* 1996; **103**: 407–412.

17. Canick JA, Kellner LH. First trimester screening for aneuploidy: serum biochemical markers. *Semin Perinatol* 1999; **23**: 359–368.

18. Wald NJ, Hackshaw AK. Advances in antenatal screening for Down syndrome. *Baillière's Best Pract Res Clin Obstet Gynaecol* 2000; **14**: 563–580.

19. Malone FD, Wald NJ, Canick JA *et al*. First- and second-trimester evaluation if risk (FASTER) trial: principal results of the NICHD multicenter Down syndrome screening study. *Am J Obstet Gynecol* 2003; **189**: s56.

20. Wald NJ, Watt HC, Hackshaw AK. Integrated screening for Down's syndrome on the basis of tests performed during the first and second trimesters. *N Engl J Med* 1999; **341**: 461–467.

21. National Collaborating Centre for Women's and Children's Health. *Antenatal Care. Routine care for the healthy pregnant women*. London: RCOG Press, 2003.

22. Model of Best Practice, 2003.

23. A report to the UK National Screening Committee. *Antenatal screening service for Down syndrome in England: 2001*. London: UK National Screening Committee Programmes Directorate, 2002.

24. Cuckle H, Aitken D, Goodburn S, Senior B, Spencer K, Standing S, UK National Down's Syndrome Screening Programme Laboratory Advisory Group. Age standardisation when target setting and auditing performance of Down syndrome screening programmes. *Prenat Diagn* 2004; **24**: 851–856.

25. Sandall J, Lewando-Hunt G, Spencer K, Williams C, Heyman B. *Social and organisational implications of one stop first trimester prenatal screening*. London: Economic and Social Research Council, 2005.

26. Spencer K, Spencer CE, Power M, Moakes A, Nicolaides KH. One stop clinic for assessment of risk for fetal anomalies: a report of the first year of prospective screening for chromosomal anomalies in the first trimester. *Br J Obstet Gynaecol* 2000; **107**: 1271–1275.

27. Department of Health. Building the information core – Implementing the NHS plan. London:Department of Health, 2001

28. RCOG. *Report of the RCOG Working Party on Biochemical Markers and the Detection of Down's Syndrome*. London: RCOG Press, 1993.

29. Appleby L. *Antenatal ultrasound screening. 2002 Ultrasound survey: an evaluation of service provision in the south west of England*. London: UK National Screening Committee Antenatal Sub-group, 2004.

30. Department of Health. *Antenatal Screening – Working Standards. National Down's Syndrome Screening Programme for England*. London: Department of Health, 2004.

31. Whittle M. Ultrasonographic 'soft markers' of fetal chromosomal defects. *BMJ* 1997; **314**: 918.

32. Gupta JK, Cave M, Lilford RJ *et al*. Clinical significance of fetal choroid plexus cysts. *Lancet* 1995; **346**: 724–729.

33. Benacerraf BR, Mandell J, Estroff JA, Harlow BL, Frigoletto FD Jr. Fetal pyelectasis: a possible association with Down syndrome. *Obstet Gynecol* 1990; **76**: 58–60.

34. Thompson MO, Thilaganathan B. Effect of routine screening for Down's syndrome on the significance of isolated fetal hydronephrosis. *Br J Obstet Gynaecol* 1998; **105**: 860–864.

35. Boyd PA, Chamberlain P, Hicks NR. 6-year experience of prenatal diagnosis in an unselected population in Oxford, UK. *Lancet* 1998; **352**: 1577–1581.

36. Stewart-Brown S, Farmer A. Screening could seriously damage your health. *BMJ* 1997; **314**: 533–534.

37. Smith-Bindman R, Hosmer W, Feldstein VA, Deeks JJ, Goldberg JD. Second-trimester ultrasound to detect fetuses with Down syndrome: a meta-analysis. *JAMA* 2001; **285**: 1044–1055.

38. Cicero S, Sonek JD, McKenna DS, Croom CS, Johnson L, Nicolaides KH. Nasal bone hypoplasia in trisomy 21 at 15-22 weeks' gestation. *Ultrasound Obstet Gynecol* 2003; **21**: 15–18.

39. Cicero S, Dezerega V, Andrade E, Scheier M, Nicolaides KH. Learning curve for sonographic examination of the fetal nasal bone at 11–14 weeks. *Ultrasound Obstet Gynecol* 2003; **22**: 135–137.

40. Cicero S, Rembouskos G, Vandecruys H, Hogg M, Nicolaides KH. Likelihood ratio for trisomy 21 in fetuses with absent nasal bone at the 11-14-week scan. *Ultrasound Obstet Gynecol* 2004; **23**: 218–223.
41. Welch KK, Malone FD. Nuchal translucency-based screening. *Clin Obstet Gynecol* 2003; **46**: 909–922.
42. De Biasio P, Venturini PL. Absence of nasal bone and detection of trisomy 21. *Lancet* 2002; **359**: 1344.
43. Cicero S, Curcio P, Papageorghiou A, Sonek J, Nicolaides K. Absence of nasal bone in fetuses with trisomy 21 at 11-14 weeks of gestation: an observational study. *Lancet* 2001; **358**: 1665–1667.
44. Murta CG, Moron AF, Avila MA, Weiner CP. Application of ductus venosus Doppler velocimetry for the detection of fetal aneuploidy in the first trimester of pregnancy. *Fetal Diagn Ther* 2002; **17**: 308–314.
45. Borrell A. The ductus venosus in early pregnancy and congenital anomalies. *Prenat Diagn* 2004; **24**: 688–692.
46. Malone FD, D'Alton ME, Society for Maternal-Fetal Medicine. First-trimester sonographic screening for Down syndrome. *Obstet Gynecol* 2003; **102**: 1066–1079.

2

Preterm labour: prediction and treatment

Spontaneous, preterm birth before 37 weeks' gestation occurs in 7–11% of pregnancies and before 34 weeks' gestation in 3–7% of pregnancies.[1,2] The latter are more likely to be due to pathological than physiological causes (Fig. 1). Preterm delivery, particularly that before 34 weeks' gestation, accounts for three-quarters of neonatal mortality and one-half of long-term neurological impairment in children, including developmental delay.[3–5] Many of the surviving infants also suffer serious morbidity such as bronchopulmonary dysplasia and retrolental fibroplasia leading, respectively, to chronic lung problems and visual abnormalities including blindness. Advances in perinatal healthcare have not reduced the incidence of preterm labour, but there are some effective interventions (see clinical context below). The decision regarding the institution of these interventions requires timely and accurate screening of pregnant women for the risk of preterm birth.

Prediction of pregnant women's risk for preterm birth both for screening or diagnosis is based on a combination of patients' characteristics, symptoms, physical signs and investigations. For the purpose of this chapter, we consider all of these variables to be 'tests'. Without accurate tests, clinicians are handicapped in the management of pregnant women. Wrong or delayed diagnosis can put mother and baby at risk of an adverse outcome, whereas correct prediction of preterm birth provides an opportunity to institute effective therapeutic interventions. There is, therefore, a need for guidance about the best strategies with which to predict and to prevent the risk of spontaneous preterm birth (Fig. 2). In this chapter, our discussion pertains to

Honest Honest MBChB (for correspondence)
Specialist Registrar in Obstetrics and Gynaecology, Birmingham Women's Hospital, Edgbaston, Birmingham B15 2TG, UK (E-mail: honest.honest@bwhct.nhs.uk)

Khalid S. Khan MRCOG MSc
Professor of Obstetrics and Gynaecology, Birmingham Women's Hospital, Edgbaston, Birmingham B15 2TG, UK

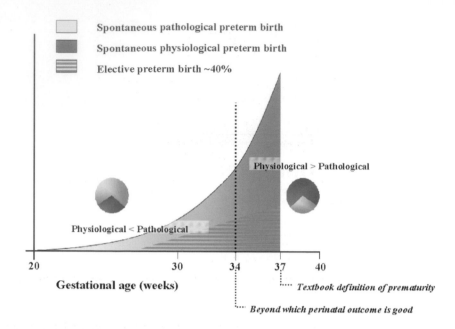

Fig. 1 Distribution of causes of spontaneous preterm birth.

singleton gestations only, excluding twins and higher order gestations. Furthermore, we do not cover the issue of iatrogenic preterm birth (delivery) or rescue cerclage.

CLINICAL CONTEXT

There are two target populations of pregnant women that need to be tested and treated for the risk of preterm birth. The first is a population of antenatal asymptomatic women having routine care. In this population, women are generally in a healthy state, anticipating a normal course of pregnancy. There might be antecedent factors or current history that might increase the risk of preterm birth. These may be evaluated in any one of the several available risks scoring systems for predicting spontaneous preterm birth.[6–9] Even when there are no apparent predisposing factors, routine antenatal tests undertaken for a different reason (*e.g.* urinalysis for urinary tract infection, multiple serum screening test for Down's syndrome risk assessment) may be utilised to uncover hitherto unknown risk of preterm birth.[10–12] Additionally, there may be specific tests (*e.g.* transvaginal ultrasonographic measurement of cervical length, cervico-vaginal fetal fibronectin detection or bacterial vaginosis [BV] screening)[13–15] which may help to identify those women at higher risk of preterm birth. If testing could predict risk of spontaneous preterm birth among these women, interventions such as antibiotics (for treatment of BV or asymptomatic bacteriuria), cervical cerclage (for short cervix on scan) and closer surveillance (to optimise antenatal care) may be considered as preventative measures.

The second population group is that of symptomatic women who present with threatened preterm labour. For these women, there is a need to delineate those among them who will go on to deliver preterm. Many tests have claimed

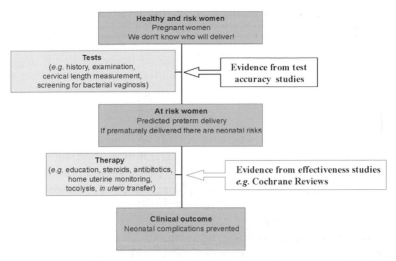

Fig. 2 Roles of test accuracy and therapeutic evidence-based management for the risk of spontaneous preterm birth.

to predict the risk of preterm delivery in this group of women (*e.g.* cervico-vaginal fetal fibronectin, corticotrophin-releasing hormone, and salivary oestriol).[16-18] If testing could predict imminent spontaneous preterm birth among these women before advanced cervical dilatation, therapies like antenatal steroids, tocolytics and *in utero* transfer (to optimise neonatal care) may be used. Antenatal steroids have maximal effectiveness among neonates delivered within 2–7 days after administration,[19] and tocolytics are known to delay birth for at least 2 days[20] effectively (to allow use of steroids[19] and *in utero* transfer[21]).

LITERATURE IDENTIFICATION

Evidence was sought through a formal search to identify existing reviews of accuracy of tests for preterm birth and those of effectiveness of relevant interventions. In addition to conventional medical literature databases (*e.g.* MEDLINE, EMBASE, BIOSIS, Pascal, and Science Citation Index), the Cochrane Library, National Research Register, Health Technology Assessment Database, and National Guideline Clearinghouse was also searched for systematic reviews of either test accuracy or effectiveness studies. Language restrictions were not applied to the searches, which were carried out from database inception to 2005. The search strategy for identifying test accuracy studies in predicting preterm birth has been previously published.[22] The search for systematic reviews of effectiveness of interventions for the prevention of spontaneous preterm birth or treatment of threatened preterm labour was based on guidance provided by the Centre for Reviews & Dissemination.[23]

MEASURING ACCURACY OF A TEST AND EFFECTIVENESS OF AN INTERVENTION

Likelihood ratio (LR) is a measure of accuracy that gauges how much the odds of disease change from the situation before testing (pre-test probability) to that after the test result becomes known (post-test probability).[24] For a test with a positive and a negative result there is a twin set of LRs, LR+ and LR−. A high LR+ (> 5) or a low LR− (< 0.2) value generally indicates a more useful test when it is positive or negative, respectively, whilst an intermediate LR+ (*e.g.* 2–5) or LR− (*e.g.* 0.2–0.5) value generally indicates a less useful test.[25] A meta-analysis of studies of test accuracy in a systematic review would generate a summary LR+ and LR− calculated from combining individual studies' LR+ and LR−, respectively.[26,27]

The odds ratio (OR) or relative risk (RR) is a measure of effectiveness of intervention.[28] Consider an example of a traditional versus an alternative treatment. If 12.5% of a traditionally treated population develop complications, then the odds of having complications following traditional treatment is 0.143 (0.125/0.875). If 10% of the alternative treatment resulted in complications, this would give odds of 0.11 (0.1/0.9). The OR would then be 1.3 (0.143/0.11), *i.e.* using traditional treatment has a 1.3 times higher odds of complications than of no complications as compared with alternative treatment. Just like summary LRs, summary ORs may be generated in meta-analysis undertaken within a systematic review of effectiveness studies.

The two values, summary LRs from test accuracy reviews and ORs from effectiveness reviews, can then be combined to provide a number needed to treat (NNT)[29] when the test is combined with an effective intervention. This method of integrating particular test(s) with intervention(s) in terms of NNT, which serves to aid clinicians in their decision making, has been illustrated previously.[16]

PREDICTION AND TREATMENT IN ASYMPTOMATIC PREGNANT WOMEN

Systematic reviews of test accuracy and effectiveness studies were available for both the prediction and treatment of asymptomatic pregnant women at risk of spontaneous preterm birth. Risk scoring,[30] maternal anthropometry,[31] ultrasound measurement of the cervical length,[32] cervico-vaginal fetal fibronectin,[16] and testing for bacterial vaginosis infection (BV)[33] have been evaluated for their utility in predicting spontaneous preterm birth in this group of women (Fig. 3). The studies on these tests generally used preterm birth before 37 weeks' gestation as the outcome. Only cervico-vaginal fetal fibronectin and cervical length were also considered for birth before 34 weeks' gestation.

Amongst these tests, ultrasound cervical length measurement was likely to be beneficial. Using a starting cut-off of 25 mm or less, between 20–24 weeks' gestation, it was found to be an accurate test in predicting spontaneous preterm birth before 37 weeks' gestation in asymptomatic pregnant women with an LR+ of 25.61 (95% CI, 8.55–76.72) and LR− of 0.47 (95% CI, 0.29–0.74).[32] Additionally, the shorter the ultrasound measurement of the cervical length, the higher the LR+. Using the same threshold of ultrasound cervical length measurement, it is also a moderately accurate test in predicting spontaneous preterm birth before 34 weeks' gestation with an LR+ of 4.4 (95% CI, 3.53–5.49). The remainder of the tests were likely to be less beneficial as tests for predicting spontaneous preterm birth for either 34 or 37 weeks' gestation.

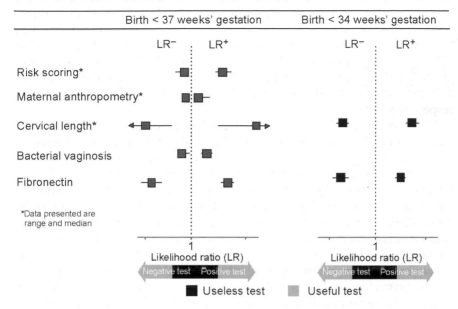

Fig. 3 Comparison of the accuracy of various tests for predicting spontaneous preterm birth in asymptomatic pregnant women.[16,30–32,52] Figures are not drawn to exact scale.

Many preventative treatments, including educational programmes of behavioural/life-style modifications,[34] bed rest,[35] home uterine monitoring,[36] antibiotics for urogenital infection,[37–43] cervical cerclage,[44,45] and progestational agents[46] have been evaluated. Amongst these, progestational agents, treatment of urogenital infection, and cervical cerclage in

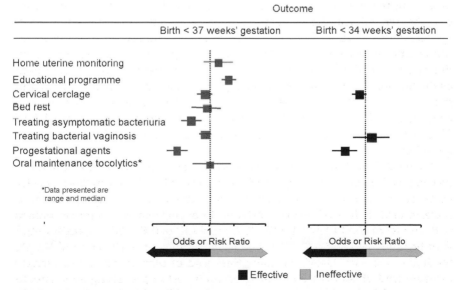

Fig. 4 Comparison of the effectiveness of interventions for preventing spontaneous preterm birth in asymptomatic pregnant women.[34–36,38,40,41 44–46,53] Figures are not drawn to exact scale.

asymptomatic women identified at risk of spontaneous preterm birth, are all possibly beneficial (Fig. 4). The remainder of the interventions, based on currently available evidence, are unlikely to be beneficial. Elective cervical cerclage may be an option in this group of women as there is evidence that the procedure is likely to be beneficial in reducing spontaneous preterm birth before 34 weeks' gestation. Nevertheless, current evidence from a systematic review of a strategy combining ultrasound measurement of cervical shortening with cervical cerclage in asymptomatic women suggests otherwise.[47]

PREDICTION AND TREATMENT IN SYMPTOMATIC PREGNANT WOMEN

Systematic reviews of test accuracy and effectiveness studies are also available for both the prediction and treatment of symptomatic pregnant women at risk for spontaneous preterm birth. These tests and treatments were used on pregnant women who presented with suspected threatened preterm labour but did not have advanced cervical dilatation, *i.e.* less than 3–4 cm dilated. Cervico-vaginal fetal fibronectin,[16] absence of fetal breathing movement on ultrasound,[48] ultrasound cervical length measurement[32] and BV testing[33] have been evaluated in test accuracy systematic reviews (Fig. 5).

Cervico-vaginal fetal fibronectin testing was found to be accurate in predicting spontaneous preterm birth before 34 weeks' gestation within 7–10 days of testing. It had an LR+ of 5.42 (95% CI, 4.36–6.74) and an LR− of 0.25 (95% CI, 0.20–0.31).[16] Absence of fetal breathing movement on ultrasound scan performed at the time of admission on women who presented with threatened

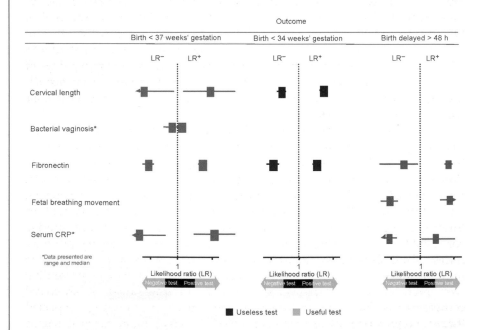

Fig. 5 Comparison of the accuracy of various tests for predicting spontaneous preterm birth in symptomatic pregnant women presenting with threatened preterm labour but before advanced dilatation.[16,32,48,52,54] Figures are not drawn to exact scale.

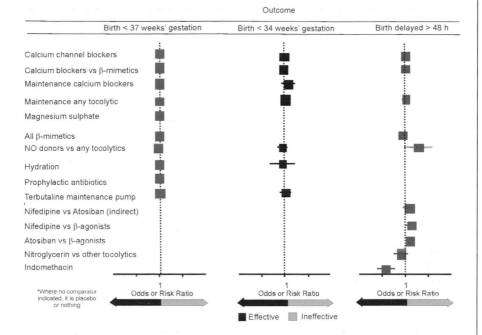

Fig. 6 Comparison of the effectiveness of interventions for preventing spontaneous preterm birth in symptomatic pregnant women presenting with threatened preterm labour but before advanced dilatation.[50,51,55–62] Figures are not drawn to exact scale.

preterm labour was also found to be an accurate test in predicting spontaneous preterm birth. It had an LR+ of 7.84 (95% CI, 1.12–54.99) and an LR− of 0.25 (95% CI, 0.13–0.48) for predicting spontaneous preterm birth within 48 h of testing.[48] It also had an LR+ of 14.80 (95% CI, 6.30–34.79) and an LR− of 0.46 (95% CI, 0.36–0.58) for predicting spontaneous preterm birth within 7 days of testing.[18] However, neither ultrasound cervical length measurement nor BV testing were found to be accurate in this group of women and therefore their use is unlikely to be beneficial.

The main aim of the management of this group of women and of those who have symptoms of spontaneous preterm labour is to optimise their neonates' birth condition thus minimising the risk and sequelae of the premature birth. This can be achieved by initiating tocolysis[20] to allow time for antenatal corticosteroids[19] and for *in utero* transfer of the fetus to a tertiary neonatal unit.[21] Intravenous fluid hydration has also been evaluated as a treatment for threatened preterm labour. Theoretically, hydration may reduce uterine contractility by increasing uterine blood flow and by decreasing pituitary release of anti-diuretic hormone and oxytocin but there is a lack of evidence to recommend the use of hydration as a specific treatment for women presenting with preterm labour.[49] However, it is the administration of antenatal corticosteroids that is an indisputable component in managing suspected threatened preterm birth as a means to accelerate fetal lung maturity. It is used to prevent respiratory distress syndrome and neonatal mortality, and its use is also associated with a significant reduction in the risk of intraventricular haemorrhage. Tocolysis (of various types; (Fig. 6) should not be given without concurrent antenatal corticosteroids as there is no clear evidence that its sole use improves outcomes in terms of perinatal and neonatal mortality or morbidity.[50]

CONCLUSIONS

Based on the currently available evidence, the preceding information on the utility of the various tests and interventions can be summarised as either likely or unlikely to be accurate and beneficial.

Testing for BV, cervicovaginal fibronectin, maternal anthropometry or risk-scoring assessment is unlikely to be beneficial in predicting spontaneous preterm birth in asymptomatic pregnant women. In this group of women, however, ultrasound cervical length measurement using a starting cut-off of 25 mm or less between 20–24 weeks' gestation, is likely to be accurate in predicting spontaneous preterm birth before 34 and 37 weeks' gestation. However, in spite of this, there is currently a paucity of clear evidence concerning effective means of intervention to benefit asymptomatic women thus identified to be at high risk with shortened cervical length on ultrasound measurement. Out of the many other interventions that have been studied, treatment of urogenital infection is likely to be beneficial. Progestational agents look promising, but interventions, such as educational programmes, behavioural changes, and home uterine activity monitoring are unlikely to be beneficial.

In symptomatic women, cervico-vaginal fetal fibronectin and absence of fetal breathing movement on ultrasound scan testing are likely to be accurate in predicting spontaneous preterm birth. Antenatal corticosteroid administration is beneficial in facilitating fetal lung maturation. Tocolytics are also likely to be beneficial if their use is combined with antenatal corticosteroid administration as a means to buy time to achieve maximal steroid effectiveness whilst undertaking, if necessary, *in utero* transfer to a tertiary neonatal unit. Other tests such as the ultrasound measurement of cervical length or the presence of BV are less likely to be accurate and unlikely to be beneficial in this group of women. Whilst intravenous hydration has theoretical potential, the available evidence suggests that its use is unlikely to be beneficial in the treatment of threatened preterm labour for the prevention of spontaneous preterm birth.

In applying the summarised evidence, women's values and the risks and benefits of the proposed interventions need to be taken into account. In an era where screening is gaining acceptance in obstetrical practice (*e.g.* for Down's syndrome, neural tube defects or fetal structural anomalies), further research will shed light on the issues of screening for the risk of spontaneous preterm birth in pregnant women. For symptomatic women who present with signs and symptoms of threatened preterm labour, testing for cervico-vaginal fetal fibronectin is gaining acceptance in practice to aid clinicians in their management of this group of women. With the increasing availability and resolution of ultrasound scanning machines, and trained personnel to use them, testing for the absence of fetal breathing movement may yet gain acceptance in the management of this group of women. Nevertheless, the challenge continues for clinicians to balance the risks and benefits of screening, testing and treating spontaneous preterm birth. Research, both basic and translational, continues in this field.

Key points for clinical practice

- In asymptomatic pregnant women, screening with ultrasound cervical length measurement is likely to be accurate in predicting spontaneous preterm birth before 34 and 37 weeks' gestation.

- There is currently a paucity of clear evidence concerning effective means of intervention to benefit asymptomatic pregnant women thus identified to be at high risk, unlike the clear benefit of treating urogenital infection.

- For women presenting with threatened preterm labour, tests and therapies exist that will aid clinicians in their management.

References

1. Maternal and Child Health Consortium. *6th Annual Report: Confidential Enquiries into Stillbirths and Deaths in Infancy*. London: CESDI, 1999.
2. Peters KD, Kochanek KD, Murphy SL. Deaths: final data for 1996. *Natl Vital Stat Rep* 1998; **47**: 1–100.
3. Paneth NS. The problem of low birth weight. *Future Child* 1995; **5**: 19–34.
4. Stewart AL, Rifkin L, Amess PN et al. Brain structure and neurocognitive and behavioural function in adolescents who were born very preterm. *Lancet* 1999; **353**: 1653–1657.
5. Wolke D, Meyer R. Cognitive status, language attainment, and prereading skills of 6-year-old very preterm children and their peers: the Bavarian Longitudinal Study. *Dev Med Child Neurol* 1999; **41**: 94–109.
6. Humphrey MD. The beneficial use of risk scoring in a remote and high-risk pregnant population. *Aust NZ J Obstet Gynaecol* 1995; **35**: 139–143.
7. Main DM, Richardson D, Gabbe SG, Strong S, Weller SC. Prospective evaluation of a risk scoring system for predicting preterm delivery in black inner city women. *Obstet Gynecol* 1987; **69**: 61–66.
8. Mercer BM, Goldenberg RL, Das A et al. The preterm prediction study: a clinical risk assessment system. *Am J Obstet Gynecol* 1996; **174**: 1885–1893.
9. Nesbitt Jr RE, Aubry RH. High-risk obstetrics. II. Value of semiobjective grading system in identifying the vulnerable group. *Am J Obstet Gynecol* 1969; **103**: 972–985.
10. Teppa RJ, Roberts JM. The uriscreen test to detect significant asymptomatic bacteriuria during pregnancy. *J Soc Gynecol Invest* 2005; **12**: 50–53.
11. Simpson JL, Palomaki GE, Mercer B et al. Associations between adverse perinatal outcome and serially obtained second- and third-trimester maternal serum alpha-fetoprotein measurements. *Am J Obstet Gynecol* 1995; **173**: 1742–1748.
12. Spencer K. Second-trimester prenatal screening for Down syndrome and the relationship of maternal serum biochemical markers to pregnancy complications with adverse outcome. *Prenat Diagn* 2000; **20**: 652–656.
13. Hassan SS, Romero R, Berry SM et al. Patients with an ultrasonographic cervical length < or = 15 mm have nearly a 50% risk of early spontaneous preterm delivery. *Am J Obstet Gynecol* 2000; **182**: 1458–1467.
14. Hellemans P, Gerris J, Verdonk P. Fetal fibronectin detection for prediction of preterm birth in low risk women. *Br J Obstet Gynaecol* 1995; **102**: 207–212.

15. Klebanoff MA, Hillier SL, Nugent RP *et al*. Is bacterial vaginosis a stronger risk factor for preterm birth when it is diagnosed earlier in gestation? *Am J Obstet Gynecol* 2005; **192**: 470–477.
16. Honest H, Bachmann LM, Gupta JK, Kleijnen J, Khan KS. Accuracy of cervicovaginal fetal fibronectin test in predicting risk of spontaneous preterm birth: systematic review. *BMJ* 2002; **325**: 301.
17. McGregor JA, Jackson GM, Lachelin GC *et al*. Salivary estriol as risk assessment for preterm labor: a prospective trial. *Am J Obstet Gynecol* 1995; **173**: 1337–1342.
18. McLean M, Smith R. Corticotropin-releasing Hormone in Human Pregnancy and Parturition. *Trends Endocrinol Metab* 1999; **10**: 174–178.
19. Crowley P. Prophylactic corticosteroids for preterm birth. *Cochrane Database System Rev* 2000; CD000065.
20. King JF, Flenady VJ, Papatsonis DN, Dekker GA, Carbonne B. Calcium channel blockers for inhibiting preterm labour. *Cochrane Database System Rev* 2002; CD002255.
21. Papiernik E. [Maternal transfer and neonatal transfer]. *Rev Prat* 1995; **45**: 1782–1783.
22. Honest H, Bachmann LM, Khan K. Electronic searching of the literature for systematic reviews of screening and diagnostic tests for preterm birth. *Eur J Obstet Gynecol Reprod Biol* 2003; **107**: 19–23.
23. Search Filters for Locating RCTs and Reviews. <http://www.york.ac.uk/inst/crd/dialogsearch.htm>. Last accessed 27/05/2005. Centre for Reviews & Dissemination, University of York, YO10 5DD, UK.
24. Deeks JJ, Altman DG. Diagnostic tests 4: likelihood ratios. *BMJ* 2004; **329**: 168–169.
25. Jaeschke R, Guyatt GH, Sackett DL. Users' guides to the medical literature. III. How to use an article about a diagnostic test. B. What are the results and will they help me in caring for my patients? The Evidence-Based Medicine Working Group. *JAMA* 1994; **271**: 703–707.
26. Honest H, Khan KS. Reporting of measures of accuracy in systematic reviews of diagnostic literature. *BMC Health Serv Res* 2002; **2**: 4.
27. Honest H, Khan KS. Systematic reviews of test accuracy studies in reproductive health. *WHO Reproductive Health Library (No. 5)*. Geneva: WHO/RHR, 2002.
28. Bland JM, Altman DG. Statistics notes. The odds ratio. *BMJ* 2000; **320**: 1468.
29. Moore A, McQuay H. Numbers needed to treat derived from meta analysis. NNT is a tool, to be used appropriately. *BMJ* 1999; **319**: 1200.
30. Honest H, Bachmann LM, Sundaram R, Gupta JK, Kleijnen J, Khan KS. The accuracy of risk scores in predicting preterm birth – a systematic review. *J Obstet Gynaecol* 2004; **24**: 343–359.
31. Honest H, Bachmann LM, Ngai C, Gupta JK, Kleijnen J, Khan KS. The accuracy of maternal anthropometry measurements as predictor for spontaneous preterm birth – a systematic review. *Eur J Obstet Gynecol Reprod Biol* 2005; **119**: 11–20.
32. Honest H, Bachmann LM, Coomarasamy A, Gupta JK, Kleijnen J, Khan KS. Accuracy of cervical transvaginal sonography in predicting preterm birth: a systematic review. *Ultrasound Obstet Gynecol* 2003; **22**: 305–322.
33. Honest H, Bachmann LM, Knox EM, Gupta JK, Kleijnen J, Khan KS. The accuracy of various tests for bacterial vaginosis in predicting preterm birth: a systematic review. *Br J Obstet Gynaecol* 2004; **111**: 409–422.
34. Hueston WJ, Knox MA, Eilers G, Pauwels J, Lonsdorf D. The effectiveness of preterm-birth prevention educational programs for high-risk women: a meta-analysis. *Obstet Gynecol* 1995; **86**: 705–712.
35. Sosa C, Althabe F, Belizan J, Bergel E. Bed rest in singleton pregnancies for preventing preterm birth. *Cochrane Database System Rev* 2004; CD003581.
36. Preventive US Services Task Force. Home uterine activity monitoring for preterm labor. Review article. *JAMA* 1993; **270**: 371–376.
37. Agency for Healthcare Research and Quality. Screening for bacterial vaginosis in pregnancy. *Guide to Clinical Preventive Services*, Rockville, MD: Agency for Healthcare Research and Quality, 2001.
38. McDonald H, Brocklehurst P, Parsons J, Vigneswaran R. Antibiotics for treating bacterial vaginosis in pregnancy. *Cochrane Database System Rev* 2005; CD000262.
39. Raynes-Greenow CH, Roberts CL, Bell JC, Peat B, Gilbert GL. Antibiotics for ureaplasma in the vagina in pregnancy. *Cochrane Database System Rev* 2004; CD003767.

40. Smaill F. Antibiotics for asymptomatic bacteriuria in pregnancy. Cochrane Database System Rev. 2001; CD000490.
41. Vazquez JC, Villar J. Treatments for symptomatic urinary tract infections during pregnancy. *The Cochrane Database of Systematic Reviews*: Reviews 2003 Issue 4. Chichester: John Wiley, DOI: 10.1002/14651858.
42. Villar J, Widmer M, Lydon-Rochelle MT, Gülmezoglu AM, Roganti A. Duration of treatment for asymptomatic bacteriuria during pregnancy. *The Cochrane Database of Systematic Reviews*: Reviews 2000 Issue 2. Chichester: John Wiley, DOI: 10.1002/14651858.
43. Walker GJ. Antibiotics for syphilis diagnosed during pregnancy. *Cochrane Database System Rev* 2001; CD001143.
44. Bachmann LM, Coomarasamy A, Honest H, Khan KS. Elective cervical cerclage for prevention of preterm birth: a systematic review. *Acta Obstet Gynecol Scand* 2003; **82**: 398–404.
45. Drakeley AJ, Roberts D, Alfirevic Z. Cervical stitch (cerclage) for preventing pregnancy loss in women. *Cochrane Database System Rev* 2003; CD003253.
46. Sanchez-Ramos L, Kaunitz AM, Delke I. Progestational agents to prevent preterm birth: a meta-analysis of randomized controlled trials. *Obstet Gynecol* 2005; **105**: 273–279.
47. Belej-Rak T, Okun N, Windrim R, Ross S, Hannah ME. Effectiveness of cervical cerclage for a sonographically shortened cervix: a systematic review and meta-analysis. *Am J Obstet Gynecol* 2003; **189**: 1679–1687.
48. Honest H, Bachmann LM, Sengupta R, Gupta JK, Kleijnen J, Khan KS. Accuracy of absence of fetal breathing movements in predicting preterm birth: a systematic review. *Ultrasound Obstet Gynecol* 2004; **24**: 94–100.
49. Stan C, Boulvain M, Hirsbrunner-Amagbaly P, Pfister R. Hydration for treatment of preterm labour. *Cochrane Database System Rev* 2002; CD003096.
50. Gyetvai K, Hannah ME, Hodnett ED, Ohlsson A. Tocolytics for preterm labor: a systematic review. *Obstet Gynecol* 1999; **94**: 869–877.
51. The Collaborative Home Uterine Monitoring Study (CHUMS) Group. A multicenter randomized controlled trial of home uterine monitoring: active versus sham device. *Am J Obstet Gynecol* 1995; **173**: 1120–1127.
52. Honest H, Bachmann LM, Gupta JK, Kleijnen J, Khan KS. Accuracy of C-reactive protein in predicting risk of spontaneous preterm birth: systematic review. *Manuscript* 2002.
53. Coomarasamy A, Knox EM, Gee H, Khan KS. Oxytocin antagonists for tocolysis in preterm labour – a systematic review. *Med Sci Monit* 2002; **8**: RA268–RA273.
54. Coomarasamy A, Knox EM, Gee H, Song F, Khan KS. Effectiveness of nifedipine versus Atosiban for tocolysis in preterm labour: a meta-analysis with an indirect comparison of randomised trials. *Br J Obstet Gynaecol* 2003; **110**: 1045–1049.
55. Crowther CA, Moore V. Magnesium maintenance therapy for preventing preterm birth after threatened preterm labour. *The Cochrane Database of Systematic Reviews: Reviews* 1998 Issue 1. Chichester: John Wiley, DOI: 10.1002/14651858.
56. Crowther CA, Hiller JE, Doyle LW. Magnesium sulphate for preventing preterm birth in threatened preterm labour. *Cochrane Database System Rev* 2002; CD001060.
57. Duckitt K, Thornton S. Nitric oxide donors for the treatment of preterm labour. *Cochrane Database System Rev* 2002; CD002860.
58. King J, Flenady V, Cole S, Thornton S. Cyclo-oxygenase (COX) inhibitors for treating preterm labour. *Cochrane Database System Rev* 2005; CD001992.
59. King JF, Flenady V, Papatsonis D, Dekker G, Carbonne B. Calcium channel blockers for inhibiting preterm labour; a systematic review of the evidence and a protocol for administration of nifedipine. *Aust NZ J Obstet Gynaecol*. 2003; **43**: 192–198.
60. Nanda K, Cook LA, Gallo MF, Grimes DA. Terbutaline pump maintenance therapy after threatened preterm labor for preventing preterm birth. *Cochrane Database System Rev* 2002; CD003933.

Penny C. McParland   David J. Taylor

3

Preterm prelabour rupture of the membranes

Preterm prelabour rupture of the fetal membranes (pPROM) is defined as rupture of the fetal membranes at least 1 h prior to the onset of labour at less than 37 weeks' gestation. It complicates about 2% of pregnancies, and thus precedes one-third of preterm births. Preterm delivery is the major cause of neonatal mortality and morbidity of normally formed infants. Therefore, pPROM can be considered the leading cause of preterm delivery and its adverse consequences.

FETAL MEMBRANES AND MECHANISM OF pPROM

The fetal membranes obtained after delivery comprise the amnion, chorion, and an attached layer of maternal decidua. The amnion comprises an epithelial layer, with underlying collagen-rich connective tissue layer. The chorion consists of a multilayered cytotrophoblast layer and collagen-rich connective tissue layer. Amnion and chorion fuse at about 12 weeks' gestation, via an intermediate layer of tissue, the spongy layer.[1] The resulting amniochorion fuses intimately to the maternal decidua parietalis at 20–25 weeks' gestation. Despite its lesser relative thickness, the greatest tensile strength of the fetal membranes lies within the amnion, the chorion possessing greater extensibility.[2,3]

The normal behaviour of the fetal membranes is to maintain their integrity throughout pregnancy, and to rupture spontaneously in the latter first stage or in the second stage of labour at term.[4] Prelabour rupture of the membranes

Penny C. McParland PhD MRCOG (for correspondence)
Reproductive Science Section, Department of Cancer Studies and Molecular Medicine, University of Leicester, Robert Kilpatrick Building, Leicester Royal Infirmary, Leicester LE2 7LX, UK
(E-mail: pcm7@le.ac.uk)

David J. Taylor MD FRCOG
Reproductive Science Section, Department of Cancer Studies and Molecular Medicine, University of Leicester, Robert Kilpatrick Building, Leicester Royal Infirmary, Leicester LE2 7LX, UK

occurs prior to 10% of deliveries at term and one-third of preterm deliveries. A number of strategies have been employed to investigate the potential mechanisms involved in pPROM, at the molecular, cellular, histological, biochemical and biophysical levels.

Collagen is the major structural component contributing to the strength of the fetal membranes. However, there is conflicting evidence regarding the level of collagen content in fetal membranes which undergo pPROM: some authors report a reduction in total collagen content, others report no difference compared to those at term.[2,4] However, increased levels of matrix metalloproteinases MMP-2, MMP-3, MMP-8, MMP-9 and neutrophil elastase within the amniotic fluid would support an increase in matrix degradation as a potential contributory factor in pPROM.[2] Breakdown of the fetal membranes may also be contributed to by an increased level of apoptosis in both amnion and chorion, which has been reported in fetal membranes from pPROM.[2]

There is no evidence from biophysical testing that fetal membranes, which undergo pPROM exhibit generalised weakness.[4] However, this does not preclude localised defects in the membranes being an underlying cause. A localised region of structural alteration (the 'zone of altered morphology') has been reported in the fetal membranes within the lower uterine segment associated with the rupture site of fetal membranes at term.[5] These structural alterations are also present prior to labour at term.[6] This region of fetal membranes has recently been demonstrated to be structurally weak,[7] and it has been hypothesised that premature generation of the zone of altered morphology may also be a potential mechanism of pPROM.

CLINICAL RISK FACTORS

A large number of clinical risk factors have been associated with pPROM. However, multivariate analysis in one of the most comprehensive analyses identified three major risk factors – cigarette smoking (odds ratio [OR] 2.08), vaginal bleeding (OR 6.44 for third trimester bleeding), and previous preterm delivery (OR 2.48).[8]

SMOKING

Cigarette smoking has been identified as a clinical risk factor for pPROM in numerous studies,[2] although paradoxically this association was not identified among the 2929 women included in the Preterm Prediction Study, 4.5% of whom delivered following pPROM.[9]

PREVIOUS PRETERM DELIVERY

A pregnancy complicated by pPROM is 6.3 times more likely to have been preceded by a pregnancy involving preterm than term delivery. This risk is greatest for women who had pPROM in their previous pregnancy, who have a 21–32% recurrence risk in subsequent pregnancies.[2]

These rates of recurrence may indicate specific endogenous maternal factors (*e.g.* cervical function or genetic factors); however, they also may indicate the persistent presence of exogenous factors within the maternal environment such as nutrition and/or behaviour.

VAGINAL BLEEDING

Vaginal bleeding has been associated with pPROM, especially if bleeding occurs later in pregnancy or in more than one trimester (first trimester OR 2.38; second trimester OR 4.42; third trimester OR 6.44; more than one trimester, OR 7.43).[8] Subclinical bleeding is also associated with pPROM, and may reflect decidual dysfunction: histological evidence of subclinical haemorrhage is found in 37% of pPROM deliveries compared to 8% of term controls.[10] The mechanism of pPROM is likely to be via activation of the blood coagulation cascade. Thrombin may act upon decidual cells, via a cascade of activation of metalloproteinases and plasminogen activators leading to degradation of the fetal membranes. This mechanism is supported by the finding of increased levels of thrombin–antithrombin (TAT) complexes, which are an index of *in vivo* thrombin generation, in the plasma of women who subsequently proceed to pPROM.[11,12]

NUTRITION

Most interest regarding nutrition and pPROM has rested upon vitamin C. Although some studies have reported low maternal plasma and leukocyte ascorbate levels in pPROM,[13] others have suggested that low ascorbate levels are found in amniotic fluid[14] or fetal serum,[15] but not maternal serum. Smoking, a major risk factor for pPROM, is known to reduce amniotic fluid ascorbate levels[16] and may be a contributory element. There is a plausible mechanism to link vitamin C deficiency and pPROM, as it acts as a co-enzyme for collagen cross-linking, and is thus required for extracellular matrix formation in the fetal membranes.[17]

INFECTION

The relationship between pPROM and infection has been long established. Micro-organisms may be cultured from amniotic fluid obtained by amniocentesis in 33% of women presenting with pPROM.[18] Infection is more commonly associated with pPROM in the early third trimester, compared to later preterm deliveries. Infection may also arise as a consequence of ascending infection during the latency period prior to the onset of labour, as this figure rises to 75% in women with pPROM at the onset of labour.[19]

In 76% of cases of pPROM, the micro-organisms isolated from the amniotic fluid are the same as those from the vagina or cervix, the commonest being *Mycoplasma* spp., *Streptococcus agalactiae* and *Streptococcus milleri*.[20] These organisms are also commonly associated with bacterial vaginosis, suggesting that abnormal colonisation of the lower genital tract may precede ascent of organisms from the vagina through the cervix into the uterine cavity. The function of the cervix, both cervical length and the nature of immune mechanisms such as IgA, secretory leukoproteinase inhibitor, lysozyme, lactoferrins, the β-defensins and sialidase may, therefore, be critical in permitting or preventing such ascent.[2]

CERVICAL DAMAGE

Most studies examining the relationship between cervical treatment for CIN and subsequent preterm delivery had demonstrated an association only with laser or cold-knife conisation of the cervix, and not with the more commonly used large-loop excision of the transformation zone (LLETZ; or loop electrosurgical excision procedure, LEEP). However, a recent larger study has demonstrated that women who had undergone LEEP had a relative risk of 1.9 for pPROM in a subsequent pregnancy, with risk greatest for those in whom a cone of > 1.6 cm in height was removed.[21]

GENETICS

Recurrence rates of pPROM in subsequent pregnancies may reflect the persistence of behavioural/environmental factors, or genetic predisposition, or a combination of both.

A number of inherited clinical conditions are associated with pPROM. Ehlers-Danlos syndrome is due to defects in collagen structure or assembly, and women carrying a fetus affected by Ehlers-Danlos syndrome have an increased risk of pPROM.[22]

Work has also identified functional genetic polymorphisms affecting the maternal immuno-inflammatory response. Polymorphisms associated with an increased risk of pPROM are shown in Table 1. Many of these polymorphisms have distinct racial distributions, which may contribute to the racial differences identified in risk of pPROM and preterm labour. More recently, the interaction of genetic polymorphisms and environmental risk factors has been examined. A recent study demonstrated that maternal carriage of the TNF-2 genotype was associated with an OR of 1.6 for preterm birth and carriage of bacterial vaginosis an OR 1.3 for preterm birth; however, a combination of both TNF-2 genotype and bacterial vaginosis had an OR of 6.0 for spontaneous preterm delivery. This study did not separate the deliveries arising from pPROM and preterm labour with intact membranes.[23]

Table 1 Genetic polymorphisms associated with increased risk of pPROM[2,54]

Polymorphism	Effect	Population studied	Maternal or fetal	Odds ratio	Reference population
IL-1RA	Increased IL-1ra and IL-1β	Hispanic American	Fetal	6.50	
TNF-α promoter (TNFA*2)	Increased TNF-α	African American	Maternal	3.18	Preterm birth
MMP-1 promoter (SNP)	Increased MMP-1	African American	Fetal	2.29	Term birth
MMP-9 promoter (14 CA-repeat)	Increased MMP-9	African American	Fetal	3.06	Term birth
IL-10 (homozygous GCC haplotype)	Increased IL-10	White Australian	Maternal	1.9	Term birth

PREDICTION

Numerous methods have been evaluated for the prediction of spontaneous preterm birth but very few differentiate between preterm delivery arising from pPROM and that from preterm labour with intact membranes. The Preterm Prediction Study identified previous pPROM, short cervix on transvaginal ultrasound, and the presence of fetal fibronectin in the cervicovaginal secretions as the strongest predictors of pPROM. Thus, a multiparous woman with all of these risk factors would have an absolute risk of pPROM at < 35 weeks' gestation of 25%.[24] Other studies have suggested that a very short cervix in the second trimester (< 10 mm)[25] and very high serum ferritin (> 64.5 ng/ml)[26] are associated with subsequent preterm delivery arising from pPROM rather than preterm labour.

PREVENTION

Our limited ability to identify women at risk of pPROM, and the multifactorial aetiopathology means that there is currently little evidence regarding effective interventions to prevent pPROM. The studies are also complicated by the failure to differentiate between preterm delivery arising from preterm labour with intact membranes, and that arising as a consequence of pPROM. However, a number of interventions have shown some benefit in prevention of pPROM.

There is some evidence that modification of behavioural risk factors such as stopping smoking may reduce the risk of pPROM.[27] Bacterial vaginosis in pregnancy is known to increase the risk of preterm delivery. Treatment of bacterial vaginosis has only been demonstrated to be of benefit in women with a previous preterm birth, in whom it reduces the risk of pPROM in the current pregnancy (OR 0.14; 95% CI, 0.05–0.38).[28] Studies are also underway to supplement vitamins C and E[29] to prevent pre-eclampsia, and it is possible that this strategy may also have an effect on the rate of pPROM.

DIAGNOSIS

Diagnosis of pPROM is straightforward when a clear history is obtained, and a large amount of amniotic fluid is observed draining from the vagina or cervix. Diagnosis of pPROM should be based on history and sterile speculum examination of the cervix. A combination of any two out of positive patient history, nitrazine testing and ferning has 93% accuracy for diagnosis of fetal membrane rupture.[30] Digital vaginal examination of the cervix should be avoided. A study by Lewis et al.[31] demonstrated a significant reduction in the latency period until the onset of labour in women who underwent digital vaginal examination on admission, in comparison to those who underwent sterile speculum examination only (2.1 days versus 11.3 days, P < 0.0001). A subsequent study has suggested that 1 or 2 vaginal examinations significantly reduced latency to onset of labour (from 5 days to 3 days; P < 0.009), but had no adverse maternal or neonatal effects.[32] However, it seems prudent to avoid digital vaginal examination in pPROM wherever possible.

Specific tests have been developed for use when the history and examination findings are equivocal. They are based upon the detection in cervicovaginal secretions of proteins normally found in high concentration in the amniotic fluid. Detection of fetal fibronectin, more recently used in the prediction of preterm labour, has a sensitivity of 90–98% and specificity of 59% for the detection of ruptured membranes.[33,34] A more recently introduced test, based upon detection of IGF-BP1, exhibits sensitivity of 81–100% and specificity of 71–95% for the diagnosis of ruptured membranes.[35,36]

NATURAL HISTORY AND CONSEQUENCES OF PPROM

There is an inverse relationship between gestational age and average latency period (Fig. 1).[37] A low amniotic fluid index on ultrasonography in pPROM is associated with a greater risk of infection and with a higher incidence of isolation of microbes from the amniotic fluid.[4] Both oligohydramnios and microbial invasion of the amniotic cavity are associated with a shorter latency period.[4,24] There is evidence that microbial invasion of the amniotic cavity is associated with a fetal inflammatory syndrome,[38] which in turn has been associated with an increased incidence of adverse neonatal outcomes including bronchopulmonary dysplasia and cerebral palsy.[39,40]

The major complication of pPROM is, therefore, that of preterm delivery and neonatal complications of prematurity. Complications associated with intra-uterine infection include chorio-amnionitis, endometritis, maternal wound infections and neonatal sepsis. Other obstetric complications include cord compression and cord accidents, increased incidence of malpresentation and increased incidence of abruption (5.5% in pPROM compared to 0.8% in the general obstetric population), with a higher incidence with a lower amniotic fluid volume.[4]

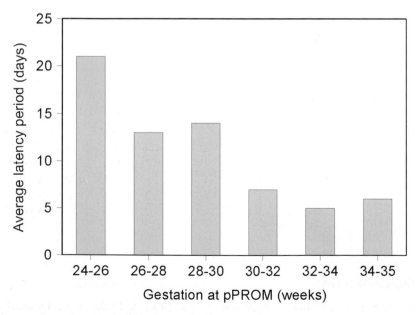

Fig. 1 Average latency period following pPROM throughout gestation (drawn from data from Lewis et al.[31]).

MANAGEMENT

ANTENATAL CORTICOSTEROIDS

The use of antenatal corticosteroids is beneficial to neonates born after pPROM. Concerns regarding potential increased risk of infective sequelae for mother and baby have not been realised. Meta-analysis suggests that corticosteroid administration to women with pPROM reduces the risk of necrotising enterocolitis (relative risk [RR] 0.21; 95% CI, 0.05–0.82), intraventricular haemorrhage (RR 0.47; 95% CI, 0.31–0.70) and respiratory distress syndrome (RR 0.56; 95% CI, 0.46–0.70).[41]

ANTIBIOTICS

A significant proportion of pPROM is infection related; as discussed above, the presence of infection after pPROM is a key factor in the duration of the latency period and the occurrence of adverse sequelae. Therefore, antibiotic therapy may be expected to improve outcomes. The ORACLE trial suggests that treatment with oral erythromycin for 10 days after pPROM will significantly delay the onset of labour and improve respiratory infections and cerebral morbidity among singletons, although no significant improvement was noted in neonatal mortality.[42] This was confirmed in a recent systematic review, which suggested that antibiotic treatment in pPROM reduced the probability of delivery within 48 h (RR 0.71; 95% CI, 0.58–0.87) and 7 days (RR 0.8; 95% CI, 0.71–0.90). Neonatal infections (RR 0.67; 95% CI, 0.52–0.85), oxygen therapy (RR 0.88; 95% CI, 0.81–0.96), need for surfactant treatment (RR 0.83; 95% CI, 0.72–0.96) and major cerebral abnormalities (RR 0.82; 95%, CI 0.68–0.99) were also reduced.[43]

TOCOLYSIS

Tocolysis has very limited value in the setting of pPROM. The majority of women have intra-uterine infection at the onset of labour with pPROM.[19] The merits of attempting to delay the onset of labour in the presence of contractions and pPROM should be weighed against the risk of adverse neonatal and maternal outcomes in the presence of chorio-amnionitis. A number of studies have examined the benefit of routine tocolysis administration to women with pPROM in the absence of contractions. A small increase in the latency period has been noted in some studies, although no benefit in neonatal outcomes was achieved.[4] There is, therefore, no evidence currently to support the use of tocolysis in the setting of pPROM.

TIMING OF DELIVERY

In the absence of evidence of intra-uterine infection, pPROM at < 34 weeks' gestation is routinely managed conservatively in order to gain fetal maturity. However, best practice if pPROM occurs at 34–36 weeks' gestation, or if a woman with pPROM occurring earlier in pregnancy reaches 34 weeks' gestation, is less certain. There is growing evidence that little benefit is gained in terms of improved neonatal mortality and morbidity in prolonging gestation beyond 34 weeks, and that delivery should be considered once this gestation is reached.[44,45]

PREVIABLE PPROM

Despite advances in obstetric and neonatal care, previable spontaneous pPROM (at 24 weeks' gestation or less) carries a very poor prognosis and is associated with risk of specific complications. Recent reviews of outcomes suggest that the median latency period achieved is 6–9 days, and that about half will deliver within a few days of presentation, although some will achieve a prolonged latency period of up to 90 days.[46,47] Overall survival rates of 26–80% have been reported, with most deaths associated with complications of extreme prematurity.[47] The occurrence of fetal membrane rupture during the canalicular phase of fetal lung development, and subsequent oligo-hydramnios, carries a specific risk of pulmonary hypoplasia even if a prolonged latency period is achieved. The greatest risk of pulmonary hypoplasia is observed if pPROM occurs at < 20 weeks' gestation, with a rate of 50% reported among neonates who subsequently delivered at > 24 weeks' gestation,[47] although pulmonary hypoplasia may occur with pPROM up to 26 weeks' gestation.

Limb restriction deformities will also occur in a small proportion of neonates (estimated at 1.5%) born after previable pPROM and prolonged period of oligohydramnios.[48]

Previable pPROM following amniocentesis carries a better prognosis, and resealing of the fetal membranes with re-accumulation of amniotic fluid will occur in a significant proportion of cases.[4]

Some work has been directed at attempting to modify the poor outcomes after early pPROM by either introducing agents into the amniotic cavity to 'reseal' the defect in the membranes, or to increase the volume of amniotic fluid by amnio-infusion and thus reduce the risk of adverse sequelae of oligohydramnios. Attempts to reseal fetal membranes in early pPROM have largely been directed at women with previable iatrogenic pPROM (e.g. following amniocentesis), in whom there is no evidence of infection. Maternal blood, platelets, cryoprecipitate, fibrinogen/thrombin, gelatin sponges and collagen grafts have all been introduced into the amniotic cavity with some degree of success.[2] However, results have been much more variable in spontaneous previable pPROM.[49,50] This suggests that women with an iatrogenic focal membrane defect without an underlying infective aetiology have a greater chance of success of treatment, in comparison to women with spontaneous pPROM in whom the immuno-inflammatory response may already be irreversibly activated.

Non-randomised studies of serial amnio-infusion in women with early pPROM have suggested a reduction in the incidence of pulmonary hypoplasia,[51] and prolongation of the latency period prior to the onset of labour.[52,53] These beneficial effects, however, may be confined to a subgroup of women who retain the infused fluid,[52,53] in whom it may be supposed the underlying membrane defect is smaller.

CONCLUSIONS

Preterm prelabour rupture of the fetal membranes remains a major cause of preterm delivery, neonatal morbidity and mortality. The underlying multifactorial aetiology, and the lack of differentiation of preterm labour with intact membranes and that following pPROM in research studies has made preventive strategies difficult to develop. Infection remains a major underlying cause, and greater understanding of the genetic basis of the immuno-inflammatory response will identify women at increased risk more accurately. Treatment strategies including antibiotic therapy and the use of corticosteroids in women who have already undergone pPROM have improved neonatal outcomes significantly. However, the prediction and prevention of pPROM remains a significant challenge in obstetrics.

Key points for clinical practice

- Preterm prelabour rupture of the fetal membranes contributes to one-third of all preterm births, and is the leading identifiable cause of prematurity and its sequelae.

- Microbial invasion of the amniotic cavity can be identified in 33% of women presenting with pPROM, and will be present in 75% at the onset of labour following a latency period. Therefore, close surveillance for evidence of infection should be the mainstay of conservative management of pPROM.

- Diagnosis of pPROM should be via speculum examination; digital vaginal examination should be avoided.

- Detection of fetal fibronectin or IGF-BP1 in vaginal secretions may aid diagnosis where history and clinical examination are equivocal.

- Routine administration of oral erythromycin to women with pPROM will significantly increase the latency period and improve neonatal respiratory morbidity.

- Administration of antenatal corticosteroids to women presenting with pPROM improves neonatal outcomes without increasing the risk of infection.

- There is no evidence regarding the safety or benefit of tocolysis in women with pPROM. It should, therefore, be used with great caution, as onset of contractions in pPROM commonly heralds the presence of intra-uterine infection.

- Conservative management to prolong gestation should be performed in the absence of evidence of infection. There is currently no evidence regarding the risks and benefits of prolongation of gestation beyond 34 weeks' gestation.

References

1. Bell SC, Malak TM. Structural and cellular biology of the fetal membranes. In: Elder MG, Romero R, Lamont RF. (eds) *Preterm Labor*. New York: Churchill Livingstone, 1997; 401–428.

2. McParland PC, Bell SC. The fetal membranes and mechanisms underlying their labour associated and pre-labour rupture during pregnancy. *Fetal Matern Med Rev* 2004; **15**: 73–108.

3. Parry S, Strauss JF. Premature rupture of the fetal membranes. *N Engl J Med* 1998; **338**: 663–670.

4. Romero R, Athayde N, Maymon E, Pacora P, Bahado-Singh R. Premature rupture of the membranes. In: Reece EA, Hobbins JC. (eds) *Medicine of the Fetus and Mother*. Philadelphia, PA: Lippincott-Raven, 1999; 1581–1625.

5. Malak TM, Bell SC. Structural characteristics of term human fetal membranes (amniochorion and decidua): a novel zone of extreme morphological alteration within the rupture site. *Br J Obstet Gynaecol* 1994; **101**: 375–386.

6. McParland PC, Taylor DJ, Bell SC. Mapping of zones of altered morphology and chorionic connective tissue cellular phenotype in human fetal membranes (amniochorion and decidua) overlying the lower uterine pole and cervix before labour at term. *Am J Obstet Gynecol* 2003; **189**: 1481–1488.

7. El Khwad M, Stetzer B, Moore RM et al. Term human fetal membranes have a weak zone overlying the lower uterine pole and cervix before onset of labor. *Biol Reprod* 2005; **72**: 720–726.

8. Harger JH, Hsing AW, Tuomala RE et al. Risk factors for preterm premature rupture of fetal membranes: A multicenter case-control study. *Am J Obstet Gynecol* 1990; **163**: 130–137.

9. Mercer BM, Goldenberg RL, Meis PJ et al. The Preterm Prediction Study: prediction of preterm premature rupture of membranes through clinical findings and ancillary testing. *Am J Obstet Gynecol* 2000; **183**: 738–745.

10. Salafia CM, Lopez-Zeno JA, Sherer DM et al. Histologic evidence of old intra-uterine bleeding is more frequent in prematurity. *Am J Obstet Gynecol* 1995; **173**: 1065–1070.

11. Chaiworapongsa T, Espinoza J, Yoshimatsu J et al. Activation of coagulation system in preterm labor and preterm premature rupture of membranes. *J Matern Fetal Neonat Med* 2002; **11**: 368–373.

12. Rosen T, Kuczynski E, O'Neill LM, Funai EF, Lockwood CJ. Plasma levels of thrombin-antithrombin complexes predict preterm premature rupture of the fetal membranes. *J Matern Fetal Med* 2001; **10**: 297–300.

13. Wideman GL, Baird GH, Bolding OT. Ascorbic acid deficiency and premature rupture of fetal membranes. *Am J Obstet Gynecol* 1964; **88**: 592–595.

14. Kim YH, Ahn BW, Yang SY, Song TB, Byun J. Antioxidant vitamins of amniotic fluid in pregnant women with preterm labor and with preterm premature rupture of membranes. *J Soc Gynecol Invest* 2000; **7 (Suppl. 1)**: 254A.

15. Eryurek FG, Genc S, Surmen E, Yalcin O. Relationship of maternal and fetal plasma ascorbic acid levels to occurrence of premature rupture of membranes. *J Clin Biochem Nutr* 1991; **10**: 225–230.

16. Barrett B, Gunter E, Jenkins J, Wang M. Ascorbic acid concentrations in amniotic fluid in late pregnancy. *Biol Neonate* 1991; **60**: 333–335.

17. Aplin JD, Campbell S, Donnai P, Bard JBL, Allen TD. Importance of vitamin C in maintenance of the normal amnion: an experimental study. *Placenta* 1986; **7**: 377–389.

18. Gomez R, Ghezzi F, Romero R et al. Premature labor and intra-amniotic infection. Clinical aspects and role of the cytokines in diagnosis and pathophysiology. *Clin Perinatol* 1995; **22**: 281–342.

19. Romero R, Quintero R, Oyarzun E et al. Intraamniotic infection and the onset of labor in preterm premature rupture of the membranes. *Am J Obstet Gynecol* 1988; **159**: 661–666.

20. Carroll SG, Papaioannou S, Ntumazah IL, Philpott-Howard J, Nicolaides KH. Lower genital tract swabs in the prediction of intrauterine infection in preterm prelabour rupture of the membranes. *Br J Obstet Gynaecol* 1996; **103**: 54–59.

21. Sadler L, Saftlas A, Wang W et al. Treatment for cervical intraepithelial neoplasia and risk of preterm delivery. *JAMA* 2004; **291**: 2100–2106.

22. Lind J, Wallenburgh HC. Pregnancy and the Ehlers-Danlos syndrome: a retrospective study in a Dutch population. *Acta Obstet Gynecol Scand* 2002; **81**: 293–300.

23. Macones GA, Parry S, Elkousy M *et al*. A polymorphism in the promoter region of TNF and bacterial vaginosis: preliminary evidence of gene-environment interaction in the etiology of spontaneous preterm birth. *Am J Obstet Gynecol* 2004; **190**: 1504–1508.

24. Mercer BM. Preterm premature rupture of the membranes. *Obstet Gynecol* 2003; **101**: 178–193.

25. Odibo AO, Talucci M, Berghella V. Prediction of preterm premature rupture of membranes by transvaginal ultrasound features and risk factors in a high-risk population. *Ultrasound Obstet Gynecol* 2002; **20**: 245–251.

26. Xiao R, Sorensen TK, Frederick IO *et al*. Maternal second-trimester serum ferritin concentrations and subsequent risk of preterm delivery. *Paediatr Perinat Epidemiol* 2002; **16**: 297–304.

27. Williams MA, Mittendorf R, Stubblefield PG *et al*. Cigarettes, coffee, and preterm premature rupture of the membranes. *Am J Epidemiol* 1992; **135**: 895–903.

28. McDonald H, Brocklehurst P, Parsons J. Antibiotics for treating bacterial vaginosis in pregnancy. *Cochrane Database System Rev* 2005; Jan 25(1): CD000262.

29. Chappell LC, Seed PT, Briley AL *et al*. Effect of antioxidants on the occurrence of pre-eclampsia in woman at increased risk: a randomised trial. *Lancet*, 1999; **354**: 810–816.

30. Friedman ML, McElin KW. Diagnosis of ruptured membranes. *Am J Obstet Gynecol* 1969; **104**: 544–550.

31. Lewis DF, Major CA, Towers CV *et al*. Effects of digital vaginal examinations on latency period in preterm premature rupture of membranes. *Obstet Gynecol* 1992; **80**: 630–634.

32. Alexander JM, Mercer BM, Miodovnik M. The impact of digital cervical examination on expectantly managed preterm rupture of membranes. *Am J Obstet Gynecol* 2000; **183**: 1003–1007.

33. Hellemans P, Verdonk P, Baeckelandt M *et al*. Preliminary results with the use of the ROM-check immunoassay in the early detection of rupture of the amniotic membranes. *Eur J Obstet Gynaecol Reprod Biol* 1992; **43**: 173–179.

34. Ericksen NL, Parisi VM, Daoust S *et al*. Fetal fibronectin: a method for detecting the presence of amniotic fluid. *Obstet Gynecol* 1992; **80**: 451–454.

35. Rutanen E-M, Pekonen F, Karkkaiinen T. Measurement of insulin-like growth factor binding protein-1 in cervical/vaginal secretions: comparison with the ROM-check membrane immunoassay in the diagnosis of ruptured fetal membranes. *Clin Chim Acta* 1993; **214**: 73–81.

36. Rutanen E-M, Seppala M. Insulin-like growth factor binding protein-1 in female reproductive functions. *Int J Gynaecol Obstet* 1992; **39**: 3–9.

37. Savitz DA, Ananth CV, Luther ER, Thorp JM. Influence of gestational age on the time from spontaneous rupture of the chorioamniotic membranes to the onset of labor. *Am J Perinatol* 1997; **14**: 129–133.

38. Gomez R, Romero R, Ghezzi F *et al*. The fetal inflammatory response syndrome. *Am J Obstet Gynecol* 1998; **179**: 194–202.

39. Yoon BH, Romero R, Kim KS. A systemic fetal inflammatory response and the development of bronchopulmonary dysplasia. *Am J Obstet Gynecol* 1999; **181**: 773–779.

40. Yoon BH, Kim CJ, Romero R. Experimentally induced intrauterine infection causes fetal brain white matter lesions in rabbits. *Am J Obstet Gynecol* 1997; **177**: 797–802.

41. Harding JE, Pang J, Knight DB, Liggins GC. Do antenatal corticosteroids help in the setting of preterm rupture of membranes? *Am J Obstet Gynecol* 2001; **184**: 131–139.

42. Kenyon SL, Taylor DJ, Tarnow-Mordi W. Broad-spectrum antibiotics for preterm, prelabour rupture of fetal membranes: the ORACLE I randomised trial. ORACLE Collaborative Group. *Lancet* 2001; **357**: 979–988.

43. Kenyon S, Boulvain M, Neilson J. Antibiotics for preterm rupture of the membranes: a systematic review. *Obstet Gynecol* 2004; **104**: 1051–1057.

44. Naef RW, Albert JW, Ross WL *et al*. Premature rupture of membranes at 34 to 37 weeks gestation: aggressive versus conservative management. *Am J Obstet Gynecol* 1998; **178**: 126–130.

45. Lieman JM, Brumfield CG, Carlo W, Ramsey PS. Preterm premature rupture of membranes: Is there an optimal gestational age for delivery? *Obstet Gynecol* 2005; **105**: 12–17.

46. Dinsmoor MJ, Bachman R, Haney EI, Goldstein M, Mackendrick W. Outcomes after expectant management of extremely preterm premature rupture of the membranes. *Am J Obstet Gynecol* 2004; **190**: 183–187.

47. Falk SJ, Campbell LJ, Lee-Parritz A *et al*. Expectant management in spontaneous preterm premature rupture of membranes between 14 and 24 weeks' gestation. *J Perinatol* 2004; **24**: 611–616.

48. Schucker JL, Mercer BM. Midtrimester premature rupture of the membranes. *Semin Perinatol* 1996; **20**: 389–400.

49. O'Brien JM, Barton JR, Milligan DA. An aggressive interventional protocol for early midtrimester premature rupture of the membranes using gelatin sponge for cervical plugging. *Am J Obstet Gynecol* 2002; **187**: 1143–1146.

50. Quintero RA. New horizons in the treatment of preterm premature rupture of membranes. *Clin Perinatol* 2001; **28**: 861–875.

51. Vergani P, Locatelli A, Strobelt N *et al*. Amnioinfusion for prevention of pulmonary hypoplasia in second-trimester rupture of membranes. *Am J Perinatol* 1997; **14**: 325–329.

52. Locatelli A, Vergani P, Di Pirro G *et al*. Role of amnioinfusion in the management of premature rupture of the membranes at < 26 weeks gestation. *Am J Obstet Gynecol* 2000; **183**: 878–882.

53. Tan LK, Kumar S, Jolly M *et al*. Test amnioinfusion to determine suitability for serial therapeutic amnioinfusion in midtrimester premature rupture of membranes. *Fetal Diagn Ther* 2003; **18**: 183–189.

54. Annells MF, Hart PH, Mullighan CG *et al*. Interleukins-1, -4, -6, -10, tumor necrosis factor, transforming growth factor-beta, FAS, and mannose-binding protein C gene polymorphisms in Australian women: risk of preterm birth. *Am J Obstet Gynecol* 2004; **191**: 2056–2067.

Mark Tattersall Siobhan Quenby

4

Dysfunctional labour

Dysfunctional labour is a common, but poorly characterised, complication of pregnancy. In order to appreciate the current problems in the management of a woman suffering from a dysfunctional labour, it is necessary to understand the terminology associated with prolonged labour, the historical development of the current management of dysfunctional labour and the current evidence for its use. Having discussed these issues, the application of recent advances in the physiology of smooth muscle to the problem of dysfunctional labour is also examined.

DEFINITION AND TERMINOLOGY

A wide variety of definitions have been given for dysfunctional labour, but the best definition is that dysfunctional labour involves a failure of either cervical dilatation or descent of the presenting part, despite the presence of uterine contractions. Such a definition would also be suggested from the term 'dystocia' which is often used interchangeably and originates from the Greek that literally means 'difficult labour'.

The term dysfunctional labour can therefore be literally seen as encompassing a clinical scenario that can result from a variety of distinct abnormalities. The simplest way of classifying these disorders is into three groups, as published by the American College of Obstetricians and Gynecologists in 1995: (i) abnormalities of the **powers** (uterine contractility or maternal expulsive effort); (ii) abnormalities involving the **passenger** (the fetus); and (iii) abnormalities involving the **passage** (the pelvis).

Mark Tattersall BMBCh
Specialist Registrar, School of Reproductive and Developmental Medicine, First Floor, Liverpool
Women's Hospital, Crown Street, Liverpool L8 7SS, UK

Siobhan Quenby MD (for correspondence)
Senior Lecturer/Honorary Consultant, School of Reproductive and Developmental Medicine, First
Floor, Liverpool Women's Hospital, Crown Street, Liverpool L8 7SS, UK (E-mail: squenby@liv.ac.uk)

'Cephalopelvic disproportion' is a term that was used synonymously with dysfunctional labour in the past. It implies that vaginal delivery has been precluded by disparity between the dimensions of the fetal head and maternal pelvis and came into usage prior to the 20th century, when the main indication for Caesarean section was pelvic contracture secondary to rickets.[1] True pelvic disproportion is now rare and it is probably more appropriate to consider the use of the term 'relative disproportion', as the majority of disproportion problems are now caused by fetal malposition. Indeed, two-thirds of women diagnosed with cephalopelvic disproportion, and therefore delivered by Caesarean section, will subsequently deliver an even larger fetus vaginally.

'Failure to progress' is a more modern term and has merit as it gives a good description of the clinical scenario, without attempting to give any suggestion as to the cause.

IS DYSFUNCTIONAL LABOUR IMPORTANT?

There has been mounting concern regarding the increasing Caesarean section rate for many years. In 1985, the World Health Organization examined national Caesarean section rates and maternal and perinatal mortality rates from various countries and concluded that there were no additional health benefits associated with a Caesarean section rate above 10–15%. The recent National Sentinel Caesarean Section Audit[2] found the Caesarean section rate in England and Wales to have risen to 21.5%. Table 1 shows the primary indications for Caesarean section in this audit of about 150,000 deliveries and clearly demonstrates that dysfunctional labour causing failure to progress is a major cause of Caesarean sections in the UK. Thus, proper understanding of the pathophysiology of dysfunctional labour and appropriate treatment will be important in any attempt to reduce the national Caesarean section rate. Although Caesarean section can be life-saving for mother or baby, it is a procedure that not only carries surgical and anaesthetic risks, but also confers significant morbidity upon women and will also influence the choice of delivery mode in any future pregnancies.

In addition to effects on the Caesarean section rate, there are a significant range of advantages of a shorter labour, as summarised in Table 2.

As well as the advantages of shorter labours, it is also important to note that there are particular risks and adverse effects of prolonged labours. Pelvic floor injury is much more common with prolonged labours and contributes to

Table 1 Primary indications for caesarean section as reported by clinicians in the National Sentinel Caesarean Section Audit[2]

Primary indication	Percentage
Fetal distress	22.0
Failure to progress	20.4
Repeat Caesarean section	13.8
Breech presentation	10.8
Maternal request	7.3
Others	25.7

Table 2 The advantages of shorter labours (*adapted from*[3])

To mother	Reduced emotional disturbance – morale has been shown to deteriorate rapidly after 12 h in labour and any emotional disturbance can last a life-time and affect subsequent pregnancies
	Elimination of need for treatment of dehydration, ketosis and salt depletion (especially a problem in tropical areas)
	Reduced need for analgesia, leading to retention of full consciousness and retention of control by the patient
	Ability of staff to provide more support
To child	Decreased exposure to trauma (instrumental delivery is more common in long labours)
To staff	Less sense of impotence and improved morale
To administrators	Greater efficiency of the delivery unit

significant morbidity for women in later life. Fistula formation is an obstetric complication that has been virtually eliminated in the Western world by avoiding extremely protracted labours. Intrapartum infection is another obstetric complication whose incidence is related to the length of labour.

PRIMIGRAVIDAE AND MULTIGRAVIDAE

In managing labour, it is imperative that one understands that there are fundamental differences in what constitutes normal labour in a primigravida and that which is normal in a multigravida. Indeed, the statement that 'primigravidae and multigravidae behave as different species' in labour[3] is undoubtedly accurate.

The most distinct feature of a first labour is its length, being much longer than any subsequent labours. This is partly due to the fact that the genital tract has not been stretched previously, but more importantly is because inefficient uterine activity is much more common in primigravidae. Indeed, inefficient uterine activity is almost entirely a disease of the first labour, being somewhat rare in subsequent pregnancies. This means that slow progress in a nulliparous women should always be assumed to be secondary to inefficient uterine action and any suggestion of obstruction should not be considered until efficient uterine activity has been achieved. In stark contrast, however, slow progress in a multiparous woman must never simply be assumed to be due to inefficient contractions and the possibility of obstruction, especially by malpresentation or malformation, must be considered. Undiagnosed obstruction can have serious consequences, as it can lead to uterine rupture, especially if oxytocin has been used. By contrast, the primigravida uterus is almost completely immune to rupture unless manipulation or instrumentation is performed.

CAUSES OF FAILURE TO PROGRESS

Although there are a variety of causes of failure to progress in labour, it is widely recognised that 'efficient uterine action is the key to normality'.[3] Steer

Table 3 Uncommon causes of failure to progress
• Incorrect diagnosis (*i.e.* patient not in labour)
• Malposition or malpresentation
• Cephalopelvic disproportion
• Other causes (*e.g.* cervical stenosis from previous cervical surgery; pelvic tumour)

and colleagues[4] studied uterine activity in 31 women progressing slowly in spontaneous labour and found that 75% had levels of uterine activity below the tenth centile for normal spontaneous labour. Thus, although the other causes of failure to progress listed in Table 3 must be considered, they can usually be excluded and treatment focused upon the problem of dysfunctional uterine activity.

DIAGNOSIS OF DYSFUNCTIONAL UTERINE ACTIVITY

The diagnosis of dysfunctional uterine activity is made by firstly recognising that the labour is failing to progress at the expected rate and then by the exclusion of any of the causes listed in Table 3. Poor labour progress is detected in most maternity units by the use of a partogram, of which there are many different types and varieties. A discussion of the partogram is given below.

THE PARTOGRAM

The concept of the partogram was first devised by Friedman and published in 1954.[5] Observations were made of cervical dilatation and the station of the presenting part and these were plotted against time elapsed in hours from onset of labour. The time of onset of labour was based on the patient's subjective perception of her contractility. Friedman found that the curves of all patients were quite similar in general shape. Plots of cervical dilatation

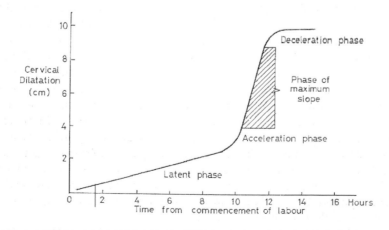

Fig. 1 Friedman's original work[5] showing the four phases of the first stage of labour.

resembled sigmoid curves and Friedman was able to define four distinct phases to the first stage of labour, as shown in Figure 1.

The first phase noted by Friedman was that of the **latent phase**. This phase had a relatively low gradient and a very wide variation in terms of length, with a mean duration of 7.3 h, but a SD of 5.5 h. The second phase was described as the **acceleration phase** and this short period was seen to lead from the minimum slope of the latent phase to the maximum slope of the third phase. The third phase, that of **maximum slope** follows this and is a linear phase during which the major portion of cervical change occurs and so its gradient is inversely related to the total duration of the first stage of labour (if the latent phase is excluded). The fourth phase of the first stage of labour is the **deceleration phase**, during which dilatation from 8.5 cm to full dilatation was seen to occur. Friedman noted that the major portion of descent of the fetal presenting part takes place during this stage, producing a hyperbolic curve when station is plotted against time.

Work published by Studd in 1972[6] further defined the characteristics of normal labour using a partogram. Studd developed 'labour stencils' which predicted the expected pattern of progress of labour. Five different stencils were developed and an important aspect of Studd's work was that the reliance on the patient's subjective perception of the onset of labour was removed. Instead, the curves were based upon the extent of cervical dilatation achieved at the time when the patient was admitted. This work meant that when a patient was admitted, the cervical dilation could be assessed and a stencil used to draw a line of expected progress on the patient's partogram. Importantly, patients crossing the expected line of progress were found to have three times the rate of instrumental delivery, compared to those that did not.[6]

Two further publications in the 1970s by Philpott and Castle[7,8] further transformed the partogram into the tool that we have today. The work introduced the concept of 'alert' and 'action' lines. Although the work was initially developed for use in African primigravidae being cared for by paramedical staff to aid in decisions as to when a patient should be transferred to a specialised tertiary care centre, these concepts have been widely accepted into Western obstetrics. The two important features of the partograph were that it was necessarily simple to use and also appeared to separate efficiently the minority of abnormal labours from the majority of normally progressing women. The alert line represented the mean rate of progress of the slowest 10% of normal African primigravid patients admitted in the active phase of labour and was drawn at a slope of 1 cm/h from the cervical dilatation measured at admission. In accordance with the findings of later studies, Philpott and Castle noted that the alert line proposed could only be used when commenced for patients with a dilatation of 3 cm or more. Philpott and Castle drew the action line 4 h to the right of the alert line, as shown in Figure 2. Crossing of the action line was the point at which Philpott and Castle argued intervention should take place. In the rural African situation, patients were managed by midwives in a peripheral unit; once the alert line was crossed, arrangements were made to transfer the patient to the labour ward of the central unit, such that within 4 h intervention could take place if required.

The choice of a delay of 4 h in the position of the action line relative to the alert line in the original work of Philpott and Castle was somewhat arbitrary,

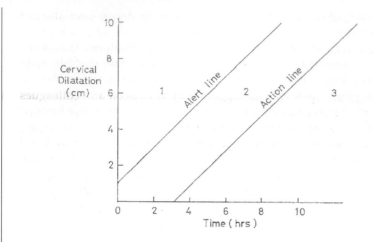

Fig. 2 Philpott and Castle's 'alert' and 'action' lines, showing the clinical subgroups: group 1, who delivered before the partograph reached the alert line; group 2, who crossed the alert line but were delivered before reaching the action line; and group 3, who crossed the action line.[7,8]

although it was influenced by the practicalities of transfer from peripheral clinics to the central labour ward. However, since then, little research has been undertaken in the form of randomised controlled trials to assess the effect of different placements of the action line. The Partogram Action Line Study[9] recently randomised nearly 1000 women to treatment using a partogram where the action line was set either 2, 3 or 4 h to the right of the alert line. Unfortunately, the results did not provide clear evidence of any difference in outcome between either an early or delayed diagnosis of dysfunctional labour. However, an important finding was that in an uncomplicated primigravid population, 44% of women had a diagnosis of prolonged labour (ranging from 52% in the 2-h group to 38% in the 4-h group). One explanation for this high proportion of women crossing the action line is that the slope of labour progression for Caucasian women in the 1990s may be different to that originally defined by Philpott and Castle[7,8] for African women in the 1970s. A steady increase in birth-weight at term, coupled with the liberal use of epidural analgesia, may also offer explanations as to why these women progressed more slowly than previously reported. Another important finding of this study was that the 2-h partogram had obvious psychological benefits. Women allocated to the 2-h group were more satisfied with their labour experience, despite receiving more intervention. This work supports an earlier randomised study[10] that found pregnant women in high-risk situations prefer active management.

MANAGEMENT

Once a diagnosis of dysfunctional labour has been made, usually via the use of a partogram to chart progress, the question arises as to how labour should be managed. Unfortunately, there is no agreed consensus answer to this question.

During the first half of the 20th century and prior to this, the duration of labour was regarded as having a very large natural variation and conservative approaches meant that attempts were rarely made to alter the duration of labour. Unless complications became obvious during labour, the main emphasis of attending practitioners was on the control of pain.

A radical change in approach was suggested by O'Driscoll and colleagues in Dublin.[11] In 1969, they produced the first publication in a series that has had much impact upon the management of dysfunctional labour since.[11] Using their technique, now known as '**active management of labour**', O'Driscoll and colleagues delivered all except one woman in a prospective study of 1000 consecutive primigravid deliveries within 24 h of the onset of labour. This was achieved with a Caesarean section rate of only 4%. The new policy also reduced the mother's requirements for analgesia and reduced the rate of forceps delivery, with a consequent reduction in the incidence of traumatic intracranial haemorrhage.

At the heart of the 'active management' protocol was the policy that once labour had started, amniotomy was performed unless dilatation of the cervix was progressive and that if this did not accelerate progress, then oxytocin infusion was commenced and continued until the placenta was delivered.

O'Driscoll et al.[11] maintained that fetal distress was the only factor that should limit the dose of oxytocin used. At the time, these proposals required the rejection of 'three popular fallacies', which were stated to be: (i) that prolonged labour in primigravidae is often an expression of cephalopelvic disproportion; (ii) that oxytocin may rupture the primigravid uterus; and (iii) that there is a valid therapeutic distinction between hypotonic and hypertonic uterine action.

A further report regarding the initial study of primigravidae[12] confirmed the first fallacy above, by showing that only 9 women (0.9%) required a Caesarean section for a diagnosis of disproportion. In addition, it was reported that in all three of these nine patients, whom had subsequently become pregnant again, normal vaginal delivery had been achieved. Furthermore, the value of X-ray pelvimetry was questioned by the finding that 4 out of 5 women, who had previously been shown to have radiological evidence of a contracted pelvis, were able to deliver vaginally.

Emphasis throughout O'Driscoll's publications has been made of his belief that an important proviso for success of active management relies upon special attention being placed upon the correct diagnosis of labour. Indeed, in a subsequent study of 1000 consecutive primigravid deliveries,[13] the Dublin team recognised the difficulty in making the diagnosis in that although the woman's diagnosis of labour was rejected on 103 occasions, the decision proved incorrect in 42 cases, as the patient returned to the delivery suite within 24 h. This mistake was the cause of 38 out of the 45 women who failed in this study to be delivered within the 12-h limit which had now been set for delivery by the team. However, the authors concluded that almost all of the 38 patients where a mistake was made in diagnosis had had a show or ruptured membranes. The conclusion from this was, therefore, that the presence of a show or ruptured membranes together with pains that caused the patient to admit herself should be considered diagnostic of labour, even in the absence of cervical changes.

Further work from Dublin has shown that clear liquor early in labour was able to virtually ensure the birth of a healthy infant, provided the length of labour was limited as per the Dublin protocol.[14] Another important point regarding the Dublin methodology is that it stresses the importance of every patient having one-to-one personal attention from a midwife/nurse, which is noted to be achieved with limited numbers of staff due to the fact that the duration of labour is limited.

The two main components of active management of labour – amniotomy and oxytocin – have become widely used in the management of labour, albeit with widely varying degrees of aggression. However, it would be useful to look at the evidence for each of these interventions.

AMNIOTOMY

A number of studies have been performed in an attempt to define the role of amniotomy in the management of dysfunctional labour. Unfortunately, limited sample sizes have reduced the ability of individual studies to assess the effects and so a recent meta-analysis provides the best data available.[15] The meta-analysis included trials where nearly 3000 women were randomised and all trials showed a reduction in labour duration with routine early amniotomy. The amount of reduction varied from 0.6–2.3 h. The meta-analysis also reported a non-significant trend towards Caesarean section, which was suggested to be due to increased intervention due to suspected fetal distress. This phenomenon was attributed to a reduction in amniotic fluid volume leading to an increase in cord compressions and a subsequent increase in fetal heart rate decelerations. However, it is important to note that the meta-analysis did not suggest that amniotomy adversely affected neonatal well-being, with routine early amniotomy producing a statistically significant improvement in the likelihood of an Apgar score of less than 7 at 5 minutes. No other indicators of neonatal depression appeared to be affected. There was no evidence for an effect of amniotomy on the likelihood of operative vaginal delivery or the use of opioid analgesia or epidural anaesthesia. A reduction in oxytocin use was observed in four of the five trials reporting on this outcome and this, together with the shortening of labour, may be responsible for the significant reduction in the proportion of women reporting severe levels of pain at some point.

OXYTOCIN INFUSION

The physiological mechanism by which oxytocin infusion might be beneficial in dysfunctional labour is best explained by the work of Steer and colleagues at St Mary's Hospital in London.[4] Initial work used oxytocin infusion in women with slow progress, whilst an intra-uterine catheter was left *in situ* to allow continuous monitoring of intra-uterine pressure.[4] Significant increases in the level of uterine activity, measured both in terms of Montevideo units and in terms of uterine activity integral (active contraction area), were seen when oxytocin infusion was commenced, compared with values obtained during a control period of measurement prior to oxytocin. Furthermore, the values obtained during the augmented period were not significantly different from the levels found in a previous study of normal spontaneous labour. It was therefore concluded that the majority of women with slow progress in labour have inadequate levels of uterine activity that can usually be corrected by oxytocin and that every uterus has an optimal level of activity (200 Montevideo units), above which increases in oxytocin infusion rate have relatively little effect.[4]

The St Mary's group later performed a small prospective randomised trial.[16] In this trial, women with slow progress were randomised to one of three groups: (i) a 'control' group where oxytocin was deferred for 8 h; (ii) a 'low-dose' group where oxytocin was only used if the uterine activity was low as measured by an intra-uterine pressure catheter and, if used, was titrated to uterine activity; and (iii) a 'high-dose' group where oxytocin was used in escalating doses, limited only by a contraction frequency of 7 per 15 min or CTG abnormality. The results showed a progressive increase in dilation rate with increasingly aggressive oxytocin use (significance was only reached in the high-dose group), together with a non-significant trend towards shorter labour. There was a trend for decreased incidence of Caesarean section (45% for the control group, 35% for the low-dose group and 26% for the high-dose group), but this was not significant. Given the small size of this study (60 patients), it would clearly be beneficial if a larger similar randomised trial were to be conducted.

ACTIVE MANAGEMENT – DOES IT WORK?

In attempting to answer the difficult question as to whether the use of active management protocols is beneficial in dysfunctional labour, it is important to establish how 'success' can be measured in this situation. The outcome measurement, which has most easily been recorded in the past, is the length of labour. Although varying definitions for this measurement have been used, it has the benefit that significant differences between groups can be demonstrated with relatively small sample sizes. Although this outcome may be important for women and those involved with the staffing of labour wards, it is widely held that the main aim of interventions in dysfunctional labour should be to reduce the Caesarean section rate without adverse effects on mother or baby.[17]

Initial work from Belfast[18] looked at 1000 consecutive primigravidae managed according to an 'active' policy. The unit was unable to match the low Caesarean section rate of the National Maternity Hospital in Dublin, producing an overall Caesarean section rate of 15.9% and with 10% of patients in spontaneous labour having a labour of longer than 12 h. However, the study showed a high rate of induction of labour of 32.5% and these patients accounted for half of the Caesarean sections performed in labour. In addition, it was found that 89% of patients with a duration of labour greater than 12 h and 72% of those in whom Caesarean sections were performed in labour were included in the group (about half) of patients in this study in whom labour was diagnosed at a cervical dilatation of 3 cm or less. Thus, it may be that the relatively poor outcomes found in this study were due to a high induction rate and the commitment to active management of patients who were not established in the active phase of labour.

Several randomised controlled trials have also attempted to assess the benefits of active management of labour, but unfortunately small sample sizes have always limited the ability of these studies to give a definitive verdict. A meta-analysis was performed,[18] which attempted to solve the problem. Ten trials were identified that met the criteria for inclusion and these were grouped into 'prevention trials' (7 trials) that accepted women with normal labour and 'therapy trials' (3 trials) that only admitted women with abnormal progress.[18] Although about 5000 women were randomised in these trials, it is unfortunate that the therapy trials only included just over 100 of these women. In terms of the main outcome variable, effects on Caesarean section rate, it was found that a policy of routine early intervention with amniotomy and oxytocin (prevention trials) did not appear to offer any significant reduction in the risk of Caesarean section or any improvement in other obstetric or neonatal outcome. However, the power of the meta-analysis was not sufficient to exclude any small beneficial effect. A trend towards a reduction in Caesarean section rate was noted in women with established slow progress (therapy trials), but unfortunately the small number of women randomised in these trials made it impossible to draw definitive conclusions. Labour was consistently shorter in duration with active management in all studies; however, in the studies that assessed subjective data from women regarding pain, it was found that active management increased the amount of pain reported. The meta-analysis also indicated that active management was associated with an increase in epidural use (as might be expected from the data regarding pain perception), but in the one study where individual one-to-one care was a component of the active intervention strategy (as advocated by Dublin), this increase in epidural use did not seem to occur.

In a subsequent small, randomised, control trial performed in Liverpool,[17] 61 patients who were making slow progress were randomised to either amniotomy and oxytocin infusion, amniotomy alone, or expectant management for 4 h. The results were in accordance with the meta-analysis, in that although there was a trend for amniotomy alone to increase dilatation rate and decrease labour length compared with expectant management, this was not significant. However, these effects were increased and became statistically significant when oxytocin infusion was added. With such a sample size, the authors did not expect to be able to determine any difference in Caesarean section rate and although there were slightly more caesarean sections performed in the oxytocin group, this was not significant. However, an important outcome from this study was the finding that satisfaction scores (determined using a validated structured questionnaire in the postnatal period before discharge from hospital) were significantly higher in the two groups where some form of intervention followed the diagnosis of dysfunctional labour. Indeed, the authors noted that 'a need to do something if things do not go according to plan' appeared to hamper recruitment to the trial, suggesting that merely the notion that action is being taken to try and correct dysfunctional labour improves mothers' perceptions of their labour.

CURRENT ADVANCES IN MYOMETRIAL PHYSIOLOGY

Research is currently on-going to improve our understanding of uterine myometrial contractility, with specific focus upon the pathophysiology that underlies the poor uterine contractility of dysfunctional labour. In the

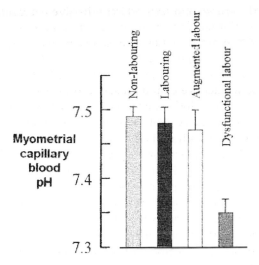

Fig. 3 There is a highly significant lower pH in myometrial blood from women undergoing emergency Caesarean section for dysfunctional labour, compared with women undergoing elective Caesarean section ('non-labouring') and those women with normal contractions undergoing emergency Caesarean section for other reasons, who have either not required augmentation ('labouring') or have required augmentation with oxytocin ('augmented labour').

myometrium, it is known that an increase in intracellular calcium is the important signal to cause a myometrial cell to contract.[20] Work in Liverpool using human myometrium obtained at elective Caesarean section has shown that both intracellular and extracellular acidification significantly reduce or even abolish phasic contractile activity and that these effects can be accounted for by changes in intracellular calcium concentration.[21]

More recent work in Liverpool[22] has provided an important new insight into the mechanism underlying dysfunctional labour. Samples of myometrial capillary blood were taken from the lower segment of the uterus in women having Caesarean sections. The results of this work were startling and significant, with the pH of the blood from women with dysfunctional labour being significantly lower ($P = 0.0009$) at 7.35, compared to that from any other group (Fig. 3). Furthermore, the lactate levels in the blood from the women

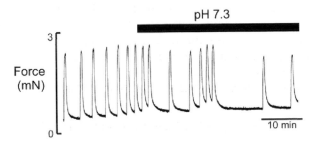

Fig. 4 The results of acidifying myometrium from women having elective Caesarean section.

with dysfunctional labour were higher and capillary oxygen saturation levels were significantly lower. In addition, when myometrium from women undergoing elective Caesarean section was isolated and perfused *in vitro*, it was shown that changing the pH of the perfusate from 7.5 to 7.3 caused 'normal' contractile patterns to change to a 'dysfunctional' appearance (*i.e.* with smaller, more irregular and less frequent contractions; Fig. 4).

The work described above, all supports the hypothesis that myometrial capillary blood is more acidic in women labouring dysfunctionally and that this causes the observed reduction in contractile activity, via a reduction in intracellular calcium. Given these results, the aim should now be to try and discover why when intermediate hypoxia occurs in all labouring women, only some become acidotic and labour dysfunctionally. It should be hoped that a better understanding of the pathophysiology of dysfunctional labour will lead to improvements in the care of women in labour. Better management could either occur by changes in practice; for example, it may be that the use of oxytocin actually increases the acidity of the myometrial blood and so 'resting' the uterus for a period might be helpful. Conversely, suggestions as to how a beneficial drug could be designed may emerge. It is also possible that methods of prediction of those women at risk of dysfunctional labour might be possible, allowing proper counselling antenatally and appropriate planning of delivery.

CONCLUSIONS

Dysfunctional labour is a common obstetric problem that causes significant distress to women. Whilst current management of this condition decreases the duration of labour there is no evidence that it decreases the Caesarean section rate. In the future, it is hoped that advances in myometrial physiology can be applied to the problem of the management of prolonged labour in order to increase the rate of vaginal delivery.

Key points for clinical practice

- Poor uterine contractility is the most common cause of poor progress in labour in the Western world.

- The established management of dysfunctional labour is diagnosis using a partogram, augmentation with oxytocin and amniotomy. However, these interventions have not been shown to decrease the Caesarean section rate.

- Advances in the understanding of the physiology of myometrium point to new therapeutic strategies in the future.

References

1. Oláh KSJ, Neilson JP. Failure to progress in the management of labour. *Br J Obstet Gynaecol* 1994; **101**: 1–3.
2. Thomas J, Paranjothy S. *RCOG Clinical Effectiveness Support Unit: National Sentinel Caesarean Section Audit Report.* London: RCOG Press, 2001.

3. O'Driscoll K, Meagher D, Boylan P. *Active Management of Labour*, 3rd edn. Mosby Year Book Europe Limited, 2003

4. Steer PJ, Carter MC, Beard RW. The effect of oxytocin infusion on uterine activity levels in slow labour. *Br J Obstet Gynaecol* 1985; **92**: 1120 1126.

5. Friedman EA. The graphic analysis of labour. *Am J Obstet Gynecol* 1954; **68**: 1568–1571.

6. Studd JWW. Graphic records in labour. *BMJ* 1972; **4**: 426.

7. Philpott RH. Graphic records in labour. *BMJ* 1972; **4**: 163–165.

8. Philpott RH, Castle WM. Cervicographs in the management of labour in primigravidae. *J Obstet Gynaecol Br Commonw* 1972; **79**: 592–598.

9. Lavender T, Alfirevic Z, Walkinshaw S. Partogram action line study: a randomised trial. *Br J Obstet Gynaecol* 1998; **105**: 976–980.

10. Hodnett ED, Hannah ME, Weston JA *et al*. Women evaluations of induction of labor versus expectant management for prelabor rupture of the membranes at term. *Birth* 1997; **24**: 214–220.

11. O'Driscoll K, Jackson RJA, Gallagher JT. Prevention of prolonged labour. *BMJ* 1969; **2**: 477–480.

12. O'Driscoll K, Jackson RJA, Gallagher JT. Active management of labour and cephalopelvic disproportion. *J Obstet Gynaecol Br Commonw* 1970; **77**: 385–389.

13. O'Driscoll K, Stronge JM, Minogue M. Active management of labour. *BMJ* 1973; **3**: 135–137.

14. O'Driscoll K, Coughlan M, Fenton V, Skelly M. Active management of labour: care of the fetus. *BMJ* 1977; **2**: 1451–1453.

15. Brisson-Carroll G, Fraser W, Bréart G, Krauss I, Thornton J. The effect of routine early amniotomy on spontaneous labour: a meta-analysis. *Obstet Gynecol* 1996; **87**: 891–896.

16. Bigwood KA, Steer PJ. A randomised control study of oxytocin augmentation of labour. 1. Obstetric outcome. *Br J Obstet Gynaecol* 1987; **94**: 512–517.

17. Blanch G, Lavender T, Walkinshaw S, Alfirevic Z. Dysfunctional labour: a randomised trial. *Br J Obstet Gynaecol* 1998; **105**: 117–120.

18. Boyle DD, White RG, Ritchie JWK. An assessment of active management of primigravid labour. *Ir J Med Sci* 1980; **149**: 465 468.

19. Fraser W, Vendittelli F, Krauss I, Bréart G. Effects of early augmentation of labour with amniotomy and oxytocin in nulliparous women: a meta-analysis. *Br J Obstet Gynaecol* 1998, **105**. 189–194.

20. Wray S, Jones K, Kupittayanant S *et al*. Calcium signalling and uterine contractility. *J Soc Gynecol Invest* 2003; **10**: 252 264.

21. Pierce SJ, Kupittayanant S, Shmygol T, Wray S. The effects of pH change on Ca^{++} signalling and force in pregnant human myometrium. *Am J Obstet Gynecol* 2003; **188**: 1031–1038.

22. Quenby S, Pierce SJ, Brigham S, Wray S. Dysfunctional labour and myometrial lactic acidosis. *Obstet Gynecol* 2004; **103**: 718–723.

Loraine Bacchus Susan Bewley

5

Domestic violence: opportunities for effective responses in maternity services

Violence against women is a major health and social problem globally. The World Health Organization states that such violence represents an infringement of human rights as it negates women's autonomy and undermines their potential as individuals and members of society.[1] The effects of domestic violence on pregnant women make it a significant issue for all midwives and obstetricians. Health services have an important role in raising awareness of the issue, facilitating discussion of abuse, documentation and signposting women to appropriate sources of help.

DEFINITION AND EPIDEMIOLOGY

The UK Department of Health[2] describes domestic violence as a 'continuum of behaviour ranging from verbal abuse through to threats and intimidation, manipulative behaviour, physical and sexual assault, to rape and even homicide'. Population-based surveys in England and Wales indicate that men perpetrate the majority of this violence and the most severe incidents are against women they know.[3,4] A review article by Shadigan *et al.*[5] states that heterosexual women are 5–8 times more likely than heterosexual men to experience violence by an intimate partner. However, men and women in gay and lesbian relationships experience partner violence at a rate comparable to women in heterosexual relationships. Studies from the UK report that between 26% and 42% of women experience some form of abuse by a current or former

Loraine Bacchus BSc MA PhD (for correspondence)
Research Associate, Kings College London, Florence Nightingale School of Nursing and Midwifery, Women's Health Academic Unit, 10th Floor North Wing, St Thomas's Hospital, Lambeth Palace Road, London SE1 7EH, UK (E-mail: loraine.bacchus@kcl.ac.uk)

Susan Bewley MB BS MA MD FRCOG
Consultant Obstetrician/Maternal Fetal Medicine, Women's Services Directorate, 10 Floor North Wing, St Thomas's Hospital, Lambeth Palace Road, London SE1 7EH, UK (E-mail: susan.bewley@gstt.nhs.uk)

partner at some point in their lives.[3,6,7] Similar rates of domestic violence have been reported in surveys from Canada[8] and the US.[9] Domestic violence accounts for 41% of female homicides in the UK compared with 8% of male homicides.[10] A report by the Metropolitan Police found that domestic violence accounts for 25% of all homicides in London and 35% in England and Wales.[11]

Although these figures are alarming, they are unlikely to reflect the true extent of the problem. On average, a woman will be assaulted 35 times before she reports the abuse to the police.[12] In the 1996 British Crime Survey, only 22% of the women who experienced chronic abuse and 9% of women with intermittent abuse had informed the police of the last incident.[3] Abused women often express feelings of shame and guilt about their situation; their self-esteem and confidence is progressively undermined. Subsequently, many women live in constant fear of their partner and are either reluctant to, or may be prevented from, confiding in others for help.[13,14]

EXTENT OF DOMESTIC VIOLENCE DURING PREGNANCY

Rather than offering respite, pregnancy may represent a period of increased vulnerability to domestic violence.[15] Between 2.5% and 3.4% of women experience partner abuse during pregnancy in the UK.[16-18] Studies from the US report the prevalence of domestic violence during pregnancy to be between 5.2%[19] and 33.7%,[20] with the greatest risk occurring postpartum[21] and amongst teenagers.[22]

A review of 56 domestic violence murders that occurred in London between 2001 and 2002 identified pregnancy as one of six risk factors for homicide.[11] Domestic violence was first mentioned as a cause of maternal death in the 1994–1996 Confidential Enquiry into Maternal Deaths (CEMD) in the UK, where six women died as a result of violence by a partner.[23] The 2000–2002 CEMD highlighted that 40% of the 391 deaths reported to the enquiry had domestic violence documented in the maternity notes.[24] Fifty-five women who died (of 391, 14%) self-reported domestic violence or were known to health professionals to have a history of violence; 12 of these women died as a result of the violence.

The report also highlighted a number of practice-related issues that increased women's vulnerability. These include the use of family members as interpreters, poor communication and co-ordination between maternity and other services involved in the women's care, failure to follow-up poor attendance actively, inappropriately questioning a woman's partner about the cause of her injuries, and failing to ask about domestic violence.

RISK FACTORS AND INDICATORS

Those most at risk of experiencing domestic violence are young women who are single, separated or divorced with children living at home.[3] Women with a prior history of victimisation also appear to be at greater risk of violence during pregnancy. Helton et al.[25] found that 87.5% of women who experienced abuse during pregnancy had also been abused prior to pregnancy.

There is a common misconception that women from lower socio-economic groups are disproportionately affected by domestic violence. However, it is suggested that social class differences in reported rates of domestic violence may reflect differences in ability to escape violent relationships. For example,

Table 1 Physical and behavioural indicators of abuse

Physical indicators	Behavioural indicators
Burns from cigarettes, appliances, rope, friction or boiling water	Beginning antenatal care late
Back, chest or abdominal pain or tenderness	Missed appointments, non-compliance with treatment regimens, discharging herself early against medical advice
Injuries to the breasts, abdomen or genitals	Frequent attendance at the antenatal clinic or emergency services; admissions with vague complaints and symptoms
Injuries to the extremities	Over-solicitous partner who answers questions directed at the woman, reluctant to leave her alone with a health professional
Head, neck or facial injuries (*e.g.* bruises, scratches, bite marks strangulation marks)	Woman appears frightened, anxious or afraid to speak in front of her partner
Premature removal and infection of perineal sutures (a possible indicator of forced sex)	Community practitioners denied access to the home for postnatal visits
Dizziness, blackouts, partial loss of hearing or vision (possible indicator of head injuries)	Delay in seeking treatment for injuries
Vaginal bleeding, genital injury, sexually transmitted infections	Distress, aggression or withdrawn behaviour during pelvic examinations, labour and delivery (pelvic examinations and labour may trigger feelings of loss of control as a result of sexual abuse)

women from lower socio-economic groups may have no alternative but to seek help from the police, refuges and healthcare settings due to a lack of access to resources.[26] A UK study found that women from higher socio-economic groups experienced domestic violence at a rate comparable to women from lower socio-economic groups, but were less likely to report the abuse to an outside agency.[27]

Table 1 presents a number of physical and behavioural indicators that may raise a health professional's index of suspicion. However, it is important to recognise that no single factor will accurately predict which women are likely to be affected by domestic violence. It is important to note that abused women may present with a range of symptoms, injuries and behaviours or none at all.

IMPLICATIONS FOR MATERNAL AND FETAL HEALTH

Domestic violence is a significant factor in maternal and perinatal morbidity.[28] Abuse during pregnancy is associated with miscarriage, placental abruption, premature rupture of membranes, premature labour, chronic pain, hyperemesis, vaginal bleeding, infections, low maternal weight gain, and the delivery of low birth weight infants.[29] The precise mechanism by which these outcomes occur is unclear as prospective studies are lacking. It is suggested that both direct (*e.g.* trauma to the abdomen) and indirect (*e.g.* exacerbation of existing conditions) causal pathways exist.[30] Fetal fractures, bruising and deformity have been reported in case studies of women presenting with trauma to the abdomen inflicted by a partner.[31] McKenna *et al.*[32] describe a case study of a pregnant woman presenting at 37 weeks with sudden onset of abdominal pain and concealed abruption. Further investigation revealed that the woman had sustained splenic injury that was actively bleeding. Post-surgery, the woman admitted to having been assaulted by her partner and had been violently punched in the left flank 8 days earlier. There is some evidence to suggest that domestic violence in pregnancy may affect infant health during the puerperium. Huth-Bocks *et al.*[22] compared 68 pregnant women who experienced domestic violence in pregnancy with 134 non-abused pregnant women. Abused women had significantly more infant-related visits to the emergency department and infant-doctor visits than non-abused women.

Research suggests that women who have been abused during pregnancy are more likely than non-abused women to be admitted with vague unresolved problems.[33] Women may use the antenatal ward for respite from the abuse[34] or present at the clinic or day-assessment unit after an assault to check that the baby is unharmed.

There has been very little work investigating the impact of domestic violence on women's mental health during pregnancy and the postpartum. However, studies of non-pregnant women have reported increased rates of depressive illness, post-traumatic stress disorder and suicidal ideation in abused women compared to non-abused women.[35] Stark and Flitcraft's[36] US study of suicide found that women who had experienced partner abuse were significantly more likely to be pregnant when they attempted suicide than non-abused women. A UK survey of antenatal and postnatal women found that increased depressive symptomatology was significantly associated with a history of domestic violence.[17]

There is also a link between abuse during pregnancy and behaviours which have an additional adverse effect on maternal and fetal health, such as increased smoking or alcohol use, illicit drug use, delayed entry to antenatal care and missed appointments.[37] Women who experience domestic violence are more likely to describe their pregnancy as unplanned or unwanted.[37] This may indicate that the woman is unable to negotiate contraceptive use within an abusive relationship or that some pregnancies are conceived out of rape.

The availability of emotional or practical support is known to serve as a buffer against the effects of domestic violence by reducing the woman's feelings of isolation, encouraging her to seek positive solutions and adopt self-care behaviours that are health enhancing.[38]

DEVELOPING EFFECTIVE RESPONSES TO DOMESTIC VIOLENCE

Before outlining the role of the health professional in supporting abused women, it is important to acknowledge that domestic violence is not a 'disease' of women, but a pervasive social problem that can cause long-term emotional and physical damage to women and children. Therefore, it cannot be approached or managed within the traditional medical framework of 'diagnosis' and 'remedy', since any support or intervention offered will not necessarily effect an immediate change in the woman's situation. However, as with other public health issues such as smoking and alcohol, health professionals have an important role in prevention and early intervention through awareness raising and offering advice and information. As is the case when dealing with other victims of crime, the attitude of professionals can make a difference to how women perceive their situation and their feelings of self-worth, which may ultimately have an impact on their recovery. This can be encapsulated in a quote from one pregnant woman suffering partner abuse: 'Not every (health professional) can deal with this problem. It's a very delicate problem...they are between destroying or helping the person because some can make you feel more foolish, or they could help you stand on your own feet'. In accepting the limitation of their actions, health professionals can avoid feelings of frustration or helplessness when they encounter an abused woman who is clearly not ready to make immediate changes to her situation. Living with abuse on a daily basis causes feelings of entrapment, isolation and disempowerment[13,14] which can lower a woman's self-esteem, making it difficult to discuss the situation with healthcare professionals or accept any help offered. Denial and minimisation of the abuse are protective behaviours that women engage in to survive.[14] Therefore, any intervention offered may only produce observable benefits for the women who are ready to disclose and accept help. But for others, it may provide important validation of their experiences and may trigger active help-seeking at a later date.

The UK Department of Health[2] published the *Domestic Violence Resource Manual* recommending that public and social care health organisations 'take every opportunity to identify those who many be subject to violence, and by offering practical and emotional support, help prevent the situation deteriorating'. Historically, health professionals have tended to treat the consequential injuries of domestic violence, but failed to offer any additional support or follow-up.[39] However, this practice is no longer considered acceptable.[34] Abused women frequently come into contact with healthcare services. A UK study of 198 women attending an accident and emergency department reported the prevalence of life-time physical abuse to be 34.8%, physical abuse in the previous year was 6.1% and life-time life-threatening abuse was 10.6%.[40] Contact with healthcare services may become more frequent as the abuse continues. Unfortunately, abused women's encounters with health services have not always been helpful, mainly due to the lack of training and awareness amongst health professionals.[41] It is possible that health professionals respond differently to women who have experienced domestic violence or other stressful life events because their presentation may send out subtle clues that the appointment will be lengthy unless managed carefully. Given that most health professionals work under pressure and feel poorly equipped to deal with domestic violence, it is not surprising that many abused women report negative experiences during their health encounters.

ROUTINE ENQUIRY FOR DOMESTIC VIOLENCE

There is no risk-management tool that health professionals can use to identify accurately which women are likely to be affected by domestic violence. Price[34] states that screening for risk markers may not be useful, due to the covert nature of domestic violence. Asking appropriate and timely questions of all women using maternity services may be effective. In the UK, there has been considerable debate between academics and activists concerning the use of the term 'screening' in relation to identification of domestic violence. Taket et al.[42] suggest that the term 'routine enquiry' is a more suitable approach for domestic violence, as in practice the questions themselves may vary, or may be asked in certain health settings or when there is a high index of suspicion. The use of routine questioning for domestic violence significantly increases the rate of identification of abused women in antenatal settings.[16] Covington et al.[43] compared enquiry for domestic violence by maternity care co-ordinators at three points during pregnancy using structured and direct questions, with a standard one-time assessment consisting of unstructured, indirect questions. The rate of documented domestic violence at the first assessment increased from 5.4% to 10.3%. Over the three time periods, the rate of documented violence increased from 5.4% to 16.2%.

WHAT DO ABUSED WOMEN FIND HELPFUL AND UNHELPFUL IN THEIR HEALTH ENCOUNTERS?

Health professionals sometimes fear that women will view the questions as an invasion of privacy and will be offended. However, it would appear that the majority of women find the practice appropriate if they are asked in a non-judgemental manner by a trained health professional.[6,44] Abused women are more likely than non-abused women to prefer specific questions about abuse as opposed to general, open-ended questions.[45]

Qualitative studies with abused women have contributed to a better understanding of the benefits of routine questioning and the factors likely to influence acceptability and willingness to discuss abuse. Key factors that facilitate disclosure of abuse are: continuity of carer; the availability of a safe, confidential environment; the degree of rapport and trust between the woman and health care provider; a sensitive approach to questioning; active listening; follow-up support; and allowing the woman to remain in control of her actions.[44,46] The health professional's body language and facial expressions can be subtle, but important, ways of showing concern and developing trust.[46]

Factors that appear to inhibit disclosure of domestic violence in health settings include: the woman's fear of escalating abuse from the partner (keeping quiet is a safety strategy); low self-esteem; the woman's sense of family responsibility; the perceived difficulties of single parenthood and the prospect of financial hardship; concerns over confidentiality and lack of time during antenatal appointments.[46] Responses that abused women find unhelpful include: blaming, judgemental and insensitive attitudes, the health professional taking control of the situation without obtaining consent (e.g. calling the police) and discussing the abuse with the perpetrator present.[45] Health professionals must strike a balance between being proactive and supportive, but accepting of the fact that leaving an abusive relationship can be a lengthy process.

Midwives caring for pregnant women are understandably concerned about what they are expected to do when they encounter abused woman. Lack of time, privacy, confidentiality, concerns about child protection and personal safety are just some of the factors identified by midwives.[47] It is important to set realistic goals when working with abused women, and to be honest and clear from the start about what can and cannot be achieved, as well as what can and cannot be kept confidential (*e.g.* with regards to concerns about children). Abused women do not expect health professionals to act as problem solvers; nor do they expect immediate solutions to their difficulties. Appropriate responses, as identified by abused women, include; information giving, making referrals to community organisations, documenting the abuse, ensuring the woman's safety, conveying positive messages to the woman (*e.g.* telling them that they are not to blame, that domestic violence is a crime), and discussing the situation in a sensitive and non-judgemental manner.[44,45] Simply asking about domestic violence may constitute a form of early intervention, in that it provides an opportunity to acknowledge and confront the issue, and to discuss the effects of abuse and options available. Documentation, both of the woman's recall of events and any physical examination, needs to be thorough and placed in confidential medical records (*i.e.* not hand-held maternity records) as it may provide vital evidence in the future. The mere act of documentation or 'witnessing' of abuse and violence may enable a woman who has very little control in her life to feel respected and taken seriously.

RESEARCH ON MATERNITY-BASED INTERVENTIONS FOR ABUSED WOMEN

There has been little systematic evaluation of maternity-based interventions for women experiencing domestic violence, particularly in terms of the long-term impact on physical and psychological health, women's and children's safety, parenting and quality of life. In addition, no studies have attempted to define or assess the potential harmful outcomes of health service interventions. To date, there are two published papers, both from the US, that evaluate interventions for pregnant women attending maternity services, using violence as the outcome measure. Parker *et al.*[48] reported a reduction in the frequency and severity of the violence at 6- and 12-month follow-up amongst women receiving a counselling intervention compared to women who received information only. McFarlane *et al.*[49] compared three types of intervention for abused pregnant women: information giving; counselling; and counselling plus outreach support. At the 2-month follow-up, the women who received information had significantly lower scores on measures of abuse (indicating a reduction in severity) compared to those receiving the more intensive interventions. This would appear to suggest that the minimum response of providing abused women with referral information is sufficient to produce a short-term reduction in the violence. However, it may be that women in different stages of the abuse trajectory benefit from different intervention approaches, although no studies have attempted to explore this as a possibility. However, these differences did not persist at the 6-, 12- or 18-month follow-up. In addition, counselling support was only provided during pregnancy, which may have limited the effects of the intervention, as prevalence studies indicate that women are most at risk of escalating abuse during the postpartum period.[21] Clearly, there is a need for further evaluative research to help inform the development of effective interventions.

Table 1 Summary of good practice for enquiring about and responding to domestic violence

Awareness and recognition of domestic violence
- Training and education for all health and non-health staff
- Displaying leaflets and posters about the extent of domestic violence and useful phone numbers

Provide a safe and confidential environment where you cannot be overheard
- Ask to see the woman alone at the beginning or end of the appointment as a routine procedure
- Have a clinic policy that woman are seen alone, and notices in the waiting rooms referring to this
- Use strategies to obtain confidential consulting time (*e.g.* directing her to another area to provide a urine sample, take a blood test, meet her at the home of a friend/family member if you are a community practitioner)
- Only use professional interpreters, preferably female

Identifying and aiding disclosure
- Start with open-ended questions such as 'How are things at home?' and 'Are you getting the support you need?'
- Explain why you ask about partner abuse. For example, 'Many of the women I see are dealing with abusive relationships. However, many are too afraid or uncomfortable to discuss it. That's why I've started to ask about it routinely'
- The following are examples of direct questions about abuse that may be used:
i. *Many women tell me that they've been hurt by someone close to them. Could this be happening to you?*
ii. *Has your partner ever physically hurt or threatened you?*
iii. *Have you ever been in a relationship where you've been hit, punched or hurt in any way? Is that happening now?*
iv. *Does your partner sometimes try to put you down or control what you do?*
v. *Are you afraid of anyone at home?*
vi. *I've noticed some bruises. Has someone hurt you? Was it your partner?*

Document the abuse meticulously – it may be used later as agencies request evidence
- Never document domestic violence in hand-held notes. Use confidential patient records
- Describe in detail how the injuries were sustained (*e.g.* Mrs A was punched in the face with a closed fist by her partner Mr B, on the 3rd September at 2:00 pm. The incident took place at her home address, *etc.*) and note frequency and severity of past and current abuse
- Describe the size, pattern and location of any injuries (use a body map picture if necessary)
- It may be necessary to provide treatment for any injuries/symptoms resulting from the abuse
- Document the help you offer, whether or not the woman accepts it

Safety assessment, information giving and on-going support
- Is it safe for the woman (and her children) to return home that day?
- Inform the woman of her options and of specialist domestic violence services in and out of her area that can provide emergency help and long-term support
- Do not work in isolation. Access the expertise of local organisations
- Offer written information about domestic violence organisations and other support services, but check that it is safe for the woman to take the information home. It may be safer to write a list of useful numbers on a piece of paper, or offer a small card with useful numbers that she can carry discretely
- Offer on-going support and monitoring of the situation

GOOD PRACTICE POINTERS FOR WORKING WITH ABUSED WOMEN

Table 2 presents an overview of good practice when enquiring about and supporting women affected by domestic violence.

CONCLUSIONS

Appropriate training, support and supervision are necessary to facilitate changes in health professionals' practice. This should be underpinned by the development of guidelines within the maternity service and the relevant resources, such as the availability of confidential consulting time with women and funds for staff training. Partnership work with local voluntary and statutory agencies is the most effective way to address domestic violence. Health professionals are not expected to work in isolation. There is a vast amount of expertise that can be accessed, for example, from Women's Aid Federation of England, Refuge, Police Community Safety Units and local specialist domestic violence agencies. Information about local domestic violence services and strategies can be accessed through local domestic violence fora. Health services can promote awareness of domestic violence amongst health staff; facilitate discussion of abuse by asking the right questions; document the abuse; signpost women to sources of help; and work in partnership with other voluntary and statutory agencies to provide co ordinated support for the woman and her children.

Although domestic violence in pregnancy has been a taboo subject and its detection is a sensitive issue, pregnancy and childbirth are life-changing times. Both the mother and developing newborn are vulnerable from the abuse. The mother who passes through maternity services needs opportunities for validation and information if she is to make meaningful adjustments to her situation. It is beholden on maternity care health providers to be aware of the prevalence of abuse, skilled in its detection and to provide appropriate support.

Key points for clinical practice

- Violence in pregnancy is common, hidden and presents a risk to both the mother's and child's life and health.

- Women do not mind being questioned sensitively about their relationships and abuse.

- Questioning must be safe, confidential and non-judgemental.

- Safety is paramount. Women may need an emergency admission or referral to a refuge, or may prefer to go home. They should at least be encouraged to consider a 'safety plan' if violence worsens.

- Maternity professionals can take women seriously, document abuse, and offer referrals onto other helping agencies (refuges, police, social services, housing, advocacy).

- Women with little self-esteem may not disclose their abuse nor be able to make immediate changes to their circumstances.

References

1. World Health Organization. *Violence against women information pack: a priority health issue.* WHO: Geneva 1997. Available online at: <http://www.who.int/frh-whd/VAW/infopack/English/VAW_infopack.htm>.
2. Department of Health. *Domestic violence: a resource manual for health care professionals.* London: DoH, 2000.
3. Mirlees-Black C. *Domestic violence: findings from a new British Crime Survey self-completion questionnaire.* Research Study 191. London: Home Office, 1999.
4. Kershaw C, Budd T, Kinshott G, Mattinson J, Mayhew P, Myhill SA. *The 2000 British Crime Survey. England and Wales.* Home Office Statistical Bulletin 18/00. London: Home Office, 2000.
5. Shadigan EM, Bauer ST. Screening for partner violence during pregnancy. *Int J Gynecol Obstet* 2004; **84**: 273–280.
6. Bradley F, Smith M, Long J, O'Dowd T. Reported frequency of domestic violence: cross sectional survey of women attending general practice. *BMJ* 2002; **324**: 271–274.
7. Richardson J, Coid J, Petruckevitch A, Chung WS, Moorey S, Feder G. Identifying domestic violence: cross sectional study in primary care. *BMJ* 2002; **324**: 274–277.
8. Johnson H, Sacco VF. Researching violence against women: Statistics Canada's national survey. *Can J Crim* 1995; **37**: 281–304.
9. McFarlane J, Christoffel K, Bateman L, Miller V, Bullock L. Assessing for abuse: self-report versus nurse interview. *Public Health Nurse* 1991; **8**: 245–250.
10. Home Office Research and Statistics Directorate. *Criminal statistics England and Wales* 1995. London: Stationary Office, 1996.
11. Metropolitan Police. *Findings from the multi-agency domestic violence murder reviews in London. Prepared for the ACPO Homicide Working Group.* London: Metropolitan Police, 2003.
12. Yearnshire S. Analysis of cohort. In: Bewley S, Friend J, Mezey G. (eds) *Violence against women.* London: RCOG Press, 1997; 45.
13. Frank JB, Rodowski MF. Review of psychological issues in victims of domestic violence seen in emergency settings. *Emerg Med Clin North Am* 1999; **17**: 657–677.
14. Landenburger KM. The dynamics of leaving and recovering from an abusive relationship. *J Obstet Gynecol Neonatal Nurs* 1998; **27**: 700–706.
15. Berenson AB, Stiglich NJ, Wilkinson GS, Anderson GD. Drug abuse and other risk factors for physical abuse in pregnancy among white non-Hispanic, black and Hispanic women. *Am J Obstet Gynecol* 1991; **164**: 1491–1499.
16. Bacchus L, Mezey G, Bewley S, Haworth A. Prevalence of domestic violence in pregnancy when midwives routinely enquire. *Br J Obstet Gynaecol* 2004; **111**: 441–445.
17. Bacchus L, Mezey G, Bewley S. Domestic violence: prevalence in pregnant women and associations with physical and psychological health. *Eur J Obstet Gynecol Reprod Biol* 2004; **113**: 6–11.
18. Johnson JK, Haider F, Ellis K, Hay DM, Lindow SW. The prevalence of domestic violence in pregnant women. *Br J Obstet Gynaecol* 2003; **110**: 272–275.
19. Torres S, Han HR. Psychological distress in non-Hispanic white and Hispanic abused women. *Arch Psychol Nurse* 2000; **14**: 19–29.
20. Huth-Bocks AC, Levendosky AA, Bogat GA. The effects of violence during pregnancy on maternal and infant health. *Viol Vict* 2002; **17**: 169–185.
21. Harrykissoon SD, Rickert VI, Wiemann CM. Prevalence and patterns of intimate partner violence among adolescent mothers during the postpartum period. *Arch Pediatr Adolesc Med* 2002; **156**: 325–330.
22. Parker B, McFarlane J, Soeken K. Abuse during pregnancy: Effects on maternal complications and birth weight in adult and teenage women. *Obstet Gynecol* 1994; **84**: 323–328.
23. Department of Health. *Why mothers die. Report on confidential enquiries into maternal deaths in the United Kingdom 1994–1996.* London: DoH, 1998.
24. CEMACH (Confidential Enquiry into Maternal and Child Health) *Why mothers die 2000–2002. The confidential enquiries into maternal deaths in the United Kingdom.* London: RCOG Press, 2004.

25. Helton A, McFarlane J, Anderson ET. Battered and pregnant: a prevalence study. *Am J Public Health* 1987; **77**: 1337–1339.
26. Hunt SC, Martin AM. *Pregnant women violent men. What midwives need to know*. Oxford: Butterworth-Heinemann, 2001.
27. Mooney J. *The hidden figure: domestic violence in North London*. London: Islington Council, 1993.
28. Jasinski JL. Pregnancy and domestic violence. A review of the literature. *Trauma Viol Abuse* 2004; **5**: 47–64.
29. Bacchus L, Bewley S, Mezey G. Domestic violence in pregnancy. *Fetal Matern Med Rev* 2001; **12**: 249–271.
30. Newberger EH, Barkan SE, Lieberman WS *et al*. Abuse of pregnant women and adverse birth outcome. Current knowledge and implications for practice. *JAMA* 1992; **267**: 2370–2372.
31. Ribe JK, Teggatz JR, Harvey CM. Blows to the maternal abdomen causing fetal demise: report of three cases and a review of the literature. *J Forens Sci* 1993; **38**: 1092–1096.
32. McKenna D, Adair S, Price J. Domestic violence in late pregnancy and splenic injury: delayed presentation. *Acta Obstet Gynecol Scand* 2003; **82**: 95–96.
33. Mezey G, Bacchus L, Bewley S, Haworth S. *An exploration of the prevalence, nature and effects of domestic violence in pregnancy*. Economic and Social Research Council, Violence Research Programme 2001. Available online at: <http://www.rhul.ac.uk/sociopolitical-science/VRP/Findings/Findings.htm>.
34. Price S. Domestic violence. In: Squire C. (ed) *The social context of birth*. Abingdon: Radcliffe Medical Press, 2003.
35. Kemp A, Rawlings EL, Green BL. Post-traumatic stress disorder (PTSD) in battered women: a shelter sample. *J Trauma Stress* 1991; **4**: 137–148.
36. Stark E, Flitcraft A. Killing the beast within: woman battering and female suicidality. *Int J Health Serv* 1995; **25**: 43–64.
37. Cokkinides VE, Coker AL. Experiencing physical violence during pregnancy: prevalence and correlates. *Fam Com Heal* 1998; **20**: 19–37.
38. Sullivan CM, Bybee DI. Reducing violence using community-based advocacy for women with abusive partners. *J Consul Clin Psychol* 1999; **67**: 43–54.
39. Kurz D. Interventions with battered women in health care settings. *Viol Vic* 1990; **5**: 243–256.
40. Sethi D, Watts S, Zwi A, Watson J, McCarthy C. Experience of domestic violence by women attending an inner city accident and emergency department. *Emerg Med J* 2004; **21**: 180–184.
41. Gerbert B, Johnston K, Caspers N *et al*. Experiences of battered women in health care settings: a qualitative study. *Women Health* 1996; **24**: 1–17.
42. Taket A, Nurse J, Smith K *et al*. Routinely asking women about domestic violence in health settings. *BMJ* 2003; **327**: 673–676.
43. Covington DL, Diehl SJ, Wright BD, Piner MH. Assessing for violence during pregnancy using a systematic approach. *Matern Child Health J* 1997; **1**: 129–132.
44. Bacchus L, Mezey G, Bewley S. Women's perceptions and experiences of routine screening for domestic violence in a maternity service. *Br J Obstet Gynaecol* 2002; **109**: 9–16.
45. McNutt LA, Carlson BE, Gagen D, Winterbauer N. Reproductive violence screening in primary care: perspectives and experiences of patients and battered women. *JAMWA* 1999; **54**: 85–90.
46. Rodriguez MA, Szkupinski S, Bauer HM. Breaking the silence. *Arch Fam Med* 1996; **5**: 153–158.
47. Mezey G, Bacchus L, Bewley S, Haworth A. Midwives' perceptions and experiences of routine screening for domestic violence. *Br J Obstet Gynaecol* 2003; **110**: 744–752.
48. Parker B, McFarlane J, Soeken K, Silva C, Reel S. Testing an intervention to prevent further abuse to pregnant women. *Res Nurs Health* 1999; **22**: 59–66.
49. McFarlane J, Soeken K, Wiist W. An evaluation of interventions to decrease intimate partner violence to pregnant women. *Public Health Nurs* 2000; **17**: 443–451.

Peter Brocklehurst Sara Kenyon

6

Group B streptococcus in pregnancy

Colonisation of the genital tract with group B streptococcus (GBS) in pregnancy is common and may lead to neonatal sepsis, which remains a major cause of neonatal death and disability. GBS is the most frequent cause of early-onset neonatal sepsis and occurs in about 0.5 per 1000 live births in the UK and has a case fatality of about 10%.

Prevention of neonatal GBS sepsis remains controversial. In the US, all women are offered antenatal screening and intrapartum antibiotic prophylaxis to try and prevent neonatal sepsis. This results in large numbers of women being treated in labour. In the UK, despite there being no systematic screening, the incidence of neonatal sepsis is the same as that in the US in the presence of universal screening.

To date, there is little evidence that universal screening for GBS in pregnancy is happening in the UK. However, this remains a topical and controversial issue. With the recent National Service Framework for Children, Young People and Maternity services[1] advocating normal birth and the NICE Intrapartum Guidelines being undertaken at present, the introduction of a universal antenatal screening programme for GBS would have a substantial impact on the configuration of maternity care. There seems little doubt that such a programme should not be introduced without thorough prior evaluation.

THE ORGANISM

The group B streptococcus (GBS), *Streptococcus agalactiae*, is a Gram-positive diplococcus. It can be divided into a number of different serotypes – Ia, Ib, Ia/c,

Peter Brocklehurst MBChB FRCOG MSc(Epidemiology) (for correspondence)
Director, National Perinatal Epidemiology Unit, University of Oxford, Old Road Campus, Headington, Oxford OX3 7LF, UK (E-mail: Peter.brocklehurst@npeu.ox.ac.uk)

Sara Kenyon RM MA (Applied Health Studies)
Senior Research Fellow, Reproductive Sciences Section, Department of Cancer and Molecular Studies, University of Leicester, Leicester LE2 7LX, UK. (E-mail: oracle@leicester.ac.uk)

II, III, IV, V, VI. The different sereotypes are important to distinguish, as they are associated with differing virulence and presentations.[2] For example, serotype III accounts for about a third of all early-onset neonatal sepsis, whilst serotype II accounts for about a quarter of all cases. In contrast, serotype III is associated with 85% of early-onset neonatal meningitis and nearly 90% of all late-onset neonatal sepsis. This contrasts with the situation in adults, where serotype II is responsible for about 60% of adult meningitis and 30% of adult bacteraemia.

EPIDEMIOLOGY

COLONISATION IN PREGNANCY

GBS is frequently isolated from the lower gastrointestinal tract, the genital tract and urinary tract. The prevalence of asymptomatic colonisation in pregnant women is similar to that in non-pregnant women and varies depending on the methods used for identifying the organism. However, despite the differing methods of isolation used, the world-wide prevalence of asymptomatic carriage in the vagina during pregnancy appears to be in the region of 15–25%, although carriage rates as low as 10% and as high as 40% have been reported. If swabs are taken from the rectum as well as the vagina, the identification of asymptomatic carriage increases; if a specific GBS culture medium is used, the prevalence of carriage will increase even further. Around 25% of mothers in the UK appear to be GBS carriers.[3] However, this estimate is based on a single study performed in the 1980s in London and it is possible that this does not reflect current carriage levels throughout the UK.

The prevalence of colonisation varies according to a number of characteristics. A higher prevalence has been found in younger women, in diabetic women and women of Hispanic or Caribbean origin. In contrast, the frequency of sexual intercourse or number of sexual partners does not appear to influence carriage rates. GBS is not considered a sexually transmitted infection and treatment of partners does not prevent re-colonisation of treated women.

MOTHER-TO-CHILD TRANSMISSION

The main concern about GBS colonisation in pregnancy is that the organism may be transmitted to the baby before or during birth.

Fetal infection
Although GBS has been reported to cross intact membranes and cause fetal infection, which may result in stillbirth, this remains an infrequent event considering the large number of women who carry GBS in the genital tract.

Transmission during birth
The usual route of neonatal exposure to GBS is at the time of birth, either through ascending infection in the presence of ruptured membranes or during passage through the colonised birth canal. A number of risk factors have been identified which increase the likelihood of the neonate being colonised. These

include increasing duration of membrane rupture prior to delivery, maternal postpartum fever or endometritis (or both), prolonged labour, and preterm birth. An increased risk of colonisation and neonatal sepsis is also associated with higher maternal bacterial load.[2]

RISK OF NEONATAL COLONISATION

It is estimated that about half of all babies born to women carrying GBS will themselves be colonised with GBS. However, the vast majority of these infants will not develop symptomatic GBS infection. Between February 2000 and February 2001, national surveillance of invasive GBS disease in infants younger than 90 days was undertaken through an active surveillance system involving paediatricians, microbiologists and parents.[4] In this study, 377 cases of confirmed early-onset GBS neonatal sepsis were identified in England, Wales, Scotland, Northern Ireland and the Republic of Ireland out of a total population of 794,037 live-births. If 25% of these women were colonised with GBS, then 198,500 babies will have been born to women who were colonised with GBS. If 80% of these neonates were exposed to GBS during labour or vaginal delivery, then about 79,400 are likely to have been colonised. As only 377 of these 79,400 colonised babies became infected, the risk of early-onset neonatal sepsis developing as a result of being colonised is about 5 per 1000. However, the likelihood of developing GBS early-onset neonatal sepsis as a result of being born to a woman who carried GBS in the lower genital tract is less than 2 per 1000.

INCIDENCE OF GBS NEONATAL SEPSIS

Until the national surveillance study of neonatal GBS infection was undertaken, there was no accurate information on the incidence of GBS neonatal sepsis in the UK. During the 1-year study period, 568 cases were identified, equivalent to a total incidence of 0.72 per 1000 live births (95% CI, 0.66–0.78). The incidence of early-onset disease was 0.48 per 1000 (95% CI, 0.43–0.53) and for late-onset disease 0.24 per 1000 (95% CI, 0.21–0.28). Risk factors were identified for 218 (58%) cases of early-onset disease, these being: preterm delivery (less than 37 weeks' gestation) in 37%, prolonged rupture of the membranes for more than 18 h in 44% or known genital carriage of GBS during pregnancy in 4%.

There is also evidence to suggest that intra-uterine fetal monitoring during labour significantly increases the risk of neonatal sepsis.[5]

Recent evidence has suggested that the incidence of culture-proven GBS neonatal sepsis is likely to underestimate the true incidence of this infection in neonates. Data collected prospectively in one centre in the UK for over a year for 413 neonates who underwent a septic screen in the first 72 h after birth have suggested that the true incidence of early-onset neonatal GBS sepsis may be as high as 3.6 per 1000 live births.[6] This was based on the presence of GBS colonisation and symptomatic neonatal sepsis without isolation of any organism from a usually sterile site such as blood or CSF.

In the US, the incidence of culture-confirmed, early-onset GBS neonatal sepsis was 2–3 cases per 1000 live births in the early 1980s.[7] Following the introduction of a national screening and treatment programme advocated by the Centers for Disease Control and Prevention,[8] the incidence of confirmed GBS neonatal sepsis has fallen to 0.32 per 1000 live births which is the lowest ever recorded (Fig. 1).[9] In contrast, the rate of late-onset GBS sepsis has remained fairly constant at 0.35 per 1000 live births over this period,[9] leading to the suggestion that nosocomical infection plays a large part in the aetiology of late-onset disease.

CLINICAL PRESENTATION AND MANAGEMENT

MATERNAL INFECTION

In the antenatal period, GBS infection rarely presents clinically. On occasion, women may present with an increased vaginal discharge which, when cultured, yields GBS. Whether GBS is the cause of the discharge is often uncertain, although antibiotic treatment may alleviate the symptoms. GBS may also cause urinary tract infections in pregnancy which may be found incidentally or may cause symptoms of dysuria and frequency.

Symptomatic women should be treated with oral penicillin.

In the postpartum period, GBS can cause maternal infectious morbidity. Clinical presentation includes endometritis, sepsis and urinary tract infection. Rarely, it can cause meningitis. Presenting signs and symptoms of pelvic infection in the mother can include fever, malaise, uterine tenderness and offensive lochia. With the advent of wide-spread use of intrapartum antibiotic prophylaxis for GBS in the US, the incidence of pregnancy-associated, culture-confirmed GBS infection (including endometritis) decreased from 0.29 per 1000 live births in 1993 to 0.23 per 1000 live births in 1998.[10] Maternal death from GBS-associated postpartum infection is extremely rare.

Postpartum endometritis is frequently a polymicrobial infection and broad-spectrum antibiotics should be used to treat these women.

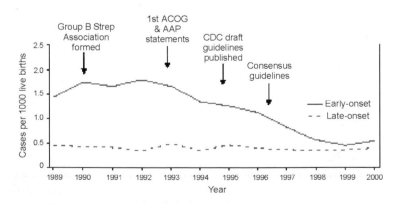

Fig. 1 Incidence of early- and late-onset invasive GBS disease – selected Active Bacterial Core surveillance areas, 1989–2000, and activities for prevention of GBS disease. ACOG, American College of Obstetricians and Gynecologists; AAP, American Academy of Pediatrics. Adapted from CDC (Early onset group B streptococcal disease, United States, 1998–1999. *MMWR* 2000; **49**: 793–796) and Schrag *et al.*[10]

INFECTION IN THE NEWBORN

Early-onset disease

This condition occurs during the first 7 days after birth with the majority of cases (about 90%) presenting during the first 24 h (Fig. 2).[4] Neonates most commonly present with septicaemia (63%) or pneumonia (26%).[4] Clinical manifestations are frequently non-specific and may include irritability, poor feeding, and lethargy. If not present at birth, the infant may present within a few hours of birth with moderate respiratory distress (closely mimicking respiratory distress syndrome on X-ray).[11]

Late-onset disease

This occurs beyond 7 days after birth and can develop up to 90 days. These babies are more likely than those who have early-onset disease to present with meningitis (43%) or focal infection (7%).[4] The clinical presentation is once again often non-specific in the first instance.

For the neonate with confirmed GBS infection, the treatment of choice is penicillin G for 10 days. As the causative organism is not always known at the onset of symptoms, broad-spectrum antibiotics are often used in the first instance which should include an agent active against GBS.

PROGNOSIS OF NEONATAL SEPSIS

In the past, the case fatality of GBS sepsis was reported as about 20% with small, preterm infants suffering the highest mortality and morbidity. Early-

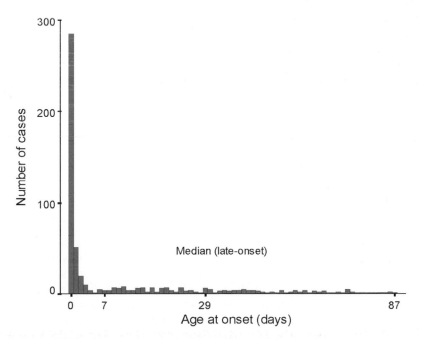

Fig. 2 Age of onset of signs of sepsis in babies with confirmed neonatal GBS sepsis. Reproduced with kind permission of Springer Science and Business Media from Pollard McCracken & Finn (2004) in *Hot Topics in Infection and Immunology in Children* (Menson & Heath, eds), figure 30.1 on page 232.

onset disease was associated with the highest mortality.[11] An incidence of 12% of major neurological sequelae was reported following GBS meningitis.[12] Improvements in the treatment of neonates has resulted in a reduction in this mortality. Overall mortality for the disease for culture-positive babies was 53 (9.7%) in the UK national surveillance study[4] with a 10.6% mortality for early-onset disease and 8% for late-onset disease. The case fatality was significantly higher in infants born prematurely with a mortality of 15.2% in babies at 33 weeks or less compared with a mortality of 6.4% for babies of 37 weeks or more.

DIAGNOSIS

The diagnosis of GBS sepsis is confirmed by culture of the organism from blood, CSF or another sterile site. Culture of GBS from surface sites, including skin or mucus membranes, will identify colonisation but will not confirm GBS sepsis.

Other methods of diagnosis are available. There are a number of antigen detection methods which have been used in an attempt to identify GBS more rapidly than standard culture techniques. The detection rate and false-positive rate associated with these antigen detection tests has not yet been sufficiently high for them to be used routinely in place of the standard culture methods.[13]

Molecular methods are also available, although not in routine clinical practice, and have very high detection rates with low false-positive rates; however, these are only used in the context of on-going research at present.

PREVENTION OF NEONATAL GBS SEPSIS

EFFECTIVENESS OF INTRAPARTUM ANTIBIOTIC PROPHYLAXIS

There have been five randomised controlled trials conducted in a total of 838 women to determine the effectiveness of intrapartum antibiotic prophylaxis at preventing mother-to-child transmission of GBS. These have been included in a Cochrane Review,[14] which concludes that antibiotic prophylaxis results in a relative risk decrease of 83% (95% CI, 61–93%) of babies with confirmed early-onset GBS neonatal infection. However, there are a number of concerns with this conclusion. The first is that all five trials were judged to be of poor quality, but perhaps the most important concern is the choice of outcomes reported in these trials. These include GBS colonisation and GBS sepsis confirmed by culture. Most neonatal sepsis is 'presumed'. This means that in less than half of all cases of neonatal sepsis is the infecting organism identified. By only measuring culture-confirmed GBS infection, the existing randomised controlled trials will underestimate the incidence of all sepsis due to GBS. Similarly, they will underestimate the incidence of any specific cause of sepsis, such as *Escherichia coli*. However, the most important issue is that if a woman is given antibiotics during labour to prevent GBS transmission and the baby then develops sepsis, it is very likely that GBS will not be isolated from the neonate because of the transplacental transfer of antibiotics. This does not mean that the baby's sepsis is not due to GBS, but that the organism cannot be isolated because of the presence of antibiotic in the sample taken. As no trials have measured the effect of intrapartum antibiotic prophylaxis on the incidence of neonatal sepsis as a whole or on other outcomes, such as neonatal death, it is not possible to be certain to what extent intrapartum antibiotic prophylaxis decreases the incidence of neonatal sepsis, neonatal death and other substantive measures of neonatal and later morbidity.

SCREENING PROGRAMMES

The evidence that intrapartum antibiotic prophylaxis may reduce the risk of neonatal sepsis has led to the development of a number of screening strategies which aim to identify women at risk of having a baby with neonatal sepsis so that intrapartum antibiotic prophylaxis can be offered.

The first strategy, and the one that is recommended by the Centers for Disease Control and Prevention for national screening in the US,[13] involves taking swabs from the rectum and vagina between 35–37 weeks from all pregnant women and offering intrapartum antibiotic prophylaxis if they are identified as GBS carriers. If women present in labour before a swab has been taken or before the results are available, then intrapartum antibiotic prophylaxis is offered.

A second strategy is a 'risk-based' approach. In this strategy, women are not swabbed antenatally but are identified as being at increased risk of having a baby who develops early-onset GBS sepsis if they present with 'risk-factors' such as preterm labour, prolonged rupture of the membranes or have a fever during labour. These women are offered intrapartum antibiotic prophylaxis. This strategy used to be advocated by the Centers for Disease Control and Prevention[8] as being equally effective as a swab-based strategy but is now felt to be inferior and is no longer recommended.

A third strategy is a combination of the previous two. In this approach, women are swabbed antenatally and if they subsequently present with a 'risk-factor' in labour, such as prolonged ruptured membranes or fever, they are offered intrapartum antibiotic prophylaxis. If no 'risk-factor' is identified, then no antibiotics are offered. This strategy has been suggested by a Canadian group but does not appear to be used anywhere in the world.

A fourth strategy is one of rapid bed-side testing in labour. Women identified as being carriers are then offered intrapartum antibiotic prophylaxis. This strategy is not yet possible because of the unknown reliability of intrapartum rapid testing. There is a randomised controlled trial currently underway in the UK testing this approach. In addition, in a UK setting, testing in labour would require women being cared for in midwife-led units to transfer in labour to consultant-led units in order for them to receive intravenous antibiotics.

Intrapartum antibiotic prophylaxis

It is recommended that intravenous benzyl penicillin 3 g be given as soon as possible after the onset of labour and 1.5 g, 4-hourly, until delivery. It has a narrow spectrum of activity and is relatively cheap. Clindamycin 900 mg should be given intravenously 8-hourly to those allergic to penicillin. Broad-spectrum antibiotics such as ampicillin should be avoided if possible, as concerns have been raised regarding increased rates of neonatal Gram-negative sepsis.[15] To optimise the efficiency of antibiotic prophylaxis, the first dose should be given at least 2 h before delivery.[16]

Management of the infant identified as being at high risk of GBS sepsis

Newborn infants with clinical signs of early-onset disease should be treated promptly with the necessary antibiotics, whether or not their mothers received intrapartum treatment. Blood cultures should always be obtained prior to the commencement of treatment.

If maternal treatment was given for at least 2 h prior to delivery, there is no reason to treat the well-infant with intravenous antibiotics, as the risk of developing disease is remote.[16] The baby should be examined and observed closely.

If maternal treatment was not received at all or for the minimum time period, there are insufficient data available to recommend a single management strategy for the neonate. Because 90% of cases of early-onset GBS sepsis present in the first 12 h of age, the risk of disease in infants who remain well without treatment beyond this time may not be substantially elevated above that of the infant with no risk factors. The argument for using prophylactic treatment in well-infants may be stronger in the presence of multiple risk factors, such as prematurity or prolonged rupture of the membranes, but is still unproven.

It is not necessary to perform routine surface or blood cultures on well-infants as the illness will usually present before the culture results are available.

For the infant whose mother had a previous infant with GBS disease, either clinical evaluation after birth and observation for at least 12 h are necessary, or blood cultures should be obtained and the infant treated with penicillin until the culture results are available.

Effects of screening

There have been no randomised controlled trials which have compared antenatal screening with no antenatal screening and none have compared different screening strategies.

Estimates of the efficacy of the screening strategies are based on observational studies. In addition, the focus of these studies has been the incidence of culture-proven GBS sepsis. In infants exposed to intrapartum antibiotic prophylaxis, it is possible that the confirmation of GBS disease is made more difficult by the presence of antibiotics effective against GBS in the neonate's blood. Studies have not measured the incidence of neonatal sepsis as a whole, a large proportion of which is culture negative (some of which will be caused by GBS). In addition, some studies have suggested that a decreased incidence of neonatal sepsis due to GBS has not been accompanied by a decrease in neonatal sepsis as a whole nor in neonatal mortality. However, findings from different studies have been contradictory.

Observational studies from the US have suggested that the introduction of a screening programme for antenatal GBS has resulted in a substantial fall in the incidence of neonatal early-onset GBS sepsis from 1.5 per 1000 births to 0.5 per 1000 births from 1996 to 2000 (Fig. 1).[13] The fact that such wide-spread use of intrapartum antibiotics may lead to selection pressure on the organisms causing early-onset neonatal sepsis has also raised concerns. It may be that wide-spread screening in pregnancy and treatment increases the rate of late-onset GBS disease, although the evidence for this is not strong.[17] There is also evidence that other causes of severe neonatal sepsis (such as *E. coli* sepsis) may be increased thereby resulting in no overall reduction in neonatal sepsis.[18,19] The Neonatal Research Network in 15 centres in North America examined babies weighing less than 1500 g over two time periods from 1991–1993 (7606 infants) and 1998–2000 (5447 infants). The overall rate of sepsis remained unchanged (19.3 per 1000 live births in the first period to 15.4 per 1000 in the second (no significant difference) but the *E. coli* sepsis rate increased from 3.2 per 1000 to 6.4 per 1000 live birth ($P = 0.004$).[15]

Several papers, on the other hand, have reported either a stable or decreasing rate of Gram-negative neonatal sepsis.[20,21] Data from the Australian Study Group for Neonatal Infections (ASGNI) suggest that from 1992 to 2001 there has been a suggestion of a trend (although not a statistically significant one) of decreasing early-onset *E. coli* sepsis in all babies and that the rate in very low birth-weight infants in Australasia is stable.[22]

As the real benefit of a screening programme can only be hypothesised from the available evidence, it is not possible to weigh explicitly the benefit against the possible harm. There are, however, two major and direct possible harms from wide-spread use of intrapartum antibiotic prophylaxis which merit further consideration:

1. **Anaphylaxis**. The incidence of severe anaphylaxis associated with the use of penicillin in labour has been estimated at 1 per 10,000 women treated. The fetal effects of severe anaphylaxis have not been well reported. Fatal maternal anaphylaxis has been estimated to occur in as many as 1 per 100,000 patients treated.[23] If 25% of the UK pregnant population is treated with penicillin, this might result in two maternal deaths per year as a consequence of penicillin anaphylaxis. In the US, maternal deaths are not systematically reported as they are in the UK[24] although there have been no reports in the literature of maternal deaths associated with the GBS screening programme.

2. **Antibiotic resistance**. GBS isolates with confirmed resistance to penicillin or ampicillin have not been observed to date.[13] Penicillin remains the agent of choice for intrapartum antibiotic prophylaxis as it has a narrower spectrum of antimicrobial activity and may be less likely to select for resistant organisms.

   The SENTRY programme was established in 30 centres in the US, Canada and South America in 1997 and gathers data on nosocomical and community-acquired infections. These laboratories contribute their first 20 bloodstream isolates to a central laboratory every month.[25] Significant geographical variation in antibiotic resistance of GBS was seen on 182 invasive GBS isolates from neonates over a 3-year period. In South America, no resistance was detected to either erythromycin (0%; 95% CI, 0–9%) or clindamycin (0%; 95% CI, 0–9%), while in Canada erythromycin resistance was 14% (95% CI, 4–34%) and clindamycin resistance was 7% (95% CI, 1–31%). Resistance to clindamycin was the same in the US (7%; 95% CI, 3–15%) but 25% of GBS was erythromycin resistant (95% CI, 17–37%).

This increasing erythromycin resistance supports the strategy advocated by the most recent CDC guidelines[13] that clindamycin be the antibiotic of choice for β-lactam allergic women. The factors influencing antibiotic resistance are numerous, and would also include the increased use of antibiotics more generally in pregnancy.[26]

If wide-spread use of intrapartum antibiotic prophylaxis is to be used, it would appear prudent to use a narrow-spectrum antibiotic, such as benzyl penicillin, rather than broad-spectrum agents such as ampicillin. This may minimise antibiotic resistance patterns.

The impact of adopting universal antenatal screening in the UK

Using data from the UK National Surveillance Study, it is possible to estimate the potential impact of a screening policy in the UK. During the year of the surveillance project, there were 794,037 births. If 25% of women carry GBS in their genital tract, this will result in 198,500 women being identified as GBS carriers during the antenatal period. If about 80% of these women go into labour, this will result in 158,800 women a year receiving intrapartum antibiotic prophylaxis. In the same delivery population, there were 377 cases of confirmed GBS early-onset neonatal sepsis. If intrapartum prophylaxis decreases this by 80% to 75 cases a year, then 526 women will be treated to prevent one case of neonatal GBS infection. Of the 377 cases of early-onset sepsis, 38 babies died as a consequence of their infection. Once again, assuming that intrapartum prophylaxis can decrease this by 80% then this may prevent 30 deaths per year in the UK out of a total number of neonatal deaths of 2519. This means that 5290 women will require intrapartum antibiotic prophylaxis to prevent one neonatal death from GBS sepsis. All of the above calculations assume that intrapartum antibiotic prophylaxis is as effective as the existing Cochrane Review suggests.[13] If intrapartum antibiotic prophylaxis is 50% effective at preventing neonatal sepsis and neonatal death, then the number of women who will require treatment to prevent one case of neonatal GBS sepsis is 840 and to prevent one neonatal death will be 8360.

Current UK practice

Practice regarding screening and intrapartum management of GBS in the UK was assessed in 1999 and 2001 by a survey of all obstetric units.[27] The response rates were 84% in 1999 and 82% in 2001. Of the responding units, six (3%) in 1999 and four (2%) in 2001 used vaginal swab based screening for GBS colonisation in the antenatal period. In 1999, intrapartum antibiotic prophylaxis was offered to women with a previous baby affected by GBS disease in 85% (176/207) of maternity units and in 2001 this had risen to 95% (193/203). Similarly, in 1999 intrapartum antibiotic prophylaxis was offered to women who were known GBS carriers in 87% (179/207) of maternity units and in 2001 this had risen to 95%(193/203). When intrapartum antibiotic prophylaxis was used, the appropriate dose of a recommended antibiotic was prescribed in 7% (9/123) units in 1999 and in 20% (35/178) in 2001.

Current UK recommendations

The Royal College of Obstetricians and Gynaecologists has produced national guidelines for the prevention of neonatal GBS infection:[16]

Intrapartum treatment is recommended if a woman is found to be colonised in her current pregnancy, has GBS bacteriuria, or has had a previously affected baby. The risk factors of prematurity (less than 35 weeks), intrapartum fever (higher than 38°C) and prolonged membrane rupture at term (longer than 18 hours) should inform discussions with women as to whether or not to advise intrapartum antibiotic prophylaxis. The argument for treatment becomes stronger in the presence of two or more risk factors.

VACCINES – A LONG-TERM SOLUTION?

The vaccination of women of child-bearing age and the provision of protection by placental transfer of specific antibody appears to be an ideal solution for the prevention of neonatal GBS sepsis. The complexity of achieving this has been highlighted by the recent publication of the entire genome of *S. agalactiae*.[28] This GBS genome contains 2082 genes and the function of 40% remain unknown, so there remain many vaccine targets yet to be explored.

The majority of vaccine strategies to date have involved conjugating capsular polysaccharide with T-cell dependent protein antigens, such as tetanus toxoid or diphtheria toxoid, which enhance immunogenicity.[29] Other groups have used novel conjugates such as the C5a peptidase which is present in most GBS isolates. Antibody to this peptidase provides serotype-independent killing of GBS.[30]

In a recent study, the risk of disease correlated with the amount of protective maternal antibody present.[31] When maternal antibodies levels were ≥ 5 μg/ml, there was an 88% risk reduction in invasive disease (95% CI, 7–98%). Therefore, it appears that not only does any vaccination have to maintain a certain level of antibody but this also has to be maintained for potentially many years when that woman could bear children.

Vaccine trials in pregnant women would also be ethically difficult and large sample sizes would be needed to show an effect on neonatal sepsis rates as GBS disease is still a relatively rare event.

In addition to potentially reducing neonatal GBS disease, vaccination could also lead to reductions in maternal GBS urinary tract infection and chorioamnioitis, and could potentially prevent preterm birth. Also, with vaccination a reality, the complications associated with intrapartum antibiotic prophylaxis such as maternal anaphylaxis, antibiotic resistance and changes in neonatal sepsis rates would no longer present the same potential problems.

References

1. Department of Health. *National Services Framework for Children, Young People and Maternity Services: Maternity.* London: DH Publications, 2004.
2. Baker C, Edwards M. Group B streptococcal infections. In: Remington & Klein. (eds) *Infectious Diseases of the Fetus and Newborn Infant*, 4th edn. Philadelphia, PA: WB Saunders, 1995; 980–1054.
3. Easmon CS. The carrier state: group B streptococcus. *J Antimicrobial Chemother* 1986; **18**: 59–65.
4. Heath PT, Balfour G, Weisnor AM *et al.* on behalf of PHLS GBS Working Group. Group B streptococcal disease in UK and Irish infants younger than 90 days. *Lancet* 2004; **363**: 292–294.
5. Adair C. Kowalsky L, Quon H *et al.* Risk factors for early-onset group B streptococcal disease in neonates: a population based case-control study. *Can Med Assoc J* 2003; **163**: 198–203.
6. Luck S, Torny M, d'Agapeyeff K *et al.* Estimated early-onset group B streptococcal neonatal disease. *Lancet* 2003; **361**: 1953–1954.

7. Zangwill KM, Schuchat A, Wengen JD. Group B streptococcal disease in the United States 1990: report from a multistate active surveillance system. *MMWR* 1992; **41** (556): 25–32.
8. Centers for Disease Control and Prevention. Prevention of perinatal group B streptococcal disease: a public health perspective. *MMWR* 1996; **45** (No. RR-7).
9. Centers for Disease Control and Prevention. Diminishing racial disparities in early-onset neonatal group B streptococcal disease. United States 2002–2003. *MMWR* 2004; **53** (23): 502–505.
10. Schrag SJ, Zywicki S, Farley MM et al. Group B streptococcal disease in the era of intrapartum antibiotic prophylaxis. *N Engl J Med* 2000; **342**: 15–20.
11. Feldman RG. *Streptococcus agalactiae* group B streptococcus. In: Greenough A, Osbourne J, Sutherland S. (eds) *Congenital, Perinatal and Neonatal Infections*. Edinburgh: Churchill Livingstone, 1992; 185–192.
12. Wald ER, Bergman I, Taylor HG, Chiponis D, Porter C, Kubek K. Long-term outcome of group B streptococcal meningitis. *Paediatrics* 1986; **77**: 217–221.
13. Centers for Disease Control and Prevention. Prevention of perinatal group B streptococcal disease. *MMWR* 2002; **51** (No. RR-11,1-23).
14. Smaill F. Intrapartum antibiotics for group B streptococcal colonisation. In: Cochrane Library, Issue 1. Oxford Update Software, 1996.
15. Stoll B, Hansen N, Farcroft AA et al. Changes in pathogens causing early onset in very low birth weight infants. *N Engl J Med* 2002; **347**: 240–247.
16. The Royal College of Obstetrics and Gynaecology. *Prevention of early onset neonatal group B streptococcal disease*. Guideline Number 36. London, RCOG, 2003. Available <http://www.rcog.org.uk>.
17. Wiseman LE, Adams KM, Lodinger BS. Is late onset group B streptococcal disease in infants increasing? *Pediatr Res* 2000; **47**: 348A.
18. Towers CV, Carr MH, Padilla G, Asrat T. Potential consequences of widespread antepartum use of ampicillin. *Am J Obstet Gynecol* 1998; **179**: 879–883.
19. Wolf H, Schaap AHP, Smit BJ, Spanjaard L, Adriannse AH. Liberal diagnosis and treatment of intrauterine infection reduced early-onset neonatal group B streptococcal infection but not sepsis by other pathogens. *Infect Dis Obstet Gynaecol* 2000; **8**: 143–150.
20. Wendel Jr GD, Leveno KJ, Sanchez PJ, Jackson GL, McIntire DD, Seigel JD. Prevention of neonatal group B streptococcal disease: a combined intrapartum and neonatal protocol. *Am J Obstet Gynecol* 2002; **186**: 618–626.
21. Reisner DP, Haas MJ, Zingheim RW, Williams MA, Lutny DA. Performance of a group B streptococcus prophylaxis protocol combining high-risk treatment and low-risk screening. *Am J Obstet Gynecol* 2000; **182**: 1335–1343.
22. Daley AJ, Garland SM. Prevention of neonatal group B streptococcal disease. Progress, challenges and dilemmas. *J Paediatr Child Health* 2004; **40**: 664–668.
23. Weiss ME, Adkinson NF. Immediate hypersensitivity reactions to penicillin and related antibiotics. *Clin Allergy* 1988; **18**: 515–540.
24. Department of Health. *Why Mothers Die 1997–99*. The fifth report of the Confidential Enquiries into Maternal Deaths in the United Kingdom. London: RCOG Press, 2001.
25. Andrews JJ, Diekema DJ, Hunter SK et al. Group B streptococcal causing neonatal bloodstream infection: antimicrobial susceptibility and serotyping results from SENTRY centres in western hemisphere. *Am J Obstet Gynecol* 2000; **183**: 859–862.
26. Mercer BM, Carr IL, Beazley DD, Crouse DT, Sibai BM. Antibiotic use in pregnancy and drug-resistant infant sepsis. *Am J Obstet Gynecol* 1999; **181**: 816–821.
27. Kenyon S, Brocklehurst P, Blackburn A, Taylor D. Antenatal screening and intrapartum management of group B streptococcus in the UK. *Br J Obstet Gynaecol* 2004; **111**: 226–230.
28. Glaser P, Rusniok C, Buchrieser C et al. Genome sequence of *Streptococcus agalactiae*: a pathogen causing invasive neonatal disease. *Mol Microbiol* 2002; **45**: 1499–1513.
29. Berner R. Group B streptococci during pregnancy and infancy. *Curr Opin Infect Dis* 2002; **15**: 307–313.
30. Cheng QI, Carlson B, Pillai S et al. Antibody against surface bound C5a peptidase is opsonic and initiates macrophage killing in group B streptococci. *Infect Immun* 2001; **69**: 2302–2308.
31. Lin F-YC, Philips JB, Azimi PH et al. Level of maternal antibody required to protect neonates against early onset disease caused by group B streptococcus type 1a: a multicentre, seroepidemiology study. *J Infect Dis* 2001; **184**: 1022–1028.

Otto P. Bleker Leonie A.M. van der Hulst
Martine Eskes Gouke J. Bonsel

7

Place of birth: evidence for best practice

There is no doubt that the optimal place of birth for high-risk pregnant women is the hospital, staffed with experienced perinatal caregivers. Specialist care and continuous fetal monitoring can be applied during labour with delivery around the clock; there is little doubt that by doing so, in most cases, possible fetal distress is noticed in due time and proper treatment modalities are readily provided.

However, in low-risk pregnant women, labour and delivery is a normal physiological process that most women experience without complications. Nevertheless, in most Western countries, the preferred place of birth is the hospital, which generally means that the responsible caregiver is a medical specialist, *i.e.* the obstetrician. Some professional guidelines even argue that because intrapartum complications can sometimes arise quickly and without warning, the hospital provides the safest setting for labour, delivery, and the immediate postpartum period.[1]

Questions have emerged about this latter reasoning. While it is generally true for all industrialised societies that their population is healthier than ever, all countries face a steady general increase of obstetrical interventions during

Otto P. Bleker MD PhD FRCOG (for correspondence)
Professor of Obstetrics and Gynaecology, Academic Medical Center, H4-210, PO Box 22700, 1100 DE Amsterdam, The Netherlands (E-mail: o.p.bleker@amc.uva.nl)

Leonie A.M. van der Hulst MA
Midwife and Sociologist, Department of Obstetrics and Gynaecology, AMC, Amsterdam, The Netherlands

Martine Eskes MD PhD
Obstetrician and Gynaecologist, Medical Advisor at the Health Care Insurance Board (CVZ), Diemen, The Netherlands

Gouke J. Bonsel MD PhD
Professor of Public Health Methods, Department of Social Medicine, AMC, Amsterdam, The Netherlands

labour and delivery, even in low risk pregnant women. In a recent report from Dublin on 1000 nulliparous women in spontaneous labour with cephalic presentation at term, epidural analgesia was given in 77.2% and other forms of pain relief in another 9.2%. Augmentation of labour (as part of active management) was undertaken in 51.9%. Spontaneous vaginal delivery was achieved by 71.8% of women.[2] These figures may or may not be considered a success. In any event, a significant proportion of these nulliparous women must have been healthy and at low-risk of obstetrical interventions including pain relief. It is intriguing to speculate on the results of such women in a non-hospital environment and in midwifery care, as this may provide a provisional clue on the dominance of 'push' (technology induced) rather than 'pull' (induced by ill health) forces.

The hospital environment is thought to be responsible for an increase in obstetrical interventions and the medicalisation of labour and delivery in healthy, low-risk women, due to a set of cumulative factors such as: (i) separation of family members; (ii) the rigid application of procedures; (iii) the lack of choice (e.g. for positions for labour), (iv) the routine implementation of continuous electronic fetal monitoring, even in low-risk cases, which is associated with a rather high false-positive rate for 'fetal distress'; etc. Apart from the hospital environment, inter-related aspects of obstetric care (e.g. personal and emotional factors) are very likely to also play an important role with respect to the course of labour. Important aspects of emotional, social, and empathic support during child-birth serve to establish a relationship based on trust. This type of care is thoroughly discussed by Keirse et al.[3] and van der Hulst.[4] These authors stress particularly that the effects of a more personal and continuous support during labour and delivery, focused on empowering women's feelings of certainty, should be the goal of future research.

At present, fewer than 2% of births in the UK, most other European countries, and the US take place at home. In contrast, in The Netherlands about 40% of all deliveries are led by independent midwives and 75% of these are home births. Obviously, among the public, the pregnant women and their families and among the professionals involved, opinions about the best place of birth differ widely.

We will discuss the literature with special emphasis on the quality of obstetric care in relation to the place of labour and delivery in an attempt to answer the question: what is the best place of birth for a healthy woman at low risk of obstetric pathology and thus low interventions, after a normal pregnancy?

Analysis will focus on the on-going selection process during pregnancy, which selects high-risk pregnancies during the antenatal period, prior to the definite choice of the place of birth, and on the incidence of referral from primary care to secondary (hospital) care during labour and delivery. The outcome of pregnancy is defined as obstetric interventions and perinatal mortality and morbidity, and the feelings of the women.

SELECTION BETWEEN LOW- AND HIGH-RISK PREGNANCIES

The Dutch system of maternity care is based upon risk management. Primary obstetric care is provided by midwives and general practitioners for low-risk pregnancies, and secondary care is provided under the responsibility of obstetricians for high-risk pregnancies. A low-risk, pregnant woman may become high-risk at any stage of her pregnancy (*e.g.* facts arising from the history taken during the first antenatal visit, because risk factors or complications become apparent during pregnancy, or during labour and even delivery). Both primary and secondary caregivers have agreed a guideline which contains a list of reasons for consultation or referral to secondary care – *The Obstetric Manual*, a report of the Obstetric Working Group of the National Health Insurance Board of The Netherlands (Appendix). The famous screening principles of Jungner and Wilson were the basis of this manual, combined with clinical reasoning where evidence was scarce. Low-risk pregnant women have free choice to deliver at home or in hospital, delivery in both settings being the responsibility of an independent midwife.

It cannot be over emphasised that to offer the opportunity to give birth at home, or give birth in home-like facilities not directly connected to hospitals, implies the presence and high-quality implementation of selection procedures distinguishing between low-risk and high-risk during pregnancy and beyond. Only pregnant women at low risk of obstetric complications should be offered the free choice of a home birth. This means, for instance, that a previous Caesarean section, a current breech presentation or twin pregnancy can never be accepted for home birth. Nevertheless, in a recent British Columbia study, 23 of 862 women who were booked for home birth had a history of Caesarean section (2.7%).[5]

The effectiveness of antenatal selection by midwives has been studied by several groups in The Netherlands, in all cases with an observational design. The first large-scale study analysed the risk selection process in Wormerveer (a small Dutch city in the urban western part of the country) between 1969 and 1983. A group of 7980 pregnant women, booked consecutively at the practice of independent midwives was studied. Perinatal mortality in the total group was low (11.1 per 1000) compared with national figures of 14.5 per 1000 between 1969 and 1983. The highest mortality (57.1 per 1000) was found in the group of 1430 infants born after maternal referral during pregnancy to a specialist obstetrician. The perinatal mortality in the group selected during pregnancy as low-risk cases was very low (2.3 per 1000).[6]

More recently, Bais analysed all 8031 consecutive pregnancies (1990–1995) in the (Dutch) Zaanstreek region (Wormerveer included).[7] In that complete cohort, 29% of all initially low-risk nulliparous women were referred to secondary care during pregnancy, the most important reasons being hypertensive disorders, post-term pregnancy, abnormal presentation, threatening preterm birth and possible retardation of fetal growth. In multiparous women that percentage was 14, especially because of 'post term pregnancy and abnormal presentation'. In the 1969–1973 Wormerveer study, these figures were much lower – 17.6% and 8.6%, respectively.[8] Obviously, referral rates have risen, very likely due to a more thorough selection procedure, more diagnostic and therapeutic possibilities and, at the same time, an increase in defensive medicine. Although the age of the mother has increased gradually, increased ill-health is very unlikely to have been a factor of importance.

REFERRAL FROM PRIMARY TO SECONDARY CARE

We need to answer the questions – what portion of low-risk pregnant women are referred to secondary care during labour and delivery, at what stage, and why. In the 1990–1995 cohort studied by Bais, 28% of the initially low-risk nulliparous women were referred due to problems raised during the first or second stage of labour, which is 40% of those who started labour under the responsibility of a midwife. The observed indications for referral, expressed as percentages of the number of low-risk women at the start of labour, are given in Table 1. Reasons for relatively acute referral in nulliparous women were 'possible fetal distress' in 4.6% of those considered low risk at the start of labour and 'failure to progress in the second stage' in 11.5%.[7]

In multiparous women, the percentage of referral was 6% of the starting cohort, and only 10% of those who were considered low-risk at the start of labour. Here, only 0.8% of those considered low-risk at the start of labour were referred to specialist care because of 'possible fetal distress' and only 1.3% because of 'failure to progress in the second stage'.

Four percent of nulliparous and 2.7% of multiparous low-risk women who started labour under the responsibility of a midwife were referred during the third stage of labour, predominantly because of abnormal blood loss.

These figures of referral to an obstetrician during labour are similar to those found in a third Dutch study carried out in 1990–1992 in the Gelderland region (eastern non-urban part of The Netherlands). Of 1640 women who started labour in primary care, 39% of primiparous women and 10.3% of multiparous women were referred to secondary care during labour.[9] Of interest, this study also retrospectively examined the feelings of the women about the unplanned transfer from a planned home birth to hospital during labour and found little influence on the experience of childbirth. Obviously, self-confident women chose home birth and were not easily disturbed by unplanned events.

Table 1 Indications for referral to secondary care during the first or second stage of labour for nulliparous and multiparous women at low risk at the start of labour

Reasons for referral	Nulliparous women ($n = 2344$)		Multiparous women ($n = 2630$)	
	No.	%	No.	%
Failure to progress during second stage	270	11.5	36	1.3
Failure to progress during first stage	209	8.9	34	1.3
Meconium-stained amniotic fluid	190	8.1	99	3.7
Premature rupture of membranes	121	5.1	48	1.8
Fetal distress	109	4.6	21	0.8
Hypertensive disorder/growth restriction	4	0.2	–	–
Abnormal presentation	15	0.6	14	0.5
Fetal death	5	0.2	3	0.1
Other	4	0.2	2	0.1
		39.5		7.6

Data are the number and percentage of the cohort of low-risk women at the start of labour and taken from Bais[7] Table 3.4, page 41.

Similar observations were made in the 1993 Newcastle-upon-Tyne study of 251 women opting for home delivery: 57% in fact delivered at home, 29% were referred to hospital before the onset of labour and 14% during labour. There were 17 (7%) Caesarean sections and no perinatal deaths. It is of interest that transfers during labour and delivery were uneventful, and that half of the mothers commented spontaneously that they still valued having spent even part of their labour at home.[10]

In a US study of 1404 women who planned for home birth, only 8.3% were transported to hospital during labour and only 0.8% after delivery. Compared with the Dutch reports cited above, these figures are relatively low. Selection bias may have played a role; for instance, most women (78%) were multiparous and 68.8% of them had had a previous out-of-hospital birth experience, a relatively very favourable group.[11] One should be also aware that only 0.6% of US births occur at home and that only about 40% of all intended home deliveries could be included in the study.

We conclude that if low-risk pregnant women opt for labour and delivery at home or in home-like settings, rigorous selection during labour carries a risk of antenatal referral to hospital care during labour and delivery, which ranges from 40% (15% relatively acute) in nulliparous women to 10% (2% relatively acute) in multiparous women. Another 4% of nulliparous and 3% of multiparous women will be transferred in the third stage of labour, the majority related to abnormal blood loss. In Dutch practice, the extra risks related to these short-distance transfers during labour are considered very low and acceptable.

In nulliparous women, referral rates have more than tripled compared to those observed in 1969–1973, a dramatic increase. It is debatable whether, besides a more rigorous selection during labour, an increase of maternal age and other factors have also played an important role. Factors involved may be: (i) non-realistic information; (ii) high expectations of women and their family members; (iii) increase in medicalisation related to defensive medicine; and (iv) a lack of continuity, guidance and support from caregivers, especially during pregnancy in the first stage of labour. Therefore, we will give more attention to the specific roles of caregivers and patients themselves.

Table 2 Home-like versus conventional institutional settings for birth, Cochrane Review, outcomes[12]

	Relative risk	95% Confidence interval
Less intrapartum analgesia/anaesthesia	1.19	1.01–1.40
Spontaneous vaginal birth	1.03	1.01–1.06
Vaginal/perineal tears	1.08	1.03–1.13
Episiotomy	0.85	0.74–0.99
Preference for the same setting next time	1.81	1.65–1.98
Satisfaction with intrapartum care	1.14	1.07–1.21
Satisfaction with breast-feeding initiation	1.05	1.02–1.09
Continuation of breast-feeding to 6–8 weeks	1.06	1.02–1.10

OBSTETRIC INTERVENTIONS

To our knowledge, no randomised controlled studies exist on obstetric outcome in terms of interventions and neonatal morbidity and mortality, directly comparing home births with hospital births. The problem is, of course, that such a trial requires informed consent from women opting for home birth, which implies willingness to accept a 50% chance to be forced to accept hospital birth instead. Low-risk, pregnant women opting for home birth are certainly a selective group who are better educated, relatively independent and self-confident, which itself may affect outcome. This group of women will not be willing to let themselves be randomised to what is in their opinion a second choice – the hospital birth. Any RCT without this group lacks generalisability.

However, home-like settings for birth versus conventional institutional settings, have been studied in randomised trials. Hodnett *et al.*[12] published a meta-analysis of six trials, involving 8677 women (Table 2). These results suggest modest benefits of home-like birth settings, including decreased medical intervention and higher rates of spontaneous vaginal birth, breast-feeding, and maternal satisfaction.

With respect to home birth versus hospital birth, only observational studies are available. In Zürich, healthy low-risk women were studied, 489 opting for home delivery and 385 opting for hospital delivery. During delivery, those having home birth needed significantly less medication and fewer obstetric interventions, whereas no differences were found in the duration of labour, in the occurrence of severe perineal lesions, and in maternal blood loss.[13]

In the 1998–1999 British Columbia study, 862 planned home births attended by midwives were compared with planned hospital deliveries attended by either midwives (571) or physicians (743). Women in the home birth group were less likely to have epidural analgesia (odds ratio 0.3; 95% CI, 0.14–0.27), to be induced, to have their labours augmented, or to have an episiotomy. The adjusted odds ratio for Caesarean section in the home-birth group compared with the physician-attended hospital births was 0.3 (95% CI, 0.22–0.43).[14]

In a recent prospective Dutch study (1998–1999) in 603 low-risk pregnant women attended by midwives at planned home births (422) or hospital births (181), referral during labour to secondary care was statistically significantly higher among multiparous women in the hospital birth group (45.1%) compared to the home birth group (22.9%); the same trend was observed in primiparous women. In agreement with these findings, in multiparous women significantly more specialist interventions occurred in the hospital birth group (28.0%) compared to the home birth group (13.1%); again, in primiparous women, the same trend was found (62.6% versus 53.8%) but this difference was not significant. The same study demonstrated that women who opt for home birth have a very much higher prior 'technology rejecting attitude' as compared to those who opt for hospital birth (82% versus 18%). We conclude that these women are more self-confident about their ability to deliver spontaneously and, indeed, perform better.[15]

These data point to a second difficulty in defining the appropriate design apart from obtaining consent from a broad enough group. The incidence of obstetric interventions during labour and delivery in a previously low-risk group of pregnant women is most likely related to both the place of birth and the discipline of the caregivers, both factors interacting. The perfect randomised controlled studies on home birth versus hospital birth (in home-like settings or not) should, therefore, stratify for the discipline of caregivers. Obviously, a more home-like approach in the hospital may lower the incidence of interventions. From observational studies, it seems likely that home birth and hospital birth, supervised by midwives, may lower the need for referral to specialist care during labour and delivery, especially in multiparous women, and may also lower the incidence of obstetric interventions.

So far, the arguments on equivalence of home birth on the outcome level, and potential superiority on the process level (less interventions given the same outcome), have been rather global focusing more on the absolute requirement for prior risk selection. We shall consider data on outcome, in particular the safety of the child. Furthermore, we will address the woman's perspective. Not only the birth setting, but also the woman's free choice of the place of birth, her attitude towards labour and delivery, the discipline of the caregiver and the quality and the continuity of care and support given throughout labour and delivery, are important if not key aspects of outcome.

MORTALITY AND MORBIDITY

Pregnant women at low risk at booking can be cared for safely in Western societies by clinical professionals who are not obstetricians (*e.g.* well-trained midwives or general practitioners with sufficient experience, say at least 20 deliveries per year). To our knowledge, in these women and under these conditions, no maternal mortality has been reported in the last decades directly related to the planned place of birth at home.

In general, reported perinatal mortality figures for home births are very low. Of course, one should be suspicious about the presence of bias, particularly of under-reporting. Below, we report on the most sizeable Dutch studies followed by four non-Dutch studies.

Dutch studies based on cohorts of consecutive patients or on regional cohorts like those in Wormerveer, Zaanstreek and Hertogenbosch have the advantage of being less vulnerable to selection bias, because they were essentially prospective and started early in pregnancy. The most difficult task is to follow these pregnant women when they move or when they are referred to extra-regional care, mainly to a tertiary centre.

The 1969–1983 Wormerveer study included 7980 pregnant women, booked consecutively at the practices of all independent midwives in that city. It showed an overall perinatal mortality of 11.1 per 1000, which was considerably lower than the national figure (14.5 per 1000) in the same period. The highest mortality (51.7 per 1000) was found in the group of 1430 infants born after referral during pregnancy to a specialist obstetrician. In the group of women still considered to be at low risk of complications at the start of labour, perinatal mortality was indeed very low (2.3 per 1000).[16] A panel of independent experts judged all perinatal mortality cases and considered 45% as inevitable. In 66 (75%) of all 89 cases, complete consensus or near consensus was reached. In this agreed group, 29 cases were judged to have avoidable factors: 12 cases concerned the skill of the obstetrician, 7 cases the skill of the paediatrician and 7 cases the skill of the midwife. In two cases, the behaviour of the patient herself and in one case the skill of the general practitioner were responsible.[17] The care of the midwife during labour and delivery and the place of delivery (in or outside the hospital) obviously had little influence on avoidable, perinatal mortality. In the Wormerveer study, perinatal morbidity was also considered. Of the 5985 infants born alive under the continuing sole care of an independent midwife, 3.8% were at one stage admitted to hospital. Emergency admission because of unexpected birth asphyxia occurred in only 23 cases (0.4%): 21 of these infants were born in the period 1969–1976 and only 2 in the period 1977–1983. Convulsions within 48 h of birth at term occurred in 7 (0.9 per 1000) of the total group and in 5 infants born in the selected low-risk group (0.8 per 1000).[16]

These Wormerveer figures, though somewhat dated, are still vital as they prove independent midwives to be able to select during the antenatal period those pregnant women at risk of obstetric interventions. As this skill is at the centre of their profession, it seems obvious that midwives are very well able to take responsibility for labour and delivery in low-risk women, whether at home or in hospital.

The Dutch 1990–1992 study in the Gelderland region, encompassed 1836 low-risk pregnant women from 54 midwifery practices. All women had deliberately planned to give birth either at home or in hospital. These data showed that the outcome of planned home births was at least equal to that of planned hospital births. In multiparous women, perinatal outcome was considered significantly better in planned home births.[18]

The Dutch 1994–1995 study in the Hertogenbosch region considered perinatal mortality in low-risk and high-risk pregnant women and 8509 newborns. It showed an overall mortality between 24 weeks of gestational age and the first week after birth of 8.6 per 1000 (perinatal mortality calculated from the 28th week of gestational age was 5.8 per 1000). According to the perinatal audit, 23 of 73 cases (31.5%) were classified as avoidable. In the low-risk group (midwives, general practitioners) only 6 out of 32 (18.7%), and in the high-risk group (obstetricians) 16 of 39 (41.0%) were judged as probably or possibly avoidable. In this study, intra-uterine growth retardation, congenital malformations and antepartum haemorrhage were found to be the most decisive factors for perinatal mortality.[19]

As previously mentioned, other published studies from non-Dutch countries consider small groups of pregnant women, gathered over a longer period of time, because in those countries few pregnant women opt or are able to opt for home birth. Nevertheless, it is of interest that the four studies that follow are consistent with the previous low perinatal mortality figures in low-risk pregnant women in general, and in those who opted for home birth.

The Northern Region Perinatal Mortality Survey Co-ordinating Group from Newcastle had access to 558,691 registered births during 1981–1994, of which only 2888 women booked for a home birth (0.5%). The estimated perinatal death rate was 4.8 per 1000, less than half of the perinatal mortality in all the pregnant women in the region. Independent review suggested that only two of the 14 deaths might have been avoided by different management. Both births occurred in hospital and in only one was management before admission of the mother judged inappropriate.[20]

In the nation-wide 1994–1995 US study among 1404 patients intended do deliver at home, of which 1302 did so, overall intrapartum fetal and neonatal mortality was 2.5 per 1000, and only 1.8 per 1000 for those actually delivering at home. Thirty-three infants (2.7%) had 1-min Apgar scores of less than 7 and only 14 had a 5-min Apgar of less than 7 (1.2%).[11] Even lower mortality was reported in a Swiss study on healthy low-risk women opting for home delivery or hospital birth. Overall perinatal mortality was 2.3 per 1000. There was no difference between groups with respect to perinatal mortality or clinical condition of the new-born.[13]

In the 1998–1999 British Columbia study, cited above, the overall perinatal mortality was 4 in 2156 or 1.8 per 1000, of which 3 occurred in the home-birth group (3.4 per 1000) and one in the hospital birth group (0.7 per 1000), a difference which is not statistically significant. In at least two of the three cases in the home-birth group, no final cause of death could be determined. Five-min Apgar scores, meconium aspiration syndrome, or need to transfer to a different hospital for specialised new-born care were similar for the home-birth group and for births in hospital attended by a physician.[14]

However, other studies raise some concerns. In 7002 planned home births during 1985–1990 in Australia, perinatal death rate in infants weighing more than 2500 g was higher than the national average (5.7 versus 3.6 per 1000; relative risk, 1.6; 95% CI, 1.1–2.4). The largest contributors to the excess mortality were underestimation of the risks associated with post-term birth, twin pregnancy and breech presentation.[21]

As discussed above, it is essential to have national and local agreement between primary and secondary caregivers as to which pregnant women are allowed or even encouraged to choose for home birth and which are not. The Dutch obstetrician Kloosterman, the inventor of the Dutch nationally accepted and applied 'list of indications for specialist care in pregnancy and labour and delivery' (now called *The Obstetric Manual*, see Appendix), always stressed that, in principle, only healthy women with an uneventful obstetric history, a normal singleton pregnancy, or a normally grown fetus in cephalic presentation are allowed to be considered low-risk and, if they wish, are allowed to have a home birth. Post-term pregnancy, twin pregnancy and breech presentation are, according to Kloosterman, classical examples of 'indications for specialist care in clinical settings' and should never be allowed to deliver at home.

Hodnett et al.[22] who reviewed 6 randomised and quasi-randomised trials involving almost 9000 low-risk women on home-like versus conventional institutional settings for birth, found a trend towards higher perinatal mortality in the home-like setting (RR, 1.83; 95% CI, 0.99–3.38). They expressed some concern about this trend towards higher perinatal mortality in the home-like setting; however the possible underlying cause for the trend is not very clear.

From these data, we conclude that well-selected low-risk pregnant women can, and for various reasons should, have free choice of primary caregivers in pregnancy, labour and delivery. Perinatal morbidity and mortality are very low, and attentive caregivers may, even during labour and delivery, contribute to low mortality. Most cases of perinatal mortality, retrospectively judged by experts, were found not to be avoidable. The contribution of primary care to potentially avoidable perinatal deaths is low compared to obstetricians.

The lower margin of 'low' itself is difficult to quantify. From current audit and registry date world-wide, we estimate that a mortality of at least 1 in 1000 in well-grown children in normal presentation is unavoidable, regardless of the care setting. Reproductive biology sometimes shows unpredictable and undetectable fetal and/or placental problems. Moreover, human error of judgement and handling can never be excluded. If we aim to increase the quality of antenatal obstetric care, we must admit that undetected poor fetal growth retardation especially is a diagnostic problem for both midwives and specialist obstetricians. Discussions on the safety of primary obstetric care and home birth should be based on these facts, and not on emotions, like the requirement of perfect safety.

CAREGIVERS' VIEWS ABOUT THE DELIVERY SETTING

The views of caregivers with respect to the optimal place of birth are very important in the context of professional discussions, public discussions, the influence on the pregnant population and their families and friends and even on the actual practice of obstetrics.

One of the most prevalent arguments in discussions on optimal care arrangements, also in perinatal care, concerns continuity of care. In this context, it is defined as the actual provision of care by the same caregiver or small group of caregivers throughout pregnancy, during labour and birth, and in the postnatal period.[22] Even in the not too remote past, continuity of care was routine practice in most settings, whether clinical or at home. Awareness was low, however, on its supportive impact for women in the prenatal period and in labour. For a long time, the Dutch health care system has supported intrapartum and post-natal care through the 'Maternity Home Help Organization', a nation-wide institute which places well-trained, maternity-aid nurses at the disposal of young mothers. Such help may be regarded as an extension of the continuity principle. The nurses assist the midwives and general practitioners during labour and delivery at home and take care of the mother and child during the first 8 days after delivery.

Current caregivers in western countries work part-time, have a partner and children, and spend time on duties besides their professional tasks. Balanced time management may interfere with the stated ideal of continuity of care. We cannot refute the suggestion that the reported increase of referrals from primary to secondary care, especially during labour, may be related to this rather dramatic change in the private situation of midwives and other caregivers. This change also effects obstetricians. Younger Dutch specialists (obstetricians included) tend to work part-time more often and opt for jobs in large specialist teams in larger clinics to bring down the frequency of on-call duties.

In our view, pregnancy and especially labour and delivery are major life events which are physically and emotionally demanding, especially in nulliparous women. For these reasons, continuity of care and personal support are critical, and should be more available than in today's practice. Apart from continuity of care, the care 'philosophy' appears to be relevant. An attitude among caregivers towards the birth process being a natural and physiological process empowers women to be able to engage in labour and delivery as a natural life event[22] Medicalisation by unnecessary interventions such as continuous electronic fetal monitoring in low-risk pregnant women and operating theatre-like conditions in the labour ward may easily interfere with the subtle process of natural birth and even destroy what has been gained by continuous support. The maternity-aid nurses can and should play a more important role in the continuity of care in home birth and low-risk hospital birth, together with involved obstetric professionals.

Hodnett published a Cochrane Review on the possible effect of continuity of care, defined as given above. She could only find two randomised controlled trials, together involving 1815 women.[23] Compared to usual care by multiple caregivers, women who had continuity of care from a team of midwives were less likely to be admitted to hospital antenatally (odds ratio, 0.79; 95% CI, 0.64–0.97), and more likely to attend antenatal education programmes. They were also less likely to have drugs for pain relief during labour (odds ratio, 0.53; 95% CI, 0.52–0.83), less likely to have an episiotomy (odds ratio, 0.75; 95% CI, 0.60–0.94), more likely to have vaginal or perineal tear (odds ratio, 1.28; 95% CI, 1.05–1.56), and were more likely to be pleased with their antenatal, intrapartum and postnatal care. There were no differences detected in Apgar scores, low birth weight, stillbirth or neonatal death rates.

Lack of continuity is a more prevalent issue in specialist care compared to midwife care. In the primary obstetric health care system for low-risk pregnant women, the attitudes of midwives towards their clients and their clinical colleagues (the obstetricians) are an additional factor for outcome. Wiegers et al.[24] observed a wide, practice-dependent variation in home birth rates among 42 midwifery practices during pregnancy in 0–44% (mean 13%) and during labour in 4–36% (mean 20%). Yet, about 64% of this variation between practices was explained by midwife and practice characteristics. Higher home birth rates were associated with a positive attitude to home birth, a critical approach to non-medical reasons for hospital birth, and good co-operation with specialist obstetricians.[24] Good co-operation with specialist obstetricians with agreed regional protocols for referral of patients during pregnancy and labour and with improved communication between caregivers solving conflicts and restoring mutual trust will take time and may deserve a phased implementation strategy. However, this can and must be achieved.[25]

Given the strong attitudes expressed by different professional groups, nations wishing to provide for low-risk pregnant women an increase in choice between home birth or clinical birth (with or without home-like settings) are warned. It will take time and deliberate effort to change medical professionals' views as well as public opinion on these matters. A most important step may be the honest intention of the caregivers involved to work together, to respect each other's role in obstetric care, to respect each other's independence, to regard the normal birth process as a physiological event and to speak with one voice to the public, to the press and to politicians. Mutual trust reflected by joint, continuous surveillance and transparency testified by combined registration and audit of regional results are milestones during this change.

CONSUMER'S PERSPECTIVE

In The Netherlands low-risk pregnant women in primary care usually are offered free choice of a home or hospital delivery. Social factors, especially the confidence of significant others (family and friends) were found to be the strongest predictors of choice. Personal factors, measured as perceived health status before and during pregnancy, the existence of minor symptoms and fear of pain or complications during birth were found to play an indirect role. Demographic variables such as age, and education showed, amazingly, no effect.[26]

In a recent Dutch study (1998–1999) into personal attitudes of pregnant women, 608 low-risk women, enrolled in 25 independent working midwifery practices, answered questionnaires at 20–24 weeks' gestation.[15] Most women (70%) opted for home birth. Parity, age, and education had no role in that choice. Women's attitudes toward the use of labour technology showed a statistically significant relationship with the choice of birthplace for both nulliparous and multiparous women. Obviously women's desire to deliver at home is not only a choice of intimacy and 'a natural birth', but also linked to a non-technological approach to childbirth. Also, those choosing home birth were more self-confident with respect to their abilities to deliver spontaneously.

Women know what they want. To follow their own choice with respect to the place of birth may even reinforce self-confidence in their ability to deliver on their own, without important obstetric interventions. From data, it appears that self-confidence is left undisturbed by unplanned, undesired events related to their own choice. Wiegers *et al.*[9] found that an unplanned transfer from a planned home birth to hospital has little influence on the experience of childbirth. They also suggest that a first-time mother's choice for a home or a hospital birth had a substantial impact on the current and even future home birth rates.[9]

The reader should place these Dutch observations against the background of a centuries' long tradition of home birth; less frequent than a century ago, but still considered a viable option among the public, among pregnant women and among caregivers, though sometimes the debate is lively. In other countries, the background is default clinical care. A UK general practitioner studied by questionnaire the opinion of 241 women, aged 20–40 years, and found that 86% expressed a preference for hospital delivery for any future children, with only 3.5% preferring home and 10.5% undecided. Most women believed that giving birth in hospital was safer than at home. Obviously, to change the public climate, further information is needed for low-risk women to make a free and informed choice of the place of birth.[27]

CONCLUSIONS

For high-risk pregnant women, the hospital staffed with able perinatal caregivers, midwives and specialist obstetricians is the optimal place of birth. The only on-going debate with respect to high-risk pregnant women is what proportion of them, for what indication and at what gestational age, should be referred to higher care in tertiary centres with high-care obstetrics and intensive neonatal care.

For healthy pregnant women at low risk of obstetric interventions, in most western countries the hospital setting for birth has become the norm. Other options, like home birth or home-like settings, are unavailable or only available in specific areas. Ample empirical evidence shows that home birth or birth in home-like settings is at least as safe as clinical birth, provided selection is careful and a continuous process, from the first antenatal visit, during pregnancy and throughout labour and delivery. Equal safety is accompanied by more spontaneous vaginal birth, less obstetric interventions, and more satisfaction for these women and their families and even their caregivers.[23]

It is clear that certain conditions need to be met if confidence in home births is to be maintained or to be re-established:

1. An appropriate selection system to distinguish between low-risk and high-risk women on the basis of the first antenatal visit, information obtained and observations made during pregnancy, and even during labour and delivery.

2. Midwives, general practitioners and obstetricians should agree on a list of indications for secondary care in a region or, preferably, nation-wide.

3. Primary caregivers should not accept any high-risk patients for home delivery.

4. The geographic infrastructure should allow for quick transport (less than 30 min after the first call) from home to hospital.

5. The availability of home-like facilities in or at a reasonable distance from the hospital, if distances from home to hospital are too long.

6. A good back up system of specialist care in the hospital, which is able to respond adequately to unexpected complications.

7. An attitude among all regional maternity caregivers which supports permanent re-evaluation of the outcome of all primary and secondary care, with the intention of learning and improving care.

8. Transparency and public awareness of data on obstetric outcomes in order to raise interest in home birth.

9. Public campaigns which raise interest and trust in home birth based on scientific evidence. These campaigns should not only aim at pregnant women, but at the general public, younger women and their partners and families.

10. The availability of continuous support during labour and personal care and attention from caregivers is the most effective way to improve obstetric results with respect to interventions, in both low-risk and high-risk women. Caregivers should be devoted to the view that labour and delivery are natural life events.

11. Open communication among professional groups.

12. The additional participation of maternity-aid nurses in the continuity of care of low-risk births.

13. Financial arrangements which provide incentives to collaborate rather than to compete.

References

1. American Academy of Pediatrics and The American College of Obstetricians and Gynecologists. *Guidelines for Perinatal Care*, 5th edn. Elk Grove Village & Washington, 2002; 125.
2. Bohra U, Donnelly J, O'Connell MP, Geary MP, Macquillan K, Keane DP. Active management of labour revisited: the first 1000 primiparous labours in 2000. *J Obstet Gynecol* 2003; **23**: 118–20.
3. Keirse JNC, Enkin M, Lumley J. Social and professional support during childbirth. In: Chalmers I, Enkin M, Keirse JNC. (eds) *Effective Care in Pregnancy and Childbirth*. Oxford: Oxford University Press, 1989; 805–14.
4. van der Hulst LAM. Dutch midwives: relational care and birth location. *Health Soc Care Community* 1999; **7**: 242–7.
5. Jansen PA, Lee SK, Ryan EM, Etches DJ, Farquharson F, Peacock D *et al*. Outcomes of planned home births versus planned hospital birth, after regulation of midwifery in British Columbia. *Can Med Assoc J* 2002; **166**: 315–23.
6. Van Alten D, Eskes M, Treffers PE. Midwifery in The Netherlands. The Wormerveer study; selection, mode of delivery, perinatal mortality and infant morbidity. *Br J Obstet Gynaecol* 1989; **96**: 656–62.
7. Bais J. Risk selection and detection. A critical appraisal of the Dutch obstetric system. University thesis, University of Amsterdam, 2004; 23–57.
8. Eskes M. Het Wormerveer onderzoek. Meerjarenonderzoek naar de kwaliteit van de verloskundige zorg rond een vroedvrouwenpraktijk. (The Wormerveer study). University thesis, University of Amsterdam, 1989; 57–8.
9. Wiegers TA, van der Zee J, Keirse JNC. Transfer from home to hospital: what is its effect on the experience of childbirth? *Birth* 1998; **25**: 19–24.
10. Davies J, Hey E, Young G. Prospective regional study of planned home births. *BMJ* 1996; **313**: 1302–6.
11. Murphy PA, Fullerton J. Outcomes of intended home births in nurse-midwifery practice: a prospective study. *Obstet Gynecol* 1998; **92**: 461–70.
12. Hodnett ED, Downe S, Edwards N. Home-like versus conventional institutional settings for birth. The Cochrane Database of Systematic Reviews 2005, Issue 1.
13. Ackermann-Liebrich U, Gunter-Wit K, Kunz I, Zullig M, Schindler C, Maurer M. Home versus hospital deliveries: follow up study of matched pairs for procedures and outcome. *BMJ* 1996; **313**: 1313–8.
14. Jansen PA, Lee SKL, Ryan EM, Etches DJ, Farquharson F, Peacock D *et al*. Outcomes of planned home births versus planned hospital births after regulation of midwifery in British Columbia. *Can Med Assoc J* 2002; **166**: 315–23.
15. Van der Hulst LAM, van Teijlingen ER, Bonsel GJ, Eskes M, Bleker OP. Does a pregnant woman's intended place of birth influence her attitude toward and occurrence of obstetric interventions? *Birth* 2004; **31**: 28–33.
16. van Alten D, Eskes M, Treffers PE. Midwifery in The Netherlands. The Wormerveer study: selection, mode of delivery, perinatal mortality and infant morbidity. *Br J Obstet Gynaecol* 1989; **96**: 656–62.
17. Eskes M, van Alten D, Treffers PE. The Wormerveer study; perinatal mortality and non-optimal management in a practice of independent midwives. *Eur J Obstet Gynecol* 1993; **51**: 91–5.
18. Wiegers TA, Keirse MJNC, van der Zee J, Berghs GAH. Outcome of planned home and planned hospital births in low risk pregnancies: prospective study in midwifery practices in The Netherlands. *BMJ* 1996; **131**: 1309–13.
19. De Reu PAOM, Nijhuis JG, Oosterbaan HP, Eskes TKAB. Perinatal audit on avoidable mortality in a Dutch rural region: a retrospective study. *Eur J Obstet Gynaecol Reprod Biol* 2000; **88**: 65–9.
20. Northern Region Perinatal Mortality Survey Coordinating Group. Collaborative survey of perinatal loss in planned and unplanned home births. *BMJ* 1996; **313**: 1306–9.
21. Bastian H, Keirse JNC, Lancaster PAL. Perinatal death associated with planned home birth in Australia: population based study. *BMJ* 1998; **317**: 384–8.
22. Hulst LAM, Teijlingen ER van. Telling stories of midwives. In: Devries R, van Teijlingen ER, Wrede S. (eds) *Birth by Design: pregnancy, maternity care and midwifery in North America and Europe*. New York/London: Routledge, 2001; 166–80.

23. Hodnett ED. Continuity of caregivers for care during pregnancy and childbirth. The Cochrane Database of Systematic Reviews 1998, Issue 3.
24. Wiegers TA, van der Zee J, Kerssens JJ, Keirse JNC. Variation in home-birth rates between midwifery practices in The Netherlands. *Midwifery* 2000; **16**: 96–104.
25. De Veer AJ, Meijer WJ. Obstetric care: competition or co-operation. *Midwifery* 1996; **12**: 4–10.
26. Wiegers TA, van der Zee J, Kerssens JJ, Keirse MJN. Home birth or short-stay hospital birth in a low risk population in The Netherlands. *Soc Sci Med* 1998; **46**: 1505–11.
27. Fordham S. Women's views of the place of confinement. *Br J Gen Pract* 1997; **47**: 77–80.

APPENDIX 1

THE OBSTETRIC MANUAL

Abstracted and translated sections from the final report of the Obstetric Commission of the Health Care Insurance Board, Diemen, The Netherlands, 2003 (www.cvz.nl).

THE LIST OF OBSTETRICAL INDICATIONS

What follows is the list of specific obstetrical indications, including an explanation of the description of the obstetrical care provider (Table A1) and guidelines on how to deal with the consultation. The list is divided into six main groups, within which reference is made to the various obstetrical and medical disorders and diseases. Where necessary, an explanation is provided about the policy related to specific indications. The right-hand column shows the most suitable care provider for each indication. The main purpose of the

Table A1 Explanation of the codes used for the care providers

Code	Description	Care provider
A Primary obstetric care	The responsibility for obstetrical care in the situation described is with the primary obstetrical care provider	Midwife/GP
B Consultation situation	This is a case of evaluation involving both primary and secondary care. Under the item concerned, the situation of the individual pregnant woman will be evaluated and agreements will be made about the responsibility for obstetrical care	Depending on agreements
C Secondary obstetric care	This is a situation requiring care by an obstetrician at secondary level for as long as the disorder continues to exist	Obstetrician
D Transferred primary obstetric care	Obstetric responsibility remains with the primary care provider, but in this situation it is necessary that birth takes place in a hospital in order to avoid possible transport risk during birth	Midwife/GP

list is to provide a guide for risk selection. The primary obstetrical care provider, midwife or GP is primarily responsible for this risk selection. The list is a consensus document showing the agreement reached by the professional groups on their decision-making structure. The following decision-tree (Fig. A1) has been designed for use in daily practice.

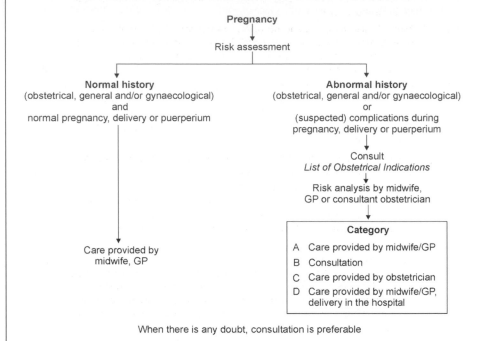

Fig. A1 Decision-tree has been designed for use in daily practice

SPECIFIC OBSTETRICAL INDICATIONS

1. PRE-EXISTING DISORDERS – NON-GYNAECOLOGICAL

In cases of pre-existing disorders that are relevant to obstetrics, care providers other than the midwife/GP or obstetrician are regularly involved with care of the pregnant woman. It is necessary to involve these additional care providers in the consultation. For this reason, in disorders given code B in this section, attention should be given to collaboration with others outside the field of obstetrics. Attention should be paid to the counselling of women who are considering the possibility of becoming pregnant.

Section 1: Pre-existing non-gynaecological disorders

1.1	Epilepsy, without medication	A
1.2	Epilepsy, with medication. Antenatal diagnostics are recommended in connection with the disorder and its medication. Optimal care requires consultation between all care providers concerned (midwife, GP, obstetrician, neurologist)	B
1.3	Subarachnoid haemorrhage, aneurysm. Care during puerperium can be at primary level	C
1.4	Multiple sclerosis. Depending upon the neurological condition, a complicated delivery and the possibility of urine retention should be taken into account. For optimal care, consultation between all care providers concerned is indicated	B
1.5	Hernia of the nucleus pulposus. This represents a C-situation in cases of a recent event or where there are still neurological symptoms. It is an A-situation after treated hernia, especially if a previous pregnancy was normal. Both the medical history and the current clinical condition are relevant	A/C
1.6	Lung function disorder/COPD. The opinion of a lung specialist should be taken into account during evaluation	A/C
1.7	Asthma. Care during pregnancy, birth and puerperium can only take place at a primary level when the asthma involves lengthy symptom-free intervals, whether or not use is made of inhalation therapy. Consultation with the GP/specialist involved is recommended	A/C
1.8	Tuberculosis, active	C
	Tuberculosis, inactive	A
	In cases of active tuberculosis and subsequent treatment, consultation should take place with the physician involved and the obstetrician regarding the clinical condition and care during pregnancy and birth. In cases of inactive tuberculosis, care during pregnancy and birth can take place at a primary level	
1.9	HIV-infection. As a result of the current possibilities of medical therapy for preventing vertical transmission, these patients should be cared for during pregnancy and birth in a hospital equipped for the treatment of HIV and AIDS	C
1.10	Hbs-Ag-carrier	A
1.11	Hepatitis C. Consultation with an obstetrician and follow-up by a paediatrician is recommended	B
1.12	A heart condition with haemodynamic compromise. Pregnancy and birth will have an effect on the pre-existing haemodynamic relationships. A cardiac evaluation is important	C
1.13	Deep-venous thrombosis/pulmonary embolism. Of importance are the underlying pathology and the presence of a positive family medical history. Preconception counselling is important	B
1.14	Coagulation disorders	C
1.15	Renal function disorders. When there is a disorder in renal function, with or without dialysis, referral to secondary care is recommended	C
1.16	Hypertension	
	Pre-existing hypertension, with or without medication, will require referral to secondary care. Preconception counselling is important for women taking medication	C
1.17	Diabetes mellitus. Preconception counselling is important	C

Continued on next page)

1.18   Thyroid disease.
In thyroid disease, measurement of TSH and free T4 is advised as soon
as possible. TSH receptor antibodies should be measured when indicated

Hyperthyroidism.
No current medication and biochemically euthyroid
     and absent TSH receptor antibodies   A
     and positive TSH receptor antibodies   C
With medication   C

Hypothyroidism
Caused by treatment of hyperthyroidism by surgery or [131I]-therapy,
euthyroid with l-thyroxine
     and absent TSH receptor antibodies   A
     and positive TSH receptor antibodies   C
Caused by Hashimoto's disease and euthyroid with l-thyroxine   A

Where l-thyroxine medication is given, direct checks are recommended
due to the frequent increase in requirements during pregnancy and
decrease just after delivery

1.19   Haemoglobinopathies   B

1.20   Inflammatory bowel disease including ulcerative colitis and
Crohn's disease   C

1.21   Systemic diseases and rare diseases. These include rare maternal disorders
such as Addison's disease and Cushing's disease. Also included are systemic
lupus erythematosus (SLE), anti-phospholipid syndrome (APS), scleroderma,
rheumatoid arthritis, peri-arteritis nodosa, Marfan's syndrome, Raynaud's
disease and other systemic and rare disorders   C

1.22   Use of hard drugs (heroin, methadone, cocaine, XTC, etc.). Attention
should be paid to actual use. A urine test can be useful even in cases
of past use in the medical history. The involvement of the
paediatrician is indicated during postpartum follow-up   C

1.23   Alcohol abuse. The fetal alcohol syndrome is important. The
involvement of a paediatrician is indicated during postpartum
follow-up   C

1.24   Psychiatric disorders. Care during pregnancy and birth will depend
on the severity and extent of the psychiatric disorder. Consultation
with the relevant psychiatrist is indicated   B

2.   **Pre-existing gynaecological disorders**

2.1   Pelvic floor reconstruction. This refers to colpo-suspension following
prolapse, fistula and previous rupture. Depending on the cause, the
operative technique used and the results achieved, the obstetrician will
determine policy regarding the birth. A primary Caesarean section or an
early primary episiotomy can be considered, to be repaired by the
obstetrician. If the chosen policy requires no special measures and no
specific operating skill, then care during birth can be at primary level   C/A

2.2   Cervical amputation   C
Cervical cone biopsy   B
Cryo- and lis-treatment   A

The practical application of obstetric policy in this field can be worked
out in local mutual agreements. If an uncomplicated pregnancy and
birth have taken place following cone biopsy then a subsequent
pregnancy and birth can take place at primary level

2.3   Myomectomy. Depending on the anatomy, the possibility of a disturbance
in the progress of the pregnancy or birth should be taken into account   C/A

2.4	Abnormalities in cervical cytology. There should be differentiation according to obstetrical versus gynaecological policy. Gynaecological consultation can be indicated even without obstetric consequences. Gynaecological follow-up is not a contra-indication to obstetrical care at primary level	B/A
2.5	DES-daughter (untreated and under supervision). There should be differentiation according to obstetrical versus gynaecological policy. Gynaecological care related to the problems surrounding DES may be necessary, while obstetric care can take place at primary level	B
2.6	IUD *in situ* Status following removal of the IUD	B A
2.7	Status following subfertility treatment	A
2.8	Pelvic deformities (trauma, symphyseal disorders). Consultation should take place at the start of the last trimester. Note that care at secondary level has not been shown to have any added value in cases of pelvic instability and symphyseal complaints	B
2.9	Female circumcision/female genital mutilation. Circumcision as such can require extra psychosocial care. Where there are serious anatomical deformities, consultation should take place in the third trimester	A/B

3. Obstetrical medical history

3.1	Active blood group incompatibility (Rh, Kell, Duffy, Kidd) ABO incompatibility. Pregnancy and birth can take place at primary care level in cases of ABO incompatibility, but one should be on the alert for neonatal problems	C A
3.2	Pregnancy-induced hypertension in the previous pregnancy (Pre)-eclampsia/HELLP-syndrome in the previous pregnancy	A B
3.3	Habitual abortion (≥ 3 times). When pregnancy is on-going, care is conducted at primary level	A

3.4	Pre-term birth (< 37 weeks) in previous pregnancy
	     Pre-term birth (< 33 weeks) in previous pregnancy
	     Pre-term birth (≥ 33 weeks) in previous pregnancy
	If a normal pregnancy has taken place subsequent to the preterm birth, then a further pregnancy can be conducted at primary level
		
		C
		A

3.5	Cervical insufficiency (and/or Shirodkar-procedure) Secondary level care during pregnancy is indicated up to 37 weeks; with a term pregnancy obstetrical attendance can take place at primary level If a subsequent pregnancy was normal, then future pregnancies and deliveries can be conducted at primary care level	C A
3.6	Placental abruption	C
3.7	Forceps or vacuum extraction. Evaluation of information from the obstetrical history is important. Documentation showing a case of an uncomplicated assisted birth may lead to the management of the present pregnancy and birth at primary care level. Consultation should take place when no documentation is available or when the previous birth has been complicated	A
3.8	Caesarean section Antenatal care Referral to obstetrician at 37 weeks Care during parturition Antenatal care can be conducted at primary care level unless complications occur	 A C C
3.9	Fetal growth restriction. A birth weight beneath the 5th centile or obvious neonatal hypoglycaemia related to fetal growth retardation	C

| 3.10 | Asphyxia. Defined as an Apgar score of < 7 at 5 min | B |

3.11 Perinatal death. Such an obstetrical history requires consultation. It is also important to know whether there was a normal pregnancy following the perinatal death. If appropriate, pregnancy and birth can be conducted at primary care level — B

3.12 Previous child with congenital and/or hereditary disorder. It is important to know the nature of the disorder and what investigations were carried out at the time. If no disorders can currently be discerned, then further care can be at primary care level — B

3.13 Postpartum haemorrhage as a result of episiotomy — A

3.14 Postpartum haemorrhage as a result of cervical tear (clinically demonstrated). The assumption is that there is a chance of a recurrence; the pregnancy and birth can be conducted at primary care level. Birth should take place in the hospital — D

3.15 Postpartum haemorrhage, other causes (> 1000 cc). In view of the chance of a recurrence, although the pregnancy and birth can be conducted at primary care level, birth should take place in the hospital — D

3.16 Manual removal of placenta in a previous pregnancy. In view of the increased recurrence risk, the following pregnancy and birth can be cared for at primary care level, but birth should take place in hospital — D
When in the previous birth a placenta accreta has been diagnosed, obstetrical care at secondary level is indicated — C

3.17 Fourth degree perineal laceration. If satisfactory functional recovery has been achieved following the 4th degree tear, then pregnancy and birth can be managed at primary care level. The possibility of performing a primary episiotomy during birth should be considered. If secondary repair surgery was necessary, then referral to secondary care is indicated. If no functional repair has been achieved following a 4th degree tear, then birth should be managed at secondary care level — A/C

3.18 Symphysis pubis dysfunction. There is no added value in managing pregnancy or birth at secondary care level in cases with a symphysis pubis dysfunction in the history or with pelvic instability — A

3.19 Postpartum depression. There is no added value in managing pregnancy or birth at secondary care level in cases with a history of post partum depression. Postpartum depression occurs so late that even the puerperium can be cared for at primary care level — A

3.20 Postpartum psychosis. It is necessary to distinguish whether there has been long-term medication. It is important to have a psychiatric evaluation of the severity of the psychosis and the risk of recurrence — A

3.21 Grand multiparity. Defined as parity > 5. There is no added value in managing pregnancy and birth at secondary care level — A

3.22 Post-term pregnancy. Previous post-term pregnancy has no predictive value for the course of the current pregnancy and birth — A

4. Conditions developing and diagnosed during pregnancy

In this section, supervision at secondary level care is necessary in situations given the code C as long as the problem described still exists. If it no longer exists, then the patient can be referred back to primary level care.

4.1 Uncertain duration of pregnancy by amenorrhoea > 22 weeks. In case of uncertain duration of pregnancy > 22 weeks, extensive fetal biometry is indicated (DBP, HC, AC, FL), combined with observations of the amount of amniotic fluid, at 2–3 week intervals. If fetal growth and amniotic fluid seem normal, gestation may determined from the 50th centile values. If fetal growth and amniotic fluid is abnormal, consultation is required — A/B

4.2	Anaemia. Further investigation is recommended (usually possible in a primary care setting) when: (i) haemoglobin < 5th centile for gestational age and MCV < 70 fl or ≥ 100 fl; or (ii) haemoglobin < 5th centile for gestational age and falls when iron supplements are given for 4 weeks	B
4.3	Urinary tract infection during pregnancy. It is important to analyse the infection by urine culture	A
	Recurrent urinary tract infections, *i.e.* when an infection has occurred more than twice. Further analysis of the infection is required. The risk of pyelonephritis and pre-term birth are important. Risks for the mother are renal dysfunction and sepsis	B
4.4	Pyelonephritis. Hospital admission is required for treatment of pyelonephritis, so care will have to be at secondary care level. After successful treatment, further care during pregnancy and birth can be at primary care level	C
4.5	Toxoplasmosis. Referral to secondary level is required both for investigation and for therapeutic policy	C
4.6	Rubella. An increased risk of fetal growth restriction, pre-term birth and visual and hearing disorders should be taken into account in the case of primary infection with rubella during pregnancy	C
4.7	Cytomegalovirus. An increased risk of perinatal death and subsequent morbidity should be taken into account	C
4.8	Herpes genitalis (primary infection)	C
	Herpes genitalis (recurrent)	A/C
	Depends on the extent of the disease. In case of frequent recurrences in pregnancy or during labour, it is recommended to carry out virus cultures from oropharynx and conjunctivae of the neonate after 24 h	
	Herpes labialis	A
4.9	Parvovirus infection. This infection can lead to fetal anaemia and hydrops. It is possible to treat these problems in most cases	C
4.10	Varicella/zoster virus infection. This refers to a maternal infection. Primary infection with varicella/zoster virus during the pregnancy might require treatment of the pregnant woman with VZV-immunoglobulin due to the risk of fetal varicella syndrome. If varicella occurs shortly before birth or early during the puerperium, there is a risk of neonatal infection. Treatment of the mother and child with an antiviral drug is sometimes indicated. If there is manifest herpes zoster (shingles), then there is no risk of fetal varicella syndrome	B
4.11	Hbs-Ag-carrier	A
4.12	Hepatitis A, B, C, D or E	B
4.13	Tuberculosis. This refers to an active tuberculous process	C
4.14	HIV-infection	
	In view of the present possibilities of medical therapy for preventing vertical transmission, care for these patients during pregnancy and birth should take place in a hospital equipped to deal with HIV and AIDS	C
4.15	Syphilis	
	Positive serology and treated	A
	Positive serology but not yet treated	B
	Primary infection	C
	Attention should be paid to collaboration between the primary and secondary care providers involved during referral. It is important to ensure perfect information exchange between the midwife, the GP, the obstetrician and the venereologist	C
4.16	Hernia of nucleus pulposus, (slipped disk) occurring during pregnancy. Policy should be determined according to complaints and clinical	

symptoms. Where there are no complaints, (further) care can take place at primary level | B

4.17 Laparotomy during pregnancy. As soon as wound healing has occurred and if the nature of the operation involves no further obstetrical risks, care for the pregnant woman can return to primary level. During hospitalisation, the obstetrician will be involved in care. If there are no further obstetrical consequences, then care for the pregnant woman can return to primary level | C/A

4.18 Cervix cytology PAP III or higher. What is important here is that further gynaecological policy (for the purpose of subsequent diagnostics) may be necessary, while the pregnancy and birth can be conducted at primary care level | B

4.19 Medication. What is obviously important here is the effect of drugs on the pregnant woman and the unborn child. Attention should also be paid to the effect on lactation and the effects in the neonatal period. In cases of doubt, consultation should take place | A/B

4.20 Use of hard drugs (heroin, methadone, cocaine, XTC, etc.). The severity of the addiction to hard drugs is important here and their effects during pregnancy and birth and in the puerperium, particularly for the neonate | C

4.21 Alcohol abuse. This involves the fetal alcohol syndrome. Obviously, the long-term involvement of the paediatrician may necessary during follow-up | C

4.22 Psychiatric disorders (neuroses/psychoses). The severity of psychiatric problems and the opinion of the physician in charge of treatment are important | A/C

4.24 Hyperemesis gravidarum. Referral to secondary care is necessary for treatment of this condition. After recovery, pregnancy and birth can be managed at primary care level | C

4.24 Ectopic pregnancy | C

4.25 Antenatal investigations. Attention should paid to the risks of congenital abnormalities. If no abnormalities can be detected, then further care can take place at primary level | C

4.26 Pre-term rupture of membranes (< 37 weeks' amenorrhoea) | C

4.27 Diabetes mellitus | C

Pregnancy-related carbohydrate intolerance | A
If blood sugar values < 7.5 mmol/l are maintained by diet alone, and no other pathology is detected, the pregnant woman can return to primary care level

4.28 Pregnancy-induced hypertension. This refers to hypertension defined by the ISSHP as: diastolic blood pressure of 90 mmHg (Korotkoff V) or more at two subsequent blood pressure measurements with an interval of at least 4 h between the two measurements in the second half of pregnancy in a previously normotensive woman, or a single event of diastolic blood pressure of 110 mmHg or more

Diastolic blood pressure 90–95 mmHg (extra care is necessary with screening for proteinuria | A

Diastolic blood pressure 95–100 mmHg (consultation is indicated and, if no other problems are detected, the pregnant woman may return to primary care level) | B

Diastolic blood pressure > 100 mmHg (referral to secondary care level is necessary) | C

4.29 Pre-eclampsia, super-imposed pre-eclampsia, HELLP-syndrome. Pre-eclampsia is a combination of pregnancy-induced hypertension and proteinuria. Super-imposed pre-eclampsia exists when there is *de novo* proteinuria during a pregnancy in a patient with pre-existing hypertension. The HELLP-syndrome is characterised by the combination of haemolysis, liver function disorder and a decrease in the number of platelets — C

4.30	Blood group incompatibility	C
4.31	Deep venous thrombosis	C
4.32	Coagulation disorders	C
4.33	Recurrent blood loss prior to 16 weeks	B
4.34	Blood loss after 16 weeks. After the blood loss has stopped, care can take place at primary care level if no significant causes were found	C
4.35	Placental abruption	C
4.36	(Evaluation of) negative size–date discrepancy	B
4.37	(Evaluation of) positive size–date discrepancy	B
4.38	Post-term pregnancy. This refers to amenorrhoea lasting longer than 294 days	C
4.39	Threat of or actual pre-term birth. As soon as there is no longer a threat of pre-term birth, care during pregnancy and birth can be continued at primary care level	C/A
4.40	Cervical incompetence. Once the pregnancy has lasted 37 weeks, further care can take place at primary care level	C
4.41	Pelvic instability. This refers to complaints that started during the present pregnancy	A
4.42	Multiple pregnancy	C
4.43	Abnormal presentation at term (including breech presentation)	C
4.44	Failure of head to engage at term. If at term there is suspected cephalopelvic disproportion, placenta praevia or comparable pathology, consultation is indicated	B
4.45	No previous antenatal care. Attention should be paid to the home situation. Lack of antenatal care can suggest psychosocial problems. This can lead to further consultation and a hospital delivery	A
4.46	Baby for adoption. The prospective adoption often goes hand-in-hand with psychosocial problems. This can lead to further consultation and a hospital delivery	A
4.47	Dead fetus. If the mother prefers to give birth at home, the care she receives should be the same as if the birth were to take place in a hospital. Attention should be paid to postmortem examination and evaluation according to protocol	C
4.48	Obstetrically relevant fibroids. Depending on the anatomy, the possibility of a disturbance in the progress of pregnancy or birth should be taken into account	B

5. Conditions occurring during birth

For the C-category in this section, when one of the items mentioned below occurs, an attempt should still be made to achieve an optimal condition for further intrapartum care, whilst referral to secondary care level may be urgent, depending on the situation. When referring from home, the risk of transporting the woman also needs to be included in the considerations.

5.1	Abnormal presentation of the child. What counts here is abnormal presentation and not abnormal position	C
5.2	Signs of fetal distress. It is important that fetal distress can be expressed in various ways (fetal heart rate, meconium staining in the amniotic fluid)	C

5.3	Intrapartum fetal death. Attention should be paid to postmortem examination	C
5.4	Pre-labour rupture of membranes. Referral should take place after the membranes have been ruptured for 24 h	C
5.5	Failure to progress in the first stage of labour	B
5.6	Failure to progress in second stage of labour	C
5.7	Excessive bleeding during birth. The degree of bleeding during birth cannot be objectively measured, but needs to be estimated. Excessive loss of blood can be a sign of a serious pathology	C
5.8	Placental abruption	C
5.9	Vasa praevia	C
5.10	Retained placenta (whole or partial). It is not always possible to be sure of the retention of part of the placenta. If there is reasonable doubt, then referral to secondary care should take place	C
5.11	Fourth degree perineal laceration	C
5.12	Meconium-stained amniotic fluid	C
5.13	Fever. It is obviously important to find out the cause of the fever. In particular, the possibility of an intra-uterine infection should be taken into account and the administration of antibiotics intrapartum should be considered	C
5.14	Analgesia. It is important to be aware of the effects on cervical dilatation and respiratory depression. The use of painkillers during birth is a subject that can be covered during local discussions with the aid of guidelines. One should attempt to achieve consensus	B
5.15	Vulval haematoma. Treatment policy is determined according to the complaints intrapartum and in the early puerperium	C
5.16	Symphyiolysis. This refers to rupturing of the symphysis. It should be distinguished from pelvic instability. The added value of consultation in cases of pelvic instability has not been proven	B
5.17	Birth with no prior antenatal care. A lack of prenatal care can be a sign of psychosocial problems and, in particular, addiction. Intrapartum monitoring, serological screening and immunisation are of the utmost importance	C

6. Conditions occurring during the puerperium

6.1	(Threat of) eclampsia, (suspected) HELLP-syndrome	C
6.2	Deep venous thrombosis	C
6.3	Psychosis. It is important to involve the GP and the psychiatrist in treating psychiatric disorders	B
6.4	Postpartum haemorrhage	C
6.5	Hospitalisation of child. It is obviously important here to involve the GP and the paediatrician. The bonding between mother and child is important in the period following birth	C

Mary C.M. Macintosh

8

Confidential Enquiries: learning lessons in maternal and perinatal health

Confidential enquiry is a unique approach, which has no equivalent amongst other bodies examining quality issues within the National Health Service. Confidential Enquiries retrospectively consider individual adverse events (usually deaths) and seek, by peer review, to evaluate whether there were any aspects of care which might have avoided the untoward outcome. The process identifies patterns of practice, service provision and public health issues that may have contributed to the deaths. The procedure involves anonymisation of information provided by health professionals and this underpins the confidential environment and the ready acknowledgement of error. From this, recommendations are made to reduce avoidable factors in care and improve future practice. The interpretation of the findings from confidential enquiries is made within a national context. In order to do this, the enquiries collaborate closely with the national registrations of births and deaths. Findings are published in reports but there is no systematic feedback from individual cases to health professionals, third parties representing the patient or hospital units.

There are a series of organisations that undertake confidential enquiry work within the UK but the one with most relevance to the discipline of maternity and perinatal services is the Confidential Enquiry into Maternal and Child Health (CEMACH). CEMACH came into being in April 2003 with the merger of its predecessor organisations the Confidential Enquiry into Maternal Deaths (CEMD) and the Confidential Enquiry into Stillbirths and Deaths in Infancy (CESDI). The remit of CEMACH includes data about children up to the age of 18 years and the challenge of enquiring into morbidity as well as deaths.

HISTORY OF CEMD AND TRENDS IN MATERNAL MORTALITY

The Confidential Enquiry into Maternal Deaths was formalised in 1952. Its origins, however, date back to the 19th and early 20th centuries. The collection

Mary C.M. Macintosh MA MRCOG MD
Medical Director, CEMACH, Chiltern Court, 188 Baker Street, London NW1 5SD, UK
(E-mail: mary.macintosh@cemach.org.uk)

of national statistics on birth and death rates commenced in England and Wales in 1837 following the introduction of the *Births and Deaths Registration Act* (1836). Nothing changed until in the 1920s when a Departmental Committee on Maternal Death and Morbidity was constituted. The committee examined 8505 deaths occurring between 1928 and 1932 and concluded that the maternal death rate could be halved. At that time, 1935, the maternal mortality figures were similar to those in the mid-19th century running at about 5 per 1000 births (Fig. 1). The work of the committee strongly supported the continuation of confidential enquiries into individual deaths and the data was published in the Chief Medical Officer's (CMO's) annual report.

In the mid 1930s, the rates fell substantially for the first time and by the 1950s the levels dropped to less than 1 per 1000. This fall was attributed primarily due the discovery of antibiotics (prontosil in 1935, sulphonamides in 1937 and penicillin in 1945) and their successful use in the treatment of puerperal sepsis, which was previously the major cause of death. By the 1950s, reporting of deaths had declined and even stopped in some areas. This success along with the desire for more detailed information led to the establishment of the CEMD in 1952.

The new CEMD system involved assessment by an experienced obstetrician at regional level in England and at national level in Wales. The assessors' reports were then sent to the CMO and reviewed centrally by two obstetric assessors. Over time, these assessors were joined by an anaesthetist, a pathologist, a physician, a midwife, a psychiatrist and an intensive care specialist reflecting changes in the service provision of maternity care. The findings were published in a triennial report. Similar systems were instituted in Northern Ireland in 1956 and in Scotland in 1965. A UK triennial report has been published since 1985–87. Death rates continued to fall and plateaued in the 1970s at about 1 per 10,000 (Fig. 1).

DEFINING MATERNAL DEATH

The International Classification of Diseases (ICD) defines **maternal death** as the death of a woman while pregnant or within 42 days of the end of the

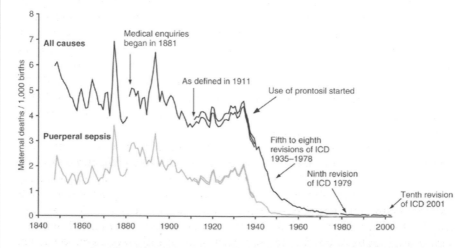

Fig. 1 Maternal mortality; England and Wales, 1847–2002. From: *Why Mothers Die*, 2000–2.[3]

pregnancy, from any cause related to or aggravated by the pregnancy or its management, but not from accidental or incidental causes (ICD 9th revision).[1] The pregnancy can be of any gestation and includes spontaneous or induced abortion and ectopic pregnancies.

The 9th revision of ICD further divided maternal deaths into a number of subgroups defined below:

1. **Direct** maternal deaths are those deaths attributed to obstetric complications of pregnancy, childbirth or the puerperium.

2. **Indirect** maternal deaths are those deaths resulting from previous existing disease or condition that developed during pregnancy and which was not due to direct obstetric causes, but which was aggravated by the physiological effects of pregnancy.

3. **Fortuitous or coincidental** maternal deaths are those deaths from unrelated causes which happen to occur in pregnancy or the puerperium. 'Fortuitous' is the term used by ICD but 'coincidental' is the preferred term used in the UK maternal death report and has now been incorporated into the 10th revision of ICD.[2]

The 42 days originally recommended in the WHO definition has become restrictive and the 10th revision of ICD[2] introduced the term 'late maternal deaths'.

4. **Late** maternal death is one which has occurred between 42 days and 1 year after abortion, miscarriage or delivery that is due to direct or indirect maternal causes.[2]

5. **Pregnancy-related deaths** are those deaths occurring in women while pregnant or within 42 days of termination of pregnancy, irrespective of the cause of death.[2]

CASE ASCERTAINMENT

Since the maternal death enquiry became part of the new CEMACH in April 2003, the day-to-day running of the enquiry has been taken over by the CEMACH central and regional offices. The CEMACH regional managers have assumed the responsibility for ascertainment of maternal deaths in their regions. They also collect all relevant clinical information and organise the regional assessment of each case. This process had been undertaken by the District Directors of Public Health but had become impractical with the successive changes in health authority boundaries. This change has led to more timely case reviews and improved case ascertainment with an increase in the numbers known to the enquiry.

Identification of maternal deaths by the enquiry also includes those identified by the Office for National Statistics (ONS) who code and collate the data on death certificates. In 2001, ONS devised a birth death record linkage study, designed to identify all deaths in women within one year of delivery to see how many unreported cases were found. The vast majority of these were late deaths and were due to coincidental causes, primarily cancer. However, a significant number were due to psychiatric causes and were classified as late indirect deaths.

Table 1 Number of maternal deaths reported to CEMD by cause, 1985–2002.[a] Adapted from: *Why Mothers Die 2000–2002*.[3]

Chapter	Cause	1985/87	1988/90	1991/93	1994/96	1997/99	2000/02
	DIRECT deaths (occurring during pregnancy and up to and including 42 days inclusive after delivery)						
2	Thrombosis and thrombo-embolism	32	33	35	48	35	30
3	Hypertensive disease of pregnancy	27	27	20	20	15	14
4	Haemorrhage	10	22	15	12	7	17
5	Amniotic fluid embolism	9	11	10	17	8	5
6	Deaths in early pregnancy – totals	22	24	18	15	17	15
	– Ectopic	16	15	8	12	13	11
	– Spontaneous miscarriage	5	6	3	2	2	1
	– Legal termination	1	3	5	1	2	3
	– Other	0	0	2	0	0	0
7	Genital tract sepsis	6[b]	7[b]	9[b]	14[c]	14[c]	11[c]
8	Other Direct deaths – totals	27	17	14	7	7	8
	– Genital tract trauma	6	3	4	5	2	1
	– Fatty liver	6	5	2	2	4	3
	– Others	15	9	8	0	1	4
9	Anaesthetic	6	4	8	1	3	6
	Total number of DIRECT deaths	**139**	**145**	**128**	**134**	**106**	**106**
	INDIRECT deaths (up to and including 42 days after delivery)						
10	Cardiac	22	18	37	39	35	44
11	Psychiatric	N/A	N/A	N/A	9	15	16
12	Other Indirect	62	75	63	86	75	90
13	Indirect malignancies	N/A	N/A	N/A	N/A	11	5
	Total number of INDIRECT deaths	**84**	**93**	**100**	**134**	**136**	**155**
14	**COINCIDENTAL deaths**	**26**	**39**	**46**	**36**	**29**	**36**
15	**LATE deaths** (42–365 days after delivery)						
	– Direct	N/A	13	10	4	7	4
	– Indirect	N/A	10	23	32	39	45
	– Coincidental	N/A	25	13	36	61	45
	Total number of LATE deaths	**16**	**48**	**46**	**72**	**107**	**94**

[a] Deaths reported to the Enquiry only and excluding deaths identified by ONS.
[b] Excluding early pregnancy deaths due to sepsis. [c] Including early pregnancy deaths due to sepsis. N/A, not available.

CALCULATING MATERNAL DEATH RATES

Reviewing trends in maternal mortality is complicated by changes in processes and definitions used to notify the deaths. In the UK, maternal mortality rates can be calculated from two different sources:

1. Through official death certification to the Register General's Office (ONS or its equivalents for Scotland and Northern Ireland).

2. Through deaths known to CEMD.

For the past 50 years, CEMD has calculated its own maternal mortality rate. The overall number and rate of direct and indirect deaths identified by CEMD has been greater than those identified through the death certification process for the last 25 years. The latter is dependent on the mention of a pregnancy-related condition on the death certificate and this is not always the case in many of the indirect causes. In addition, the criteria used to define indirect maternal deaths in the UK are more inclusive than those used in other countries, in particular the inclusion of all cases of cardiac disease, asthma, epilepsy and suicide (unless obviously related to long-standing previous psychiatric disorder). Case ascertainment is also lower in most other countries thus limiting the ability to draw valid international comparisons.

Late deaths are classified by ICD 10 (and thus ONS) as direct or indirect whereas the UK CEMD also includes coincidental deaths in this category. Late maternal deaths are described in detail by CEMD but they are not included in the numerator for determining maternal mortality rates. Over half of these deaths are identified via record linkage exercises rather than from direct reporting to the enquiry.

DIRECT MATERNAL DEATHS – TRENDS

Direct deaths have been the major category of deaths reported to the enquiry until recent years. In 1997/99, indirect deaths have become the more frequent category (Table 1). The reduction in this type of death reflects improvements in the safety and quality of the provision of emergency obstetric services over the last 50 years. The number of maternal deaths reported to the enquiry in from 1985 to 2002 by cause of death is shown in Table 1.

THROMBOSIS AND THROMBO-EMBOLISM

Since the 1950s, there has been a substantial reduction in the number of maternal deaths in all categories including venous thrombo-embolism (VTE) which remains the leading cause of direct deaths. The major decline followed the advocating of mobilisation after delivery in the 1960s. More recently, there have been some concerns regarding the increased proportion of deaths in this category following Caesarean section.

The vast majority of mothers who die from this condition have known specific risk factors and in just over half the cases the care given was substandard with delays or inadequate management in diagnosis, treatment or thromboprophylaxis. Further improvements are likely with adherence to the RCOG guidance on thromboprophylaxis especially in relation to risk assessment and appropriate therapeutic regimens.[4]

PREGNANCY-INDUCED HYPERTENSION

This was the leading cause of death in the 1950s and although the deaths declined rapidly up to the mid-1960s it remains one of the major causes of direct deaths. In the 1980s, there was increasing use of intensive care and more aggressive management and deaths from complications of the treatment itself became an issue. The 1985–87 CEMD Report highlighted the dangers of excessive infusion leading to acute respiratory distress syndrome. Careful monitoring of fluid balance, fluid restriction and central monitoring is now recognised as essential in severe pre-eclampsia. Diazepam was also criticised as an anticonvulsant and the evaluation of magnesium sulphate and phenytoin was recommended. Subsequent clinical trials demonstrated that magnesium is the anticonvulsant of choice in the treatment of eclampsia and severe pre-eclampsia.[5,6]

Today, cerebral haemorrhage is the main cause of death and is due to uncontrolled rises in systolic pressure. Obstetricians have traditionally focused on controlling the diastolic blood pressure; the need for careful observation of systolic levels as well as the diastolic is called for in the 2000/2 report. Management protocols should include the need to avoid very high systolic blood pressure and to provide guidance on thresholds above which urgent and effective treatment is required (160 mmHg is suggested).

HAEMORRHAGE

As with the other categories of direct maternal deaths, the actual numbers dying from this condition have dramatically declined. Despite this, haemorrhage continues to be the second leading cause of direct deaths. The reduction was most marked during the 1950s to the 1980s with the introduction of hospitalisation for delivery of the woman at risk, increasing use of blood transfusion, and active management of coagulopathy. Rates have remained steady since but the 2000/02 report showed a slight increase due to postpartum haemorrhage. The report advised that consultant obstetricians should not hesitate in involving surgical or radiological colleagues. Women at high risk of haemorrhage are still delivering in units ill-equipped to sudden life-threatening emergencies, that is without rapid access to specialist consultant care, blood products or intensive care.

EARLY PREGNANCY DEATHS

One of the most prominent changes in the last 50 years has been the virtual disappearance of deaths attributed to abortion and miscarriage following the implementation of the 1967 *Abortion Act*. The majority of early pregnancy deaths in recent triennial reports are due to ectopic pregnancy and half of these deaths occurred in women from an ethnic minority. Cornual pregnancies are rare but particularly dangerous; clinicians need to be aware of the difficulties of clinical and ultrasound diagnosis in these cases. Presenting symptoms may be atypical and may mimic gastrointestinal disease or urinary tract dysfunction. Clinicians in primary care and accident and emergency departments need to be aware of this.

SEPSIS

Puerperal sepsis was the leading cause of maternal death until the discovery of antibiotic treatment in the 1930s. By the time the CEMD commenced, sepsis had become one of the less frequent causes of direct maternal deaths. Since the 1980s, however, there has been a small but definite rise. Sepsis may be insidious in onset and have a fulminating course with some cases being moribund on presentation to primary care or hospital. Presentation may be similar to gastroenteritis; in the severe sepsis, there may be an absence of pyrexia. The importance of prompt, aggressive treatment of suspected sepsis is stressed.

OTHER DIRECT DEATHS

Deaths due to uterine rupture associated with the highly parous woman delivering at home and as a complication of oxytocics were seen in the first 30 years of the enquiries; latterly, genital tract trauma is a very infrequent cause of death and in the 2000/02 report accounted for one death. An emerging surgical complication seen is bowel perforation following Caesarean section. Signs of peritonism are difficult to detect in the puerperium and failures to diagnose ileus can be fatal.

Other rare causes include unpredictable conditions such as acute fatty liver and amniotic fluid embolism. Recently, a register for the latter condition has been set up; early indications are that the mortality rate is around 25% and that the chance of survival may be improved with early transfer to intensive care.

INDIRECT MATERNAL DEATHS – TRENDS

Indirect deaths since 1997 have become the major cause of maternal deaths and within this group psychiatric problems and heart disease emerge as the most frequent causes (Table 1).

CARDIAC DISEASE

The numbers and rates of maternal deaths in these categories are more frequent than those relating to thrombo-embolism, the commonest cause of direct maternal deaths.

Cardiac causes can be divided into congenital (about 20%) and acquired (about 80%). Deaths from congenital disease were not counted before 1961/63. The specific causes are outlined in Table 2.

Peripartum cardiomyopathy, the commonest category, is seen in the last months of pregnancy or within 6 months of delivery in the older obese multiparous woman with hypertension in pregnancy.

Aortic aneurysm and dissection, accounting for a fifth of the cardiac deaths, should be considered in pregnant women presenting with atypical chest pain and features of pulmonary embolus. If Marfan's syndrome is diagnosed, the family needs to be screened for this.

Myocardial infarction is the third major category of deaths from heart disease and in two-thirds coronary artery dissection had occurred. There should, therefore, be a low threshold for angiography in these circumstances as demonstration of dissection allows the possibility of intervention

Table 2 Causes of maternal deaths from heart disease 1991–2002

Cause of death	Numbers (1991–2002)
Cardiomyopathy and myocarditis	34
Aortic aneurysm and dissection	28
Myocardial infarction	27
Pulmonary hypertension	22
All other heart disease	39
Valve/endocarditis	12
Other congenital	9
Sudden adult death syndrome	6
Myocardial fibrosis	4
Other acquired	8
Total	150

Adapted from *Why Mothers Die 2000–2002*.[3]

Pulmonary hypertension is the major congenital cause and has a high proportion of women from a minority ethnic group. The risk of maternal death quoted at 40% has remained unchanged over the last 40 years.[3] Prepregnancy counselling needs to include a discussion concerning this increased risk of death or severe morbidity.

All pregnant women with known congenital heart disease should be supervised during and after pregnancy by a cardiologist/physician with an interest in heart disease in pregnancy.

PSYCHIATRIC DEATHS

In 2000/2, suicide has been identified as the leading cause of maternal death. Psychiatric deaths include deaths from substance misuse, physical illness, accidents and other misfortunes which would not have occurred in the absence of a psychiatric disorder. The huge increase in problem drug use that has occurred world-wide since the 1980s has resulted in an increase in the numbers of pregnant, drug-using women and consequently deaths related to this.

Many of the suicides or deaths recorded under an open verdict associated with pregnancy had not been reported to the enquiry but were identified through the ONS birth maternal death linkage study in 2001. Most women who die as a result of puerperal psychosis do so following the first 6 weeks of delivery, the time usually taken to define a maternal death. Reviews of these deaths have been undertaken since 1997. A picture is emerging of the women involved who are older, white and have a previous psychiatric disorder. The risk of recurrence was frequently neither identified nor managed. Because of the importance of learning lessons from deaths from psychiatric causes, CEMACH is introducing a system of Regional Psychiatric Assessors to enable better and more detailed case assessment.

COINCIDENTAL MATERNAL DEATHS

Although most coincidental deaths are considered unrelated to pregnancy, it has long been standard practice to include them in the report. These deaths which include murder, road traffic accidents and malignancies have important lessons for the management of certain non-pregnancy-related conditions, and identify wider public health issues such as domestic violence and the use of car seat belts during pregnancy.

THE INTERNATIONAL ROLE OF THE CEMD

The risks of pregnancy to women in different parts of the world are extremely variable. More than 99% of all maternal deaths occur in the non-industrialised countries of the world, where a woman's life-time risk of dying from a pregnancy-related complication can be up to 200 times higher than in many industrialised countries.[7] More than 50% of the women in the world give birth without antenatal care and without a skilled attendant. It is estimated that more than 80% of maternal deaths could be prevented or avoided even in resource-poor countries. The highest mortality rates are in Africa, followed by Asia and Latin America.

In contrast to the UK, around 80% of maternal deaths globally are due to direct obstetric causes and 20% due to indirect causes. Infectious disease is a rising cause of maternal death and HIV/AIDS is now the leading cause of maternal death in most African countries.[8] In addition, more than 30 million women in Africa are at risk of malaria infection which also increases the risk of dying from malaria-related severe anaemia, the presence of which also contributes to death from haemorrhage.[8]

The work of the CEMD in the UK has long been recognised as a gold standard in professional self-audit and its methods are included in the WHO publication *Beyond the Numbers*[9] which is part of the *Making Pregnancy Safer* initiative. To date, at least 15 countries, mainly in Africa and Asia, have approached CEMD to adapt their methodology to help plan services to improve maternal and child health.

HISTORY OF CESDI

The Confidential Enquiry into Stillbirths and Deaths in Infancy (CESDI) was set up in 1992 in response to the high infant mortality rates noted in the mid-1980s. Prior to this, some but not all regions had developed perinatal mortality surveys. The remit of CESDI was to look into the causes of stillbirths, neonatal and infant deaths and, in particular, to identify aspects of care that might have contributed to the outcome. To achieve a greater understanding of the causes of these deaths, CESDI set up a notification system to identify and record clinical details on all fetal deaths between 20 weeks' gestation and 1 year of life, around 10,000 deaths annually in England, Wales and Northern Ireland. Not all could be investigated, so a rolling programme of topics was chosen and enquiries were held on these predefined subsets of deaths. The notification and enquiry functions were served originally by the CESDI regional co-ordinators and a central office and, from 2003, a similar arrangement has continued under the auspices of CEMACH. CEMACH collects perinatal deaths between 22 weeks gestation and 28 days of life.

The enquiries are conducted at regional level by a multidisciplinary panel which reviews the anonymised medical record. The members of the panel are independent, *i.e.* not involved with the case and not from the associated unit. The panels task includes noting and grading any suboptimal care and providing an opinion regarding its contribution to the death of the baby.

TRENDS IN PERINATAL AND INFANT DEATHS

Stillbirths have been described from 1928 following the requirement to register stillbirths introduced by the *Birth and Deaths Act* (1928). At that time, the stillbirth rate was approximately 40 per 1000 total births. By the time CESDI was set up, the stillbirth rate had fallen to 4 per 1000 total births. Co-incident with the start of CESDI was a change in the law regarding the gestation at birth for registering a stillbirth, from 28 weeks to 24 weeks; thus the stillbirth rate appeared to increase but this was due to the change in definition. Following this, stillbirth rates continued to decline achieving relative stability from 1997 onwards at 5.3 per 1000 total births (Fig. 2).[26] Of concern is an upturn in this rate observed for the first time in 2001, which has continued in 2002 and 2003.

Neonatal mortality rates have paralleled falls in stillbirth rates from 35.3 per 1000 live births in 1921 to 7.7 per 1000 live births in 1980 when their decline continued at a greater rate than that of stillbirths to 3.8 per 1000 in 1998. This level has remained stable since then.

INFANT MORTALITY

Infant mortality rates for England and Wales have declined since the beginning of the twentieth century. The high levels were a cause of public health concern then and interestingly many of the questions asked then are the same as those

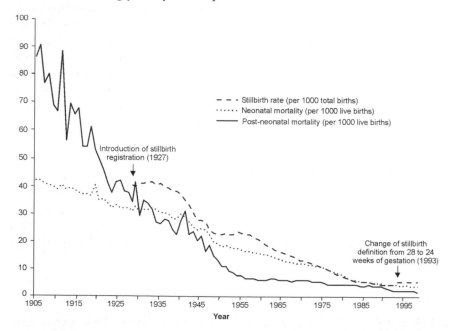

Fig. 2 Stillbirths and neonatal and postnatal deaths in England and Wales, 1910–1998. *Source*: General Register Office, OPCS and ONS mortality statistics. [Reproduced from data from *Birth Counts,*[26] Table A3.3.1]

being asked a century later.[26] The post neonatal mortality rate has declined more dramatically than the steadier decline seen in neonatal mortality (Fig. 2).[26] The wide fluctuations seen in the first half of the twentieth century were mainly due to infections. It is generally considered that improvements in housing, diet and sanitation have been major contributions to this decline.

Since 1992, as with maternal deaths, perinatal and infant deaths are reported in two ways: (i) through official death certification to the Register General's Office (ONS or its equivalents in Northern Ireland and Scotland); and (ii) through deaths reported to CESDI[17] and to CEMACH from 2003. CEMACH reports cover England, Wales and Northern Ireland and include neonatal but not post-neonatal deaths.

CLASSIFICATION OF CAUSE OF DEATH

CESDI and subsequently CEMACH use a three-level classification of perinatal deaths comprising:

1. The pathophysiological classification of Wigglesworth.[10]

2. The fetal and neonatal classification.[11]

3. The revised Aberdeen (obstetric) classification.[12,25]

Stillbirths account for about two-thirds of perinatal losses; unexplained antepartum stillbirths account for 72% of the causes of stillbirths and, even when this is further classified using the Aberdeen obstetric classification, 81% of these remain unexplained demonstrating the limitations of the current classification systems for understanding the underlying causes of death (Fig. 3).[19]

Classification of perinatal deaths ideally should include intrauterine growth restriction (IUGR). This is difficult as IUGR is not an easily defined entity and is often erroneously thought to be synonymous with small for gestational age (SGA). However, the majority of SGA infants are constitutionally small rather than IUGR[20] and a fetus with IUGR is not necessarily SGA.[21] The challenge remains as to how to accurately diagnose IUGR both antenatally and at post mortem. CEMACH plans to review the existing classification systems to improve the understanding of the causes of stillbirths.

PERINATAL ENQUIRY PROGRAMME

The purpose of undertaking confidential enquiries is to recognise trends, to understand the contributory factors to adverse events and, from this, to improve future clinical practice. Because of the large numbers of deaths reported annually, CESDI undertook a rolling programme of enquiries on predefined subsets (Table 3).

INTRAPARTUM DEATHS

In 1994 and 1995, CESDI enquired on the deaths of 875 normally formed babies weighing at least 1.5 kg dying after the onset of labour and before 28 days of life. This was equivalent to 1 in every 1561 births in England, Wales and

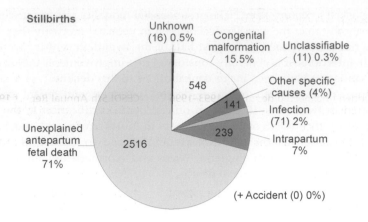

Stillbirths

Unknown (16) 0.5%
Congenital malformation 15.5%
Unclassifiable (11) 0.3%
548
Other specific causes (4%)
141
Infection (71) 2%
239
Intrapartum 7%
Unexplained antepartum fetal death 71%
2516

(+ Accident (0) 0%)

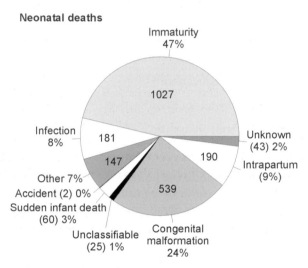

Neonatal deaths

Immaturity 47%
1027
Infection 8%
181
Unknown (43) 2%
190
Intrapartum (9%)
147
Other 7%
Accident (2) 0%
Sudden infant death (60) 3%
539
Unclassifiable (25) 1%
Congenital malformation 24%

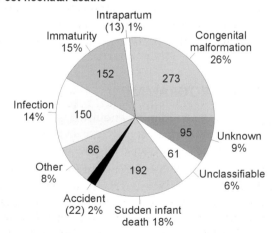

Post-neonatal deaths

Intrapartum (13) 1%
Immaturity 15%
152
Congenital malformation 26%
273
Infection 14%
150
95
Unknown 9%
86
61
Other 8%
192
Unclassifiable 6%
Accident (22) 2%
Sudden infant death 18%

Fig. 3 Deaths reported to CESDI by cause according to Wigglesworth classification, 2002. Adapted from: CEMACH *Stillbirth, neonatal and post neonatal mortality 2000–2002 England, Wales and Northern Ireland.*[19]

Table 3 Enquiry topics undertaken by CESDI (1993–2003)

Enquiry topic	Year of occurrence	Findings reported
Intrapartum deaths > 1.5 kg	1994–1995	CESDI 4th Annual Report 1997[13]
Sudden unexpected deaths in infancy	1993–1996	CESDI 5th Annual Report 1998[24] Sudden Unexpected Deaths in Infancy (SUDI)[14]
1 in 10 sample of all deaths > 1 kg	1996–1997	CESDI 6th Annual Report 1999[15]
Deaths > 4 kg	1997	CESDI 6th Annual Report 1999[15]
Premature babies at 27–28 weeks' gestation	1998–2000	CESDI 8th Annual Report 2000[16] Project 27/28 2003[17]
Pregnancies to women with diabetes	2002–2005	Publications due 2005/6

Northern Ireland.[13] Major or moderate suboptimal care was noted in 78% of cases and in just over half (52%) it was concluded that the death could have reasonably been avoided. The findings highlighted wide-spread concerns regarding the quality of maternity care, especially with regard to the service provided on labour wards. It was rare for a single factor to be regarded as critical in isolation but the most frequent failures were due to problems with clinical skills and communication rather than resource issues. There were two particular problems:

1. Interpretation and use of fetal heart recording. Health professionals of every grade demonstrated a considerable lack of interpretative skills in fetal heart recording.

2. Risk recognition and its communication. Failures in upward transfer of responsibility were common. Criticisms of obstetricians were divided equally into recognition problems and failures to seek more senior advice whereas those relating to midwives were more likely to be due to failure to ask for medical or more senior midwifery assistance.

CESDI recommended that the training assessment, supervision and practice of obstetricians and midwives of all grades needed to be re-appraised critically by their parent bodies. It also called for the introduction of a regular training programme in the use of cardiotochographs for all professionals involved in intrapartum care and emphasised the need for national and local guidelines in this area. The Clinical Negligence Scheme for Trusts, which oversees clinical negligence claims in England and Wales, includes maternity standards derived from the CESDI and CEMD reports, and has included training requirements in fetal heart rate recording. In May 2001, the National Institute for Clinical Excellence issued a national guideline on the use of electronic fetal monitoring.[18]

Between 1994 and 2002, the numbers and the rates of intrapartum related deaths weighing above 1 kg have fallen to levels of around 350 and 0.55 per 1000 total births compared to 630 and 0.95 per 1000 total births in 1994.[16,19]

ONE-IN-TEN SAMPLE OF ALL DEATHS

This was the major programme that ran between 1996 and 1997 sampling 1 in 10 of all reported deaths to CESDI after excluding post-neonatal deaths, late fetal losses, babies weighing less than a kilogram and known congenital malformations at birth. Its purpose was to scope the range of reported deaths to identify areas for future enquiry. The relationship between the various causes of death and the overall grade of care was examined to identify which types of deaths had the greatest proportion of suboptimal care. Intrapartum-related deaths were the group with the greatest proportion of poor care followed by deaths of babies due to prematurity.[15] Mothers with pre-existing diabetes were also noted to be particularly poorly managed with 75% receiving moderate or severe suboptimal care. These observations supported the choice of the subsequent two enquiry programmes.

The most frequent perinatal death sampled was a stillbirth and around 70% were classified as 'unexplained' signifying the limitations of these classifications (see above) for the current issues and causes of perinatal mortality. 'Unexplained' does not equate with unavoidable as moderate or severe suboptimal care was reported in 45% of stillbirth reviews. This indicates that improvements in care may reduce stillbirth rates. The patterns of failures were similar to those observed in the intrapartum death enquiries – problems of risk recognition and acting on high risk situations. Diagnosing intra-uterine growth restriction (IUGR) and poor management of this condition was particularly commented on, as was failure to advise or act on changes in fetal movements. The variety of comments reflected the substantial variation in opinion and practice in these clinical areas and point to the need for evidence based guidance.

PREMATURE BABIES BORN AT 27–28 WEEKS' GESTATION[17]

Prematurity (birth prior to 37 weeks' gestation) accounts for 13% of births in the UK[22] and is the major cause of neonatal deaths. Project 27/28[17] had two aims: (i) to measure survival figures for babies born at 27–28 weeks' gestation' and (ii) to identify patterns of practice or service provision that might contribute to the deaths of babies at this gestation. The range 27–28 weeks was chosen because most babies born at this stage were expected to survive and so it was anticipated that care issues would have a significant role. As gestation is not routinely notified at birth, gestation-specific survival rates required setting up a project specific notification system. The CESDI regional network in England, Wales and Northern Ireland was notified of all babies born between 26 and 30 weeks' gestation over a 2-year period (1998–2000). The survival rates at 27–28 weeks' gestation of 88% was considerably higher than anticipated at the outset of the project.[16]

Survival figures at day 28 do not measure quality of survival nor do they give insight into quality of care issues. Thus, behind these excellent survival figures, the enquiries revealed several areas for future improvement. Project 27/28 was the first national enquiry programme to include findings from a controls group.

There were three specific areas relating to obstetric care in which faults were more prevalent in the mothers of babies who died: (i) assessment of fetal well-being (26% versus 18%); (ii) efforts to administer corticosteroids (16% versus

11%); and (iii) failures to transfer to an appropriate delivery unit for delivery (9% versus 1%). These findings reinforce the '1-in-10' findings that there is substantial scope for improvement in the approach to the assessment of fetal well-being.

There were three specific areas in which failures to meet standards of neonatal care were more frequent in the babies who died: (i) temperature control (73% versus 59%); (ii) ventilation (18% versus 7%); and (iii) cardiovascular support (15% versus 7%).

As with any case control study, there is the potential for bias and this was particularly problematic for the comparisons of neonatal care as the babies who died were inherently sicker at birth, more likely to weigh less than the 5th centile and to be male. However, the differences remained after these factors were adjusted for. The most commonly cited issues included: (i) allowing the temperature to fall unnecessarily; (ii) poor management plans and failures to respond to blood gas analysis in relation to ventilation; and (iii) delay or failure to use inotropes in relation to cardiovascular support.

In general, poor care was associated with higher mortality rates and the effect of care was greatest in the babies born in good condition emphasising the importance of skilled care for the well-being of the premature baby at this gestational age.

SUDDEN UNEXPECTED DEATHS IN INFANCY (SUDI)

CESDI undertook the largest study on sudden unexpected deaths in infancy.[19] The work covered five CESDI regions between 1993 and 1996 and included review of 456 cases. All such deaths are reported to a coroner who makes arrangements for the examination of the child. The final diagnosis of sudden infant death syndrome (SIDS) or 'cot death' is reached only after exclusion of other causes. The CESDI review categorised 363 (80%) as SIDS and the remaining 93 (20%) as having an underlying cause. Half of those with a specific cause were considered to be potentially avoidable.

The diagnosis of SIDS by definition is one of exclusion and this relies on the quality of the autopsy. The findings demonstrated significant problems with the quality of autopsies, a failure which has serious consequences within society. A paediatric pathologist performed the post mortem examination in only 32% of cases and there was wide variation in the proportion of cases that were attributed to a cause of death other than SIDS.

The CESDI SUDI report[19] recommended that all relevant information should be collected ideally within 24–48 h of the death and post mortem examination should only be carried out by a paediatric pathologist or a pathologist with special training.

These recommendations were re-iterated in 2004 by a joint working group from the Royal Colleges of Paediatrics and Child Health and of Pathology.[23] Practice and outcomes are dependent on the coroner's system and specialist pathologists undertaking the associated work. Changes to the coronial system are currently under discussion.

Although this area of care may at first not seem directly relevant to maternity services, midwives in particular have a key educational role in the provision of advice on the sleeping environment and sleep position for the baby.

THE FUTURE FOR CONFIDENTIAL ENQUIRIES

For over 50 years, confidential enquiry has provided national overviews and insights into issues contributing to maternal deaths. Over the last decade, confidential enquiry has achieved the same for the baby and infant. This unique approach has managed to combine confidentiality with national epidemiological overviews on a scale that is unknown elsewhere. The need for confidentiality has been, and will continue to be, challenged. Fair and objective assessments, however, will be required especially since obstetric care continues to be the major contributor to legal costs in the health service. Confidentiality is also needed in a climate in which there are increasing demands to meet health targets and provide quality care. Gaps between reported practice and guidance will need to be explored objectively.

In the UK, maternal deaths are currently so infrequent that mortality rates now provide a poor measurement of the quality of care because the factors related to an individual death may not necessarily be extrapolated to other circumstances. The natural extension of the enquiry work is to explore severe obstetric morbidity. The challenge lies in defining and identifying relevant morbidity cases in the absence of national denominator data. CEMACH with its clinically integrated network is well placed to respond to this challenge.

Continuing to count maternal deaths in the UK will contribute to saving lives elsewhere. Globally, maternal death rates are a manifestation of an enormous health inequality of our time. The existence and experience of the UK CEMD will promote the implementation of maternal death and disability audits and reviews around the world.

Perinatally, a challenge lies with introducing a new classification of perinatal deaths more relevant to the understanding of contributory factors to the cause of stillbirths. Improved access to specialist paediatric pathology services is a current major issue with autopsy rates being at an all time low.[19]

The development of effective interventions, such as surfactant and improvements in intensive care techniques, have resulted in increased survival rates for premature babies. This, however, does not equate with improved morbidity and the enquiries have an important potential role in the future addressing quality of care issues and their relationship with long-term disability in the child.

Finally, the remit of CEMACH now includes children as well as mothers, babies and infants. Exploring why children die will be a significant task to undertake in the next few years. Work is underway addressing how to best identify and then enquire into child deaths up to the age of 18 years.

Key points for clinical practice

- Venous thrombo-embolism is the leading cause of direct maternal deaths. In just over half the cases, there is substandard care particularly in relation to risk assessment and implementation of thromboprophylaxis.[4]

- In severe pre-eclampsia, the main cause of death is cerebral haemorrhage due to uncontrolled systolic blood pressure.

Key points for clinical practice *(continued)*

Management protocols should include the need to control very high systolic blood pressure and to provide guidance on thresholds above which urgent and effective treatment is required (160 mmHg suggested).

- Cardiac disease is the commonest cause of indirect maternal death. Women with known cardiac disease should receive thorough prepregnancy counselling.

- Psychiatric death is the leading cause of late indirect maternal death. Systematic enquiries about previous psychiatric history, its severity, care received and clinical presentation should be routinely made at the antenatal booking visit. Women who require psychiatric admission following childbirth should be admitted to a specialist mother-and-baby unit, together with their infant.

- Stillbirths are the largest proportion of perinatal deaths and within this group the unexplained are the greatest category. Of mothers of stillborn babies, 45% had received moderate-to-severe suboptimal care and the most frequently cited problem was failure to act appropriately in a high-risk situation.

- The commonest fault cited in relation to intrapartum-related death relates to misinterpretation of electronic fetal heart monitoring. Midwives and obstetricians of all grades need to train and update this skill regularly.

- Nearly two-thirds of all premature babies at 27–28 weeks' gestation had a temperature below 36°C on admission to the NICU. The temperature of the delivery room should be at least 25°C and simple methods such as occlusive wrapping of the baby in the delivery room should be used.

References

1. World Health Organization. *International Classification of Diseases Manual of the International Statistical Classification of Diseases, Injuries and Causes of Death.* Ninth revision, vol 1. Geneva: WHO, 1977.
2. World Health Organization. *International Classification of Diseases and Related Health Problems.* Tenth revision, vol 1. Geneva: WHO, 1992.
3. Confidential Enquiry into Maternal and Child Health. *Why Mothers Die 2000–2002.* London: RCOG Press, 2004.
4. Royal College of Obstetrics and Gynaecology. *Thromboprophylaxis during pregnancy, labour and after vaginal delivery.* RCOG Guideline No 37. London: RCOG, 2004.
5. Magpie Trial Collaborative Group. Do women with pre-eclampsia, and their babies, benefit from magnesium sulphate? The Magpie Trial: a randomised placebo controlled trial. *Lancet* 2002; **359**: 1877–1890.
6. Duley L, Henderson-Smart DJ. Magnesium sulphate versus phenytoin for eclampsia. *Cochrane Database System Rev* 2004 (2).
7. World Health Organization. *Maternal Mortality in 2000: Estimates Developed by WHO, UNICEF and UNFPA.* Geneva: WHO, 2003.
8. World Health Organization Regional Office for Africa. *Reducing Maternal Deaths: The*

Challenge of the New Millennium in the Africa Region. Brazzaville, Congo: WHO, 2002.

9. World Health Organization. *Beyond the Numbers; Reviewing Maternal Deaths and Disabilities to Make Pregnancy Safer.* Geneva: WHO, 2004.

10. Wigglesworth JS. Monitoring perinatal mortality – a pathophysiological approach. *Lancet* 1980; **2**: 684–686.

11. Bound JP. Classification and causes of perinatal mortality. *BMJ* 1956; **ii**: 1191–1196, 1260–1265.

12. Baird D, Thomson AM. The causes and prevention of stillbirths and first week deaths. *J Obstet Gynaecol Br Emp* 1954: **61**: 433–448.

13. Confidential Enquiry into Stillbirths and Deaths in Infancy, 4th Annual Report, 1997.

14. Fleming P, Blair P, Bacon C, Berry J. (eds) *Sudden Unexpected Deaths in Infancy.* London: Stationery Office, 2000.

15. Confidential Enquiry into Stillbirths and Deaths in Infancy, 6th Annual Report, 1999.

16. Confidential Enquiry into Stillbirths and Deaths in Infancy, 8th Annual Report, 2001.

17. Project 27/28. *An Enquiry into quality of care and its effect on the survival of babies born at 27–28 weeks.* Confidential Enquiries into Stillbirths and Deaths in Infancy. London: Stationery Office, 2003.

18. National Institute for Clinical Excellence. *The use of electronic fetal monitoring: The use and interpretation of cardiotocography in intrapartum fetal surveillance* (Guideline C). London: NICE, 2001.

19. Confidential Enquiry into Maternal and Child Health (CEMACH). *Stillbirth, neonatal and post neonatal mortality 2000–2002 England, Wales and Northern Ireland*, London: ACOG Press, 2005.

20. Ott WJ. The diagnosis of altered fetal growth. *Obstet Gynecol Clin North Am* 1988; **15**: 237–263.

21. Chard T, Costeloe K, Leaf A. Evidence of growth retardation in neonates of apparently normal weight. *Eur J Obstet Gynecol Reprod Biol* 1992; **45**: 59–62.

22. Perinatal Survey Office. *All Wales Perinatal Survey 1999.* Cardiff: University of Wales College of Medicine.

23. Royal College of Pathologists. *Sudden unexpected death in infancy: a multi-agency protocol for care and investigation.* London: Royal College of Pathologists, 2004.

24. Confidential Enquiry into Stillbirths and Deaths in Infancy, 5th Annual Report, 1998.

25. Cole SK, Thomson AM. Classifying perinatal death; an obstetric approach. *Br J Obstet Gynaecol* 1986; **93**: 1204–1212.

26. Macfarlane A, Mugford M, Henderson J, Furtado A, Stevens J, Dunn A. *Birth Counts. Statistics of pregnancy and childbirth*, vol. 2. London: The Stationery Office, 2000.

James J. Walker

9

Risk management in obstetrics

In the year 2000, the UK Department of Health (DH) published a document called *An Organisation with a Memory (OWAM)*, [1] which highlighted the high incidence of medical error and the importance of learning from mistakes in the National Health Service (NHS). *Building a Safer NHS for Patients* followed this acting on the recommendations of OWAM.[2] These documents emphasised the importance of understanding the errors made and the appropriate assessment in order to learn and produce solutions. It emphasised that this had to be within a 'no blame environment' with the aim of increasing patient safety by 'reducing unintended harm or injury from healthcare treatment; rather than from disease process'.[3]

It may seem strange that patient safety needs to be on the agenda for doctors. 'First do no harm' has been a mantra from the time of the Hippocratic Oath. Surely no doctor sets out to cause harm intentionally? However, the US Institute of Medicine reported that impact of healthcare error upon patient safety was 'a national problem of epidemic proportions'.[4] Similar statistics were found in the UK (Table 1).[1] Obstetrics is no more likely to produce error than any other specialty but the potential for damage makes litigation costs considerable.

Currently, the NHS reporting systems provide an incomplete picture of the scale and nature of serious failures in the NHS.[1] However, it is clear that there is a significant financial cost as well as patient morbidity and mortality associated with medical error which involves about 10% of all admissions with a cost to the NHS of around £2 billion a year.[1] Vincent *et al.*[5] suggested that, of the 10% of patients suffering an adverse event, it is preventable in around 50% of cases. These figures are similar to those quoted in the *Why Women Die*.[6] Internationally, the rates vary from under 2.9% to over 16% depending on the

James J. Walker MD FRCP(Edin) FRCPS(Glas) FRCOG
Professor of Obstetrics and Gynaecology, Level 9, Gledhow Wing, St James's University Hospital,
Beckett Street, Leeds LS9 7TL, UK (E-mail: j.j.walker@leeds.ac.uk)

Table 1 Errors within the NHS as estimated in OWAM[1]

- 400 people die or are seriously injured in adverse events involving medical devices
- 10,000 people are reported to have experienced serious adverse reactions to drugs
- 1150 people who have been in recent contact with mental health services commit suicide
- 28,000 written complaints are made about aspects of clinical treatment in hospitals
- The NHS pays out around £400 million a year settlement of clinical negligence claims, and has a potential liability of around £2.4 billion for existing and expected claims.
- Hospital acquired infections – around 15% of which may be avoidable – are estimated to cost the NHS nearly £1 billion.

definitions used. Iatrogenic disease is not the same as patient safety incidents or adverse events, although definitions tend to overlap. Similarly, expected complications of disease are not errors, but inappropriate care in the event of the complication could be.

No matter what the definition, error in medical practice is common. Although we try our best, 'to err is human'.[4] Errors can be those of commission (we do the wrong thing) or omission (we do not do the right thing). However, in the majority of situations, it is a system failure which is the root cause in which the individual is only one part of the error matrix. Human error cannot be eliminated and the removal or punishment of the individual does not change the environment that produced the error in the first place. It is by appropriate error management that adverse events can be reduced.[7,8]

Risk management is a collective term covering the assessment, reduction and moderation of adverse events. In industry where this is more widely used, it has largely been directed towards a reduction in litigation costs and the organisation's liability. As such, the effort is not to protect the individual but the organisation. Therefore, to operate effectively, this has to be carried out in a 'no blame environment'.[3] In healthcare, the approach is similar but the aims are ultimately to improve patient safety. This is part of clinical governance, which covers event reporting, error analysis, risk management, risk prediction and prevention, and appraisal.

EVENT REPORTING

The mainstay of risk management is error reporting. This needs to be part of every-day practice. Within the airline industry, routine error (near miss) reporting followed by root-cause analysis and risk management, has led to a 4-fold reduction in major airline incidents.[4] The airline industry has many similar features to obstetric practice requiring concentration during long periods of little activity, sudden emergencies requiring instant decision-making, and a close working team which is interdependent. Root-cause analysis of major airline events found that factors that contributed to the events were:

- Failure to follow accepted procedures
- Misinterpretation of instruments
- Incorrect decisions
- Ignoring advice from colleagues
- Failure of team working
- Equipment failure
- Pilot error.

Those working within the obstetric environment will easily recognise these factors and their role in medical error. Therefore, it is the acceptance of medical error that is the first step in event reporting. However, doctors are poor in reporting error, particularly their own, as they are afraid of disciplinary action. Midwives are better at reporting error, but these are often of the 'trips and falls' variety or equipment or staffing issues. To allow a true reporting culture requires a 'no blame' environment.[3] It is the appreciation that although it is the individual that makes the error, it is the system within which they work that has produced the environment. The importance of error reporting is highlighted by the formation of the National Patient Safety Agency (NPSA).

THE NATIONAL PATIENT SAFETY AGENCY

The NPSA is a special health authority working across England and Wales. It was formed after OWAM to help implement changes that would lead to an open reporting culture. One of its statutory functions was to set up a National Reporting & Learning System (NRLS), to collect reports of patient safety incidents from individual trusts and to learn from them to help develop solutions to enhance patient safety.

The NRLS was developed to promote event reporting and a comprehensive national learning about patient safety incidents. The NRLS is now connected to all the acute trusts in England and Wales and receives a copy of reports about patient safety incidents that are reported to the local risk management system. In the future, individuals, including staff and members of the public, will be able to report over the internet independently. These reports are anonymised and collected into a specially designed, confidential national database. This allows regular interrogation of the data set to look for trends and any repeated problems. Although the NPSA defines a patient safety incident (PSI) as any unintended or unexpected incident, which could have or did lead to harm for one or more patients receiving NHS-funded care, what is reported is widely varied and requires much sifting. A limited amount of analysis can be made looking for underlying contributory factors. These data, along with others, are used for the development of solutions and feedback to care providers to enhance learning across the NHS.

However, one of the important roles of the NRLS is to assess the rate of incident reporting. It is one of the strange paradoxes of the system that incident reporting of a certain level is good and under-reporting bad. However, if the errors are too common, the organisation may be seen as dysfunctiona.

The main type of incidents reported in obstetrics fall into the following categories:

- Patient accident (trips and falls)
- Errors in treatment, procedure or medication
- Access, admission, transfer, discharge (between carers, wards and hospitals)
- Infrastructure (including staffing, facilities, environment)
- Documentation (including records, identification)
- Clinical assessment (including diagnosis, scans, tests, assessments)
- Medical device/equipment
- Implementation of care and ongoing monitoring/review.

These will come as no surprise to the majority of clinicians but it allows quantification for the first time and a guide to where risk management should be directed. Although it is the process that should be being assessed, the classification of the adverse event allows the appropriate assessment response and risk categorisation. This is based on the 'degree of harm' resulting from the event. It is categorised as no harm, low, moderate, severe and death.

Since its conception, the NPSA has tried to encourage a safety culture within the NHS with emphasis on the importance of reporting and analysis. There is no benefit from reporting in itself if the appropriate analysis and intervention is not carried through.

ERROR ANALYSIS

The traditional way to manage human error is the person approach where the individual involved is questioned and the problem tackled at that level.[7] However, there is increasing realisation that there is more to error management than this and that tackling the individual does not remove the pre-existing risk of error from clinical practice (the error trap). There has to be a move towards a system approach of error management which is wider in its remit, more open, and based on concept of system failures. This approach produces a completely different outcome for the individual concerned and is more likely to produce solutions that reduce the chance of recurrence. However, it requires a trusting environment and a 'no blame' approach.[7]

PERSON APPROACH

This remains the norm in clinical practice and concentrates on the errors carried out by midwives and doctors working at the sharp end. It assumes blame for the error due to forgetfulness, inattention, poor motivation, carelessness, negligence, and recklessness.[7] The solutions implemented solve the immediate problems by stopping the individual from doing it again. These include disciplinary measures, including suspension or sacking, retraining or writing another guideline (or adding to existing ones). The errors are treated as judgemental issues, assuming that bad things are done by bad people. This is called 'the just world hypothesis'.[8] However, this generates fear in the staff, reduces the chances of errors being reported and papers over the cracks. More importantly, the institution and the other staff learn little from the process apart from increasing fear.

SYSTEM APPROACH

The system approach accepts that humans are fallible and errors occur, even in the best organisations. The error is seen as a consequence, rather than a cause, of the problem. It assumes that there are pre-existing systemic factors that have contributed. These include recurrent 'error traps' and the processes that give rise to them. The solutions to these errors are based on the assumption that we cannot prevent human error but we can change the conditions under which humans work. This is done by producing defences within the system. When an adverse event occurs, the question is not 'who made a mistake', but 'how and why have the defences failed'.[7]

WHY IS THE SYSTEM APPROACH BEST?

For the organisation, there is much to commend the person approach. Blaming individuals is emotionally more satisfying and rewarding than looking within. It also appears logical. Since individuals can choose between safe and unsafe acts, the individual (or group of individuals) must have been responsible. The institution can distance itself from this unsafe act. Patients similarly see this as a satisfactory outcome and it is more convenient in the medicolegal environment. However, this is not the best approach for the health care system and will slow the development of a safe patient-environment. The majority of errors are not due to individual mistakes. Usually, around 90% of errors are associated with system failures and no one individual should be blamed.[9]

If errors are to be managed successfully, it has to be within a reporting culture.[10] Without this, the organisation will not discover the recurring problems due to error traps. This means that although specific incident may be 'dealt' with, the error trap that helped produce it is still there and the error will be repeated in time. This is a serious weakness of the person approach. It also ignores two important features of human error – errors are made by all and mistakes are not random and tend to recur. Therefore, it is important that any investigation looks at the root cause of the error to seek out and remove the environmental factors that helped produce it. Removal of the individual does not do that. In order to achieve this, there has to be a trusting relationship between the organisation and its staff to encourage incident reporting. It must be within a 'no-blame' environment and the staff must feel that reporting is to their benefit from a learning and safety aspect.

THE SWISS CHEESE MODEL OF SYSTEM FAILURE

The system approach to error reduction requires defences, barriers, and safeguards.[7] These defensive layers can be technical (alarms, physical barriers,

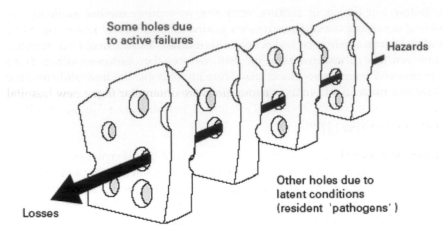

Fig. 1 Swiss cheese model of accident causation.[10]

automatic shutdowns, *etc.*), human (doctors, midwives, administrators, *etc.*), and documentation (guidelines, standard operating procedures, *etc.*). They all act to either prevent error or protect the patient if one occurs. These defences are mostly successful, but not infallible. They are more like slices of Swiss cheese, having many holes, though unlike cheese, these holes vary in their existence and location (Fig. 1). The presence of a hole in any one 'slice' will not normally lead to an error as the next layer should be intact and block its progress. However, if the holes align, the error can be perpetuated leading to an incident. These holes arise due to either active failures or latent conditions which are present in virtually all adverse events (Fig. 3).[7]

ACTIVE FAILURES

Active failures are the errors committed by people who are in direct contact with the patient. They take a variety of forms: slips, lapses, fumbles, mistakes, and procedural violations.[11]

Slips, lapses, fumbles and mistakes

An error occurs when a planned action fails either due to a deviation from the intended execution of that action (slips, lapses or fumbles) or an error of the planned action itself (mistake). In the first instance, the plan is correct but it is not carried out successfully. Slips usually relate to failures of concentration (*e.g.* failure to remove a vaginal swab after episiotomy repair), lapses are failures of memory (forgetting two drugs interact) and fumbles are where the actions are performed incorrectly (*e.g.* damage of a ureter at hysterectomy). Mistakes are when actions go as planned but the plan is inadequate to achieve the outcome (*e.g.* pulling too strongly on the baby's head at a shoulder dystocia). These are failures of intention. Therefore, all errors involve some kind of deviation but, whereas with slips, lapses, and fumbles the actions deviate from the intention at the level of execution, in the case of mistakes, the failure lies at the higher level of problem assessment and solving and the formulating of the plan. Slips and lapses are more common during routine tasks, usually in familiar surroundings. They are usually due to attention failures, either from distraction from the immediate surroundings or pre-occupation, and are more likely in situations where the surroundings are unfamiliar (*e.g.* a new hospital or locum appointment).[11] Unlike slips, lapses and fumbles, mistakes are either rule- or knowledge-based.

Rule-based mistakes

Rule-based mistakes occur when an individual is acting in a familiar situation for which he/she is well trained. This is where a common pattern of signs, indicating a particular problem, leads to routine response. This process can go wrong in two ways. The plan instigated is a good course of action, but wrong in the given situation; or the wrong plan is instigated due failure to update errors.

Knowledge-based mistakes

Knowledge-based mistakes occur when the situation lies outside the experience of the individual and they have no learned solution. The individual has to resort to reasoning and problem solving. This makes errors very likely since humans are only able to solve a limited number of problems at any one time. Also, because of unfamiliarity, the assessment of the problem is often incomplete and may be wrong. This leads to a tendency to fix on a particular hypothesis and look for signs that confirm this and ignore those that contradict. This is called 'confirmation bias' or 'cognitive lock-up' and is often seen in industry when individuals are attempting to recover from an emergency.[12]

Violations

Violations are actions that deviate from accepted practice or guideline. These are either deliberate actions (intended deviation) or erroneous (being unaware what is expected). Erroneous actions are common when people are working in unfamiliar surroundings. Deliberate violations are often associated with motivational problems relating to low morale, lack of supervision and an apparent lack of concern or consequence. This is where individuals 'cut corners' or act to get rid of the problem to someone else.

Whereas errors occur due to wrong actions of a well-meaning individual, violations are purposeful and relate to the working environment. Appropriate training and feedback of information can reduce errors but violations usually require changes within the organisation to improve the working environment and individual motivation.[13]

LATENT FAILURES

The difference between active and latent failures is best illustrated by Mr Justice Sheen's comments in his report into the capsize of the *Herald of Free Enterprise*.[14]

At first sight the faults which led to this disaster were the...errors of omission on the part of the Master, the Chief Officer and the assistant bosun. But a full investigation into the circumstances of the disaster leads inexorably to the conclusion that the underlying or cardinal faults lay higher up in the Company. From top to bottom, the body corporate was infected with the disease of sloppiness.

The active failures were those that directly led to capsize and were committed by the ship's officers and crew. However, it was clear that the *Herald of Free Enterprise* was a 'sick' ship long before it sailed from Zeebrugge on 6 March 1987. These are due to problems in the organisation itself. Therefore, active failures are committed by those at the 'sharp end' (*e.g.* anaesthetists, obstetricians, midwives) and have immediate effect. Latent failures exist within the organisation because of failure in correct attitude, supervision and safety culture and lie dormant and unnoticed for a long time, only appearing when they are associated with active failures or other errors resulting in an incident. This is like a smoke alarm without a battery; it does no harm until required, when its failure will make a problem into a worse disaster. Active failures are generally short-lived and are usually dealt with by the person approach to error management. This provides scapegoats but ignores the latent failures that allowed the error to happen. Since most violations are associated with latent failures, failure to act on them means that they will remain, leading to similar errors in the future.

These latent conditions are the inevitable 'resident pathogens' within the system. They can arise from decisions made by managers, guideline writers, supervisors, rota managers and anyone else that influences the work environment. All changes within a system can lead to such latent conditions. They can produce immediate problems such as time pressures, understaffing, inadequate equipment, fatigue, and inexperience or more subtle weaknesses in the defences such untrustworthy alarms and indicators, unworkable procedures, design and construction defects. Unlike active failures, which are hard to predict, latent conditions should be sought and corrected before an adverse event occurs. This is pro-active rather than reactive risk management. In obstetrics, an active failure may be an inexperienced SpR carrying out a Caesarean section for a placenta praevia leading to severe haemorrhage. Rescue action is possible each time this occurs, but the best solution is to create a more effective defence and make sure a consultant is present. Failure to do so means the problem will recur.

RISK MANAGEMENT

Risk management aims to limit the occurrence of errors and to place defences that limit the resultant damage. Various tools have been developed to help achieve this. There has been a move away from the person approach (which directs resources to education and training) towards the system approach which is more comprehensive covering the person, team, procedure, environment and the organisation.[7] Most high-reliability organisations, which operate in hazardous conditions, have fewer adverse events. These are usually resilient systems with intrinsic 'safety health' which allows them to withstand the operational dangers but still achieve their objectives.

THE APPROACH IN HIGH-RELIABILITY ORGANISATIONS

In the past, safety experts mostly studied why errors happen. More recently they have started to study safety successes and the reasons behind them.[7] These successes are found in high-reliability organisations such as nuclear aircraft carriers, air traffic control systems, and nuclear power plants. Many of their important cultural characteristics could be copied within medicine. Unlike traditional thinking which believed that human variability was a source of error, they recognise that human variability, such as the ability to adapt to changing events, could be an important safeguard. They see reliability as 'a dynamic non-event'.[7] It is dynamic because safety is achieved by timely human actions but it is a non-event because successful outcomes do not attract attention. These organisations can adapt themselves to the changing environment. Normally, they follow routine practice but, in emergencies, control is taken over by experts on the spot. After the crisis, routine practice resumes. Unfortunately, in medicine, the experts are often not present at the time of crisis (a latent failure). For this flexibility to work, all workers need to support the fundamental aims of the organisation which, in turn, needs to produce the environment and trust to allow its workers to act appropriately. They both expect and encourage variability of human action as well as maintaining a consistent intelligent wariness. The workers must be constantly aware of the possibility of failures and be prepared to recognise and recover from them. This is helped by rehearsing familiar scenarios (drills) and assessing possible risks (risk assessment).[7] Many failures are generic and instead of making specific changes, there should be system reforms. Effort should not be made to prevent isolated failures, either human or technical, but to attempt to make the system as robust as possible. This does not prevent all adverse events but, when they occur, they should be used to improve the process. This requires systems of incident analysis to look for errors at all levels and the implementation of solutions to prevent the error occurring again. This is done by using root-cause analysis (RCA).

ROOT-CAUSE ANALYSIS

The root cause is the earliest point or points at which action could have been taken that would have reduced the chance of the incident occurring. Root-cause analysis is methodology that questions the 'how' and 'why' in a structured and objective way to investigate all the influencing and causal factors that have led to the incident. This is by the analysis of systems, rather than focusing on individuals. The aim is to learn how to prevent similar incidents happening again, not to apply blame. An independent, trained facilitator co-ordinates the RCA and the team should involve all levels of staff involved to identifying causes and solutions, promoting a positive attitude to the management of incidents and moving towards a fair and learning culture. The people who were actually involved in the incident should be involved by providing statements or by being interviewed. It is also important to consider how patients and their families may be involved in the process.

The team should be multiprofessional, which helps to prevent specialty bias and allows open debate surrounding clinical care. This encourages team

Table 2 The five 'whys' in error assessment

A patient required a Caesarean hysterectomy:

Why? There was a bad angle tear

Why? It was a Caesarian section at full cervical dilatation

Why? The operator was an inexperienced SpR

Why? Failure of adherence to The Royal College of Obstetrics and Gynaecology guidelines about the presence of a senior doctor

Why? There is an organisational acceptance that the consultants are not disturbed overnight.

building. The facilitator is neutral, nurturing and empowers people to contribute freely to the review and gain agreement that the group signs up to an open and non-judgemental approach. There is no allocation of personal blame.

The process starts with a chronology of the events. Then the management of the case is discussed using various techniques including brainstorming, five 'whys' (Table 2), change analysis and fishbone diagrams. All these help to elucidate the contributing factors of the incident.

The important end-point is the production of a report. This should include a summary of the key issues and solutions agreed at the meeting. Each solution or recommendation requires a person-allocated responsibility for the implementation and a time scale for action. This then requires auditing.

RISK PREDICTION AND PREVENTION

Once the risk and cause of error have been identified, safeguards (barriers) need to be developed to reduce the chances of recurrence and the associated damage. These solutions are often the result of an RCA. Whenever a risk is identified, the effect it may have on the organisation can be assessed using a risk matrix (Fig. 2). This looks at the expected frequency of the potential event and the likely outcome. This is then compared to the efforts required to reduce the risk. Depending on the results of this assessment, the organisation has to decide what action to take. If the effort required is big, the frequency low, and the damage minor, it may be decided to absorb the risk and the consequences. However, if the event is common and the damage significant, significant time and effort is justified to reduce the risk.

Risk reduction is not a new concept. Since the industrial revolution there have been various developments to reduce the risk to the workers involved and, in turn, the organisation. Canary cages and then Davey lamps were designed to warn of methane gas in mines. Victorian railway signalmen used flagsticks to mark signal levers to remind them that a train is waiting to proceed and prevent changing the signal in error. Pilots use checklists prior to take off, descent, and landing to minimise the omission of important procedural steps. In medicine, scrub nurses do swab and instrument counts before and after surgery to check that nothing has been left in the patient. These techniques tend to be developed by individuals for specific situations rather than part of a planned organisation

Frequency

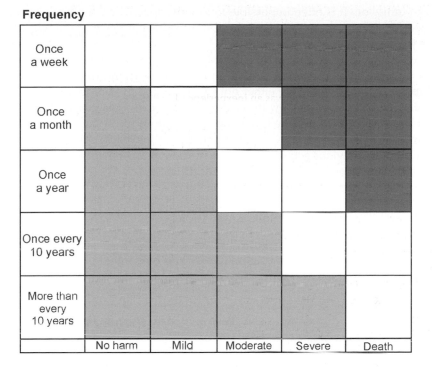

	No harm	Mild	Moderate	Severe	Death
Once a week					
Once a month					
Once a year					
Once every 10 years					
More than every 10 years					

Fig. 2 The risk matrix.

approach. They ignore systemic causal factors and are not implemented in other similar situations. An example of this is the general failure to carry out swab counts after episiotomy repair leading to regular errors of leaving swabs in the vagina. These methods are aimed at error reduction, but error containment is also required. These are measures aimed at the detection and recovery of errors in order to minimise the damage that occurs.

The most common form of human error is omission.[15] This is due to the diverse mental processes required in the implementation of an action. These involve four main stages – planning, intention storage, execution, and monitoring. An error of thought in any one or more of these processes can lead

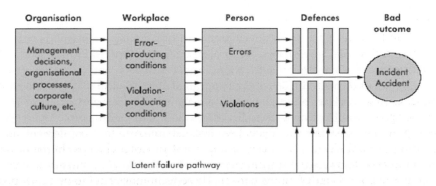

Fig. 3 Process of error production.[13]

to an omission. It is often impossible to identify where or why the error took place and even those who made the error, often have no memory of why they did it. To reduce these, it is important to focus on the structure of the tasks and what part of it is most likely to encourage omissions (termed 'affordances'). The factors that increase the chance of omissions are: (i) information overload; (ii) procedural steps that are either not related to the preceding actions or are repeated; (iii) steps that follow the achievement of the initial goal and, near the end of procedure, unexpected interruptions leading to the individual losing their place in the task; and (iv) where there is poor feedback, either mechanical or human, to previous actions.[15] Obviously, more than one of these factors can occur in any procedure producing an additive effect. These can exist as a recurrent error trap. An example of this is the use of the photocopier where the most common error is leaving the last page in the machine.[15]

Therefore, risk prediction and prevention has to:

- Identify the concerns, risks and the 'risk owners'
- Evaluate these risks as to frequency and outcome
- Assess how the risk can be accommodated
- Prioritise the risk to act on
- Develop the solutions and those responsible to implement
- Audit the implementation and outcome.

To achieve these ends, it is necessary to involve all staff, understand the environment in which they work, listen to any concerns expressed, reduce the organisational factors that increase the chances of error and improve the support, training and morale of all individuals in the organisation.[10]

Audit of practice, particularly the implementation of guidelines, is an important part of this for various reasons. There is little point in writing and having a guideline in place if there is no record of its use or the benefit of its development. Human nature is such that, if actions are not audited, they are likely not to be used in times of stress but, if audited, compliance increases. Also, if audit demonstrates benefit, it becomes accepted and supported by all the staff involved.[16] Overall, about 50% of audit projects within a hospital should be used to support the risk management process directly.

APPRAISAL

Appraisal has been a parallel development to risk management and is part of the overall clinical governance. With appraisal, the individual has to show involvement in continued education, audit projects and learning from complaints or errors. With 360 degree appraisal, the individual asks a selection of those that work with him/her to assess their behaviour and practice. This allows good feedback on personality flaws and leadership skills. Again, the individual is expected to respond to these comments and implement any required improvements. Not everyone can change, but awareness of flaws can help them and those around them to fit into the system and reduce errors that might develop. A similar process for the organisation is also required but this is less common and more difficult to implement.

CONCLUSIONS

Risk management is to some extent a rebadging of what went before. Obstetrics has a long history of audit of problems. The *Confidential Enquiry into Maternal Death* is now 50 years' old. It has seen a dramatic drop in the numbers of women dying. However, repeatedly, error is seen as a major contributor. We cannot be complacent. We must not simply react to bad outcomes but be pro-active to assess risk and design systems to reduce it. Individuals have to accept that they will make errors, but the organisation also has to accept this and that it produces the environment that encourages these errors. If error is to be reduced, and patient safety is to be maximised, it requires a partnership between the organisation and the individual to study the errors that have occurred and produce solutions that will reduce them.

Key points for clinical practice

- Accept that you will make errors.
- Be prepared to report errors freely and honestly.
- Learn from errors made.
- Managers need to develop a 'no blame' environment to encourage reporting and learning.
- The organisation needs to take responsibility for error occurrence and not blame individuals.
- The organisation needs to be pro-active in assessing the risk of error and establishing methods of prevention.
- Errors need to be assessed by some form of root-cause analysis to allow full assessment of cause and formation of appropriate solutions.

References

1. CMO. *Organisation with a memory*. London: Department of Health, 2000.
2. CMO. *Building a Safer NHS for Patients*. London: Department of Health, 2002.
3. Brennan TA, Laird NM, Lawthers A *et al*. Hospital characteristics associated with adverse events and substandard care. *JAMA* 1991; **265:** 3265–3269.
4. Kohn LT, Corrigan JM. *To Err is Human*. Washington DC: National Academy Press, 2000.
5. Vincent C, Neale G, Woloshynowych M. Adverse events in British hospitals: preliminary retrospective record review. *BMJ* 2001; **322:** 517–519.
6. The Royal College of Obstetrics and Gynaecology. *Why Mothers Die. Report on Confidential Enquiries into Maternal Deaths in the United Kingdom 2000—2002*. London: RCOG Press, 2004.
7. Reason J. Human error: models and management. *BMJ* 2000; **320:** 768–770.
8. Lerner MJ. The desire for justice and reactions to victims. In: McCauley JB. (ed) *Altruism and Helping Behaviour*. New York: Academic Press, 1970.
9. Marx D. Discipline: the role of rule based violations. *Ground Effects* 1997; **2:** 1–4.
10. Reason JT, Carthey J, de Leval MR. Diagnosing 'vulnerable system syndrome': an essential prerequisite to effective risk management. *Qual Health Care* 2001; **10 (Suppl 2):** ii21–ii25.

11. Reason J. *Human Error*. New York: Cambridge University Press, 1990.
12. Woods DD. Some results on operator performance in emergency events. *Institute of Chemical Engineers Symposium Series* 1984; **90:** 21–31.
13. Reason J. Safety in the operating theatre – Part 2: human error and organisational failure. *Qual Safety Health Care* 2005; **14:** 56–60.
14. Sheen MJ. *MV Herald of Free Enterprise. Report of Court No 8074 Formal Investigation*. London: Department of Transport, 1987.
15. Reason J. Combating omission errors through task analysis and good reminders. *Qual Safety Health Care* 2002; **11:** 40–44.
16. Tuffnell DJ, Jankowicz D, Lindow SW *et al*. Outcomes of severe pre-eclampsia/eclampsia in Yorkshire 1999/2003. *Br J Obstet Gynaecol* 2005; **112:** 875–80.

Lucia M. Dolan Paul Hilton

10

Deciding on the appropriate surgery for stress incontinence

A common experience when restoring stress continence by surgery is that it can often be at the expense of developing new symptoms, or exacerbating pre-existing lower urinary tract symptoms. The recent World Health Organization (WHO) international consultation on incontinence stated that: 'there is now recognition that outcome from surgery for stress incontinence is not simply an issue of cure of stress incontinence'.[1] However, the meaning of 'outcome' and the statistical methods used to quantify it are in themselves controversial.[2] Before deciding on the most effective surgical intervention for stress urinary incontinence, a consensus is needed on how outcome should be defined, and the clinical circumstances in which a given outcome may be applied. Further research has been proposed to determine the optimal outcome measure and interaction between symptoms, objective measures of outcome and quality of life.[1] Many surgical procedures have been described to treat stress urinary incontinence, indicating that none is optimal in all circumstances. The introduction of minimally invasive mid-urethral tapes has led to a dramatic change in operative treatment over the last decade, and thus it is timely to address the question 'what is the most appropriate surgery for women with stress urinary incontinence'.

HOW DOES SURGERY RESTORE STRESS CONTINENCE?

Surgical techniques for stress urinary incontinence have evolved over the last 150 years. The 'pressure transmission theory', proposed that re-positioning the bladder neck and proximal urethra in a high intrapelvic position allowed equal

Lucia M. Dolan MB BCh MRCGP MRCOG
Consultant Gynaecologist and Sub-specialist in Urogynaecology, Edinburgh Royal Infirmary, Edinburgh, UK

Paul Hilton MD FRCOG (for correspondence)
Consultant Gynaecologist, Directorate of Women's Services, 3rd Floor, Leazes Wing, Royal Victoria Infirmary, Newcastle upon Tyne NE1 4LP, UK (E-mail: paul.hilton@ncl.ac.uk)

pressure transmission to the bladder and proximal urethra, and resulted in stress continence. In the 1960s and 1970s, surgical success was widely attributed to this passive mechanical effect. Subsequently, it became apparent that maintenance of stress continence was not a purely passive process, and several studies examined the effect of continence surgery on mid-urethral function and urethral anatomy. Continence was found to be dependent on efficient pressure transmission during rises in intra-abdominal pressure to the proximal three-quarters of the functional urethral length.

In the 1990s, interest moved to studying the co-ordinated action of muscular, fascial and visceral components within the pelvic floor as described in the 'Integral Theory' of Petros and Ulmsten,[3] and DeLancey's 'Hammock Theory'.[4] The concept of restoring urethral support rather than urethral position was the foundation for the development of the mid-urethral tape procedures whose design embraces the concept that the mid-urethra is the focal site for surgical correction of stress incontinence. In a recent editorial *The Emperor's New Clothes*,[41] the author questions the existence of anatomical structures that are fundamental to concepts of stress incontinence. He does, however, recognise that 'it is possible that operations for stress incontinence are effective even though the principles on which they are based are faulty'.

WHEN TO OPERATE?

In continence surgery, the methods of patient selection for surgery and the appropriate surgery for individual patients are key factors in achieving a successful outcome.

ROLE OF CONSERVATIVE TREATMENT

Surgical treatment for stress urinary incontinence is usually undertaken only when physiotherapy has proved to be ineffective. Success rates of 65–75% are commonly reported following pelvic floor muscle exercises, and these results are maintained in the long term.[5] Age, symptom severity, previous surgery, and intensity of exercise regimen have been shown to be significant predictive factors in some, though not all, studies. Berghmans undertook a systematic review of 24 randomised trials of physiotherapy (22 treatment and two prevention trials).[6] He concluded that pelvic floor exercise was effective, albeit less so than surgery; he also found that pelvic floor exercise with adjunctive biofeedback, electrical stimulation or vaginal cones, was no more effective than exercise alone.[6] A recent Cochrane Review found insufficient evidence to conclude whether pelvic floor exercise was better or worse than other treatments.[7]

Clinical experience suggests that many women with stress urinary incontinence present with the expectation of being offered an operation, but one small study reported that two-thirds of women favour physiotherapy as first-line treatment. Our current practice is to arrange hospital physiotherapy as the first-line treatment for all women with stress urinary incontinence who do not require surgical correction of prolapse and in women who have not yet completed their family. Physiotherapy may be offered without prior urodynamic investigation, as subjective success following physiotherapy is independent of whether urodynamics has been performed.

The recent introduction of the drug duloxetine for the treatment for stress incontinence may provide an additional modality to treatment. Initial studies have claimed symptomatic improvement but the place of this drug in clinical practice remains to be clarified as the treatment effect over and above the placebo effect would seem limited.

SYMPTOMATIC AND URODYNAMIC EVALUATION

Traditionally, the surgeon decided on the goal of surgery in women with urinary incontinence, yet surgeons have been found to be more optimistic than patients in reporting outcome. Mixed urinary incontinence may occur in up to a third of cases of stress incontinence, and stress urinary incontinence may present as a symptom complex, or with genital prolapse. Before undertaking diagnostic tests, it is important to establish the patient's perception of which symptoms are troublesome and their impact on her quality of life[1,8] and there are now several validated incontinence-specific questionnaires for the purpose. Recommendations produced from the WHO and the American Urological Association conclude that assessment of the patient's expectations on outcome from surgery is essential.[1,8,9]

We recommend pre-operative urodynamic investigation should be undertaken prior to surgical treatment and particularly in women with mixed urinary symptoms and in women with a history of neurological disease, voiding difficulties, or previous failed surgery. Whether urodynamics are essential in women with pure stress urinary incontinence remains controversial, and neither clinical effectiveness nor cost effectiveness of pre-operative investigation has been proven.[9] Black, following up women one year after surgery for stress incontinence, of whom almost one-third had not had pre-operative urodynamics, found that the proportion of women cured was similar, with or without pre-operative investigation.[10] In their advice on Clinical Standards, The Royal College of Obstetricians and Gynaecologists nevertheless endorsed the use of urodynamic investigation before any surgery for stress urinary incontinence.[11]

WHICH PRE-OPERATIVE FACTORS INFLUENCE CHOICE?

PREVIOUS STRESS CONTINENCE SURGERY

Although several studies have failed to demonstrate a significant difference between primary surgery and that for and recurrent incontinence, systematic reviews have reported a higher operative success with primary procedures.[12,13] Factors which might contribute to lower success in secondary procedures include operative difficulties due to haemorrhage, peri-urethral fibrosis and immobility of the urethra and vaginal tissues and denervation from previous surgical dissection, delayed healing in devascularised tissues and loss of urethral mucosal coaptation.

Management of recurrent stress urinary incontinence is complex and the surgeon should carefully consider the previous surgery including: (i) duration of continence following surgery; (ii) early and late complications; (iii) clinical examination; and (iv) personal ability to undertake technically more challenging surgery. Consideration should be given to the likelihood of achieving continence with a given procedure. However, failure for authors to include separate information on outcome in primary and recurrent cases has limited comparison and prediction of outcome in recurrent cases.[8,13]

Traditionally, the sling procedure has been indicated for recurrent cases where a fixed, scarred or excessively shortened urethra would make a colposuspension technically more difficult. The risk of denervating the urethral sphincter during dissection at the time of sling procedure has been cited as a reason for using it only as a secondary procedure. In cases where the vagina is narrowed or where there has been previous radiotherapy, the sling may be indicated as a primary procedure. Sling procedures are popular as primary procedures among urological colleagues, even where other procedures might be feasible.

Several studies report on the outcome of sling procedures using a variety of natural and synthetic materials in recurrent cases, with cure rates in secondary cases ranging from 61–100%.[14] The sling procedure appears to offer the highest chance of achieving continence in recurrent cases and, with cure rates exceeding 80%, it has been suggested as being the most successful procedure for either primary or secondary stress incontinence.[13] However, newer minimally invasive sling procedures, such as the Tension-free Vaginal Tape (TVT), have been introduced since the systematic reviews cited above.[8,12,13] A few studies have reported on the outcome of TVT procedure in recurrent cases with cure rates of over 80% in the short term.

Two studies have reported on success of colposuspension as a secondary procedure after the same has been performed as a primary operation[15,16] and both reported over 80% subjective cure and over 70% objective cure. The question of surgical technique of the primary surgeon has been questioned by some, but there is no consistent evidence that the experience of the operating surgeon affects outcome.[1]

In deciding what procedure to undertake in recurrent stress incontinence, surgeons should consider the likely reasons for failure of the primary procedure. In particular, this should include: (i) whether the initial indication was correct; (ii) whether the appropriate primary procedure was undertaken; (iii) whether failure was for technical reasons; and (iv) whether additional functional abnormalities have developed following surgery to compromise symptom improvement (*e.g.* detrusor overactivity or voiding dysfunction).

DETRUSOR OVERACTIVITY

Traditional wisdom says that stress incontinence surgery should not be undertaken in the presence of detrusor overactivity. Several early studies reported lower cure rates following continence surgery in women with pre-operative detrusor overactivity, although more recent studies have reported cure rates of 76% after colposuspension,[17] and 92% following pubovaginal sling.[18]

Cure rates for stress continence surgery in the presence of detrusor over-activity may be lower than with stable detrusor function. The finding of overactivity in itself should not contra-indicate surgery and symptomatic improvement may occur in many patients. There is, however, little evidence on the best operation for women with mixed incontinence. We advocate medical and behavioural therapy in an attempt to stabilise the detrusor before embarking on surgical treatment in such cases. For women with mixed incontinence without proven detrusor overactivity, there is similarly little evidence on which to base the choice of operation, although some evidence suggests that the majority of such women may be relieved of their urgency up to 2 years following either TVT or colposuspension.[19] In all cases of mixed symptoms or mixed urodynamics, women should be carefully counselled that whilst their urge-symptoms may improve, they may not and could deteriorate postoperatively.

INTRINSIC SPHINCTER DEFICIENCY

Intrinsic sphincter deficiency (ISD) has not been clearly defined. Evidence is conflicting on whether this classification of urethral function meaningfully influences the type of surgical treatment or its outcome.[1] The International Continence Society (ICS) in its recent standardisation report stated that there is a spectrum of urethral characteristics and any delineation into categories such as 'urethral hypermobility' and 'intrinsic sphincter deficiency' may be simplistic and arbitrary and requires further research.[20]

Unsuccessful surgery for stress incontinence has been associated with a low maximum urethral closure pressure (MUCP) at rest; 65–75% of women with previous unsuccessful surgery may have MUCP less than 20 cmH$_2$O, and surgical success has been shown to be significantly lower in this group.

In primary urodynamic stress incontinence with urethral hypermobility, a retropubic urethropexy may be the procedure of choice;[13] however, in the presence of a 'low pressure urethra', a cure rate of less than 50% has been reported. Therefore, where there is ISD, a sling procedure or an artificial urethral sphincter might be considered.[13] Although the use of peri-urethral injections has also been advocated in ISD, long-term follow-up cure rates are disappointing. In one study, a 26% overall subjective improvement was reported at 5 years and women with pre-operative MUCP less than 20 cmH$_2$O were found to have even lower chance of cure.[21]

Given the long-term durability of the sling compared to injectables and the morbidity of the artificial urinary sphincter, the sling procedure is probably the preferred first-line treatment in women with ISD.

WHAT ARE THE CHANCES OF SUCCESSFUL CURE OF CONTINENCE?

The ideal continence procedure is one that achieves a high rate of relief of incontinence with a low rate of complications. The randomised comparative trial is the optimum trial design for comparing cure and complication rates following a surgical intervention, although even this is not without shortcomings,[2] and few exist in this area. Meta-analyses may improve the statistical power of numbers of small studies but may introduce bias from a heterogeneous population. A number of recent systematic reviews of surgery for stress incontinence may help to inform our clinical practices.[1,8,9,12,13] More specific reviews of individual procedures are available from the Cochrane Incontinence Group, including open colposuspension,[22] laparoscopic colposuspension,[23] needle suspension,[24] anterior colporrhaphy,[25] suburethral slings,[26] and peri-urethral injections.[27]

Black and Downs in a systematic review on the effectiveness of surgery for stress incontinence reported on 11 randomised and 20 non-randomised trials and 45 retrospective series.[12] They reported that only 800 women had ever been randomised to surgical treatment and highlighted the methodological weaknesses of the existing studies. Jarvis analysed six groups of surgical interventions in 213 papers involving 20,481 surgical procedures.[13] As primary procedures, only Marshall Marchetti Krantz (MMK), colposuspension, endoscopic bladder neck suspension and sling had objective cure rates in excess of 85% with sling and colposuspension having the narrowest confidence intervals.[13] The American Urologic Association (AUA) reviewed 282 articles on the surgical treatment of stress urinary incontinence.[8] It published data on cure and complications for retropubic suspension, needle suspension, anterior colporrhaphy and sling procedures. Long-term success based on the 'cure/dry' rate was highest with retropubic surgery including sling procedures, although these procedures also had slightly higher complication rates and longer convalescence. The AUA panel reported that if a patient accepted these risks for the sake of a longer term cure then these procedures were appropriate choices.[8]

OPEN COLPOSUSPENSION

Until recently, the open colposuspension has been the first line surgical procedure for primary stress incontinence throughout Europe and North America. Several prospective studies have reported subjective cure rates for stress incontinence between 44% and 96% and objective cure rates between 66% and 92%. In his systematic review, Jarvis reported a subjective cure rate of 90% in 1736 patients undergoing colposuspension and an objective cure rate of 84% (by cystometrogram, pad test, or ultrasound) in 2300 patients.[13] More recently, a review of 33 trials involving 2403 women reported an overall cure rate of 69–88% after the open retropubic procedure.[22]

The cure of continence following colposuspension has been found to be time dependent, although the majority of recurrences seem to occur within 5 years following surgery. The Cochrane Review reported an overall cure/dry rate of 70% at 5 years,[22] and studies with a median follow-up of over 5 years have reported cure of continence rates between 50% and 90%. The longest follow-up after colposuspension found that cure appeared to plateau at 69% at around 10–12 years (although less than a third of the original cohort of 366 women were re-studied).[28]

LAPAROSCOPIC COLPOSUSPENSION

Eight prospective studies have compared laparoscopic and open colposuspension; cure rates have been between 57% and 93%. Three reported no differences in the cure rates between procedures, four reporting a lower cure, and one reporting a higher cure in the laparoscopic group. A meta-analysis of four RCTs, which have compared laparoscopic and open colposuspension, whilst suggesting a trend towards lower cure and higher complications from the laparoscopic procedure, showed no statistically significant difference in outcomes.[29] The inconsistency in reported results makes it difficult to assess reliably at the present time the place of laparoscopic colposuspension.[1,23]

MARSHALL MARCHETTI KRANTZ (MMK) PROCEDURE

In a review of 56 articles on the MMK procedure, an overall success rate of 86% was reported in 2712 cases with 92% in primary and 85% in repeat procedures.[30] However, many of these studies were retrospective and included only subjective outcomes. Jarvis reported an overall objective cure rate of 89% following MMK and 93% subjective cure rate.[13] Five studies have compared Burch colposuspension with the MMK procedure, with no significant differences up to after 3 years.[12] In a study reporting long-term follow-up, an initial 99% subjective cure at 1 month was followed by 86% at 5 years, 72% at 10 years, and 75% at 15 years.[31]

Despite previous popularity and similar cure rates, the MMK procedure has largely been superseded by colposuspension; the incidence of osteitis pubis following MMK may have contributed to the loss of popularity.[30]

ANTERIOR COLPORRHAPHY AND BLADDER NECK BUTTRESS

Jarvis reported an overall subjective cure rate of 81% following bladder neck buttress with an objective cure rate of 72%.[13] However, the long-term success is disappointing when compared to open colposuspension. In a prospective randomised study of 107 women undergoing either anterior colporrhaphy with Kelly plication, revised Pereyra or Burch colposuspension, the colposuspension had a significantly higher success rate than the other procedures at 12 months; the cure rate for anterior colporrhaphy was 82% at 3 months, 65% at 12 months and 37% at 5 years.[32] In a Cochrane Review of eight trials comparing anterior colporrhaphy with open colposuspension, the subjective failure rates were 29% and 14%, respectively, at 1 year, and 41% and 17%, respectively, beyond 1 year.[25]

These results suggest that the medium-to-long-term outcome from colporrhaphy with bladder neck plication is poor. On the other hand, the associated morbidity is also low, and some women may prefer a reduced cure rate and a lower complication rate.[1,13]

MID-URETHRAL TAPE PROCEDURES

In a survey of members of the International Urogynecology Association, the minimally invasive mid-urethral tape procedures such as the Tension-free Vaginal Tape (TVT™) were the preferred choice of operation in primary stress incontinence.[33] The Hospital Episode Statistics data from the UK show TVT to be the most frequently undertaken procedure for stress incontinence. In the largest randomised trial comparing TVT with open colposuspension in primary cases of urodynamic stress incontinence, objective cure was not significantly different at 6 months (66% versus 57%)[19] nor at 2 years (63% versus 51%).[34] However, length of hospital stay and return to normal activities were shorter in the TVT group and postoperative complications including voiding difficulty were less in the TVT arm. Three randomised studies have compared TVT with laparoscopic colposuspension; the largest, which included 72 patients, found higher objective (97% versus 81%) cure rates in the TVT group at 1 year,[35] and the others, whilst showing no difference in cures, found shorter operating time and reduced voiding difficulty in the TVT arm.

The continuing popularity of TVT will depend on whether it proves durable in the long term, without latent mesh complications. To date, the longest published follow-up of patients undergoing TVT is 7 years, with objective and subjective cure rates of 81%.[36] The longest comparative follow-up showed no difference in re-operation rates for stress incontinence between TVT and colposuspension after 2 years, although there was a higher rate of operation for pelvic organ prolapse and need for self-catheterisation in the colposuspension arm.[34] Until more long-term evidence is available on both procedures, women with primary stress incontinence can be offered an informed choice between the two.

OTHER MID-URETHRAL TAPE PROCEDURES

Several other mid-urethral tape procedures using a modification on the original technique and/or device have been developed since the introduction of Gynecare TVT™ as the first commercially available device. In many cases, there is only anecdotal evidence on performance or data from small case series with short-term follow-up. The newest devices have been designed to avoid the retropubic space and are inserted via the transobturator foramen. Despite the large number and variety of devices, only one small randomised study has included a transobturator procedure. In a prospective randomised trial of 61 women, comparing TVT and transobturator tape cure rates (84% versus 90%) and rates of bladder outlet obstruction were similar at 1-year; the mean operative time was significantly shorter in the transobturator tape group because concurrent cystoscopy was performed only in the TVT group.[37] A reduction in complications might be anticipated from the transobturator approach but reports of urethral injury are of concern, and any reduction in postoperative voiding difficulties might be balanced by decreased efficacy. Much larger comparative studies are required to resolve these issues before widespread use could be recommended.

CONVENTIONAL SLINGS

Jarvis has reported an overall 82% subjective cure rate and an 85% objective cure rate following bladder neck sling with cure rates of 94% as a primary procedure and 86% as a secondary procedure.[13] The AUA have reported similar outcome with cure/dry rates of 83% and dry/improved rates of 87% at a minimum of 48 months.[8] Due to the inadequacy of existing studies, Black and Downs felt unable to comment on the differential success between different sling materials.[12] More recently, it has been suggested that autologous materials are associated with higher cure and lower complication rates than cadaveric or synthetic materials.[14] Long-term follow-up has shown that cure rates are durable with an 88% overall cure rate beyond 4 years.[38] The long-term risks posed by allografts and xenografts are unknown and it is important that women are counselled about potential long-term health risks when these materials are being used.

Cure rates are similar in trials with colposuspension.[12] Although traditionally sling procedures have been viewed as highly obstructive, Jarvis found them to be less obstructive than colposuspension with the range of voiding difficulties between 2% and 37% (mean 13%).[13] The more recent trend for performing a 'tension-free' sling may further reduce this incidence. While the sling procedure has recently been gaining in popularity, it has traditionally been indicated in primary cases where the vagina is narrow or in recurrent cases where ISD is suspected or where there is lack of vaginal mobility.

NEEDLE SUSPENSIONS

Pereyra described the first needle suspension procedure in 1959, and with the Raz modification, encouraging initial success rates were reported. Black and Downs reviewed 13 RCTs comparing the needle suspension with colposuspension;[12] nine reported no difference in cure, and four found a higher success with colposuspension. Overall, colposuspension achieved an 80% cure rate after 1 year compared to 50–70% cure with needle suspension.[12] In the long term, the result appears to decay more rapidly than colposuspension, with one series reporting only 20% of women as dry at 10 years. Few, if any, indications now exist to perform a needle suspension procedure.[1]

PERI-URETHRAL INJECTIONS

Bulking agents such as glutaraldehyde cross-linked bovine collagen (GAX-collagen), polytetrafluoroethylene (PTFE), autologous fat and silicone polymers have all been used to improve urethral mucosal coaptation and increase outflow resistance. However, there has been little long-term controlled study of the technique. Furthermore, any comparison of the various bulking agents between existing studies is hampered by a lack of consistency in patient selection, surgical approach, volume of agent used, number of repeat injections and length of follow-up.

Jarvis reported an overall subjective cure of 82% and objective cure of 60% in a review of 452 cases following injectables.[13] In one of the largest studies to date, a 50% continence rate was reported after trans-urethral PTFE at 2.5 years' postoperatively. However, other studies have reported much lower cure rates following PFTE, and some concerning complications such as peri-urethral granuloma, and distant chronic foreign body reaction. The use of autologous fat has given disappointing long-term results and carries a risk of fat embolism. Smith et al.[1] reviewed 15 articles on the use of GAX-collagen with follow-up between 3 months and 2 years and reported an overall cure rate of 48% (range, 13–83%) and a success rate defined as 'dry/improved' of 76% (range, 52–100%). The durability of the method is in doubt,[21] and a high re-injection rate should be anticipated. Similar decline in cure rates are reported with the newer silicone polymers, with only 40% of women reporting subjective cure or improvement at 4 years.[39]

Bulking agents would appear to be indicated for those who are either unfit or unwilling to undergo surgery and the lower risk of long-term voiding difficulties makes them suitable for those at high risk of outlet obstruction following alternative surgical interventions.

ARTIFICIAL URINARY SPHINCTER (AUS)

In a systematic review of the AUS, an 80% cure rate and 90% improvement rate has been suggested when performed as a primary procedure,[1] although continence rates of up to 100% have been reported. Complications include a recognised risk of cuff erosion especially in the irradiated pelvis although design improvements have reduced the need for removal due to malfunction. In a 10–15 year follow-up after AUS implantation, 61% of patients were continent although 58 major complications had occurred and 49 patients had undergone at least one revision procedure.[40] An overall implant removal rate of 25% has been estimated.[1]

The AUS has been usually indicated in cases of ISD as an alternative to sub-urethral sling and peri-urethral bulking agents. Jarvis was unable to include the artificial urethral sphincter in his review, as there were no studies with appropriate assessment of patients with a stable bladder and urodynamic stress incontinence.[13] He suggested that, in the absence of greater evidence, only patients with previous surgery, pure urodynamic stress incontinence and a low MUCP should be considered for an artificial sphincter.[13] Given the lower likelihood of voiding difficulties after the AUS, it may be an alternative to sling in patients who have pre-operative voiding problems and in particular for those who might be unable to self-catheterise postoperatively but who would be able to use a labial cuff.

CONCLUSIONS

Urinary incontinence is a non life-threatening condition, and consideration should always be given to conservative measures before surgical treatment. Women should be adequately counselled about possible outcomes in terms of cure, complications and change in quality of life before they decide to proceed with surgery. The paucity of high quality surgical trials of adequate power has now been recognised. Future trials should facilitate comparison by use of consistent outcome measures which reflect the impact of stress incontinence itself and the surgical intervention on the patient's quality of life.

Key points for clinical practice

- The quality of evidence in this area is poor, and further large, well-designed trials of surgery for stress incontinence are required.

- Physiotherapy should be offered as first-line treatment for all women presenting with stress or mixed urinary incontinence.

- Urodynamic investigation is recommended prior to surgical treatment of stress incontinence particularly in women with mixed urinary symptoms and with a history of neurological disease, voiding difficulties, or previous failed surgery.

- Patients should be carefully counselled on outcomes of surgery. The patient's expectations from surgery and trade-offs that they

Key points for clinical practice *(continued)*

are prepared to make in balancing success rate, recovery period, morbidity, and longevity of cure, *etc.* should form a vital part of the decision-making process.

- The choice of operation is guided by the likelihood of achieving stress continence and developing or aggravating other symptoms.

- Open colposuspension and retropubic mid-urethral tape procedures appear to have comparable success rates up to 5 years in patients with primary stress incontinence. Most patients favour the minimally invasive nature of the latter, but some give priority to the availability of longer term data for the former. Until more robust long-term data become available, patients should be given the option of both procedures.

- Conventional sling procedures seem to offer the optimal results in patients with recurrent stress incontinence. Retropubic mid-urethral tapes may have slightly lower success, and unproven longevity; but, as in primary cases, the minimally invasive nature of the procedures may make them an acceptable alternative for many patients.

- The cure rate from even repeated treatments using peri urethral injections is poor in comparison to other procedures. Patients undergoing such procedures should understand that short-term improvement in symptoms may be the best they can anticipate.

- The place of several interventions, including laparoscopic colposuspension and the newer retropubic and transobturator tape procedures, cannot yet be defined. Commercial pressure for their adoption should be resisted until more robust data are available. Clinicians considering undertaking these procedures should take special care over clinical governance and consent issues.

References

1. Smith A, Daneshgari F, Dmochowski R *et al*. Surgical treatment of incontinence in women. In: Abrams P, Cardozo L, Khoury S, Wein A. (eds) *Incontinence; 2nd WHO International Consultation on Incontinence*. London: Health Publications, 2002; 823–863.
2. Hilton P. Trials of surgery for stress incontinence – thoughts on the 'Humpty Dumpty principle'. *Br J Obstet Gynaecol* 2002; **109**: 1081–1088.
3. Petros PEP, Ulmsten UI. An integral theory of female urinary incontinence. Experimental and clinical considerations. *Acta Obstet Gynecol Scand* 1991; **153 (Suppl)**: 7–31.
4. DeLancey JOL. Structural support of the urethra as it relates to stress urinary incontinence: the hammock hypothesis. *Am J Obstet Gynecol* 1994; **170**: 1713–1723.
5. Cammu H, Van Nylen M, Amy JJ. A 10-year follow-up after Kegel pelvic floor muscle exercises for genuine stress incontinence. *Br J Urol Int* 2000; **85**: 655–658.
6. Berghmans LCM, Hendriks HJM, Bø K, Hay-Smith EJ, De Bie RA, Van Waalwijk van Doorn ESC. Conservative treatment of stress urinary incontinence in women: a systematic review of randomized clinical trials. *Br J Urol* 1998; **82**: 181–191.
7. Hay-Smith E, Bø K, Berghmans L, Hendriks H, de Bie R, van Waalwijk van Doorn E. Pelvic floor muscle training for urinary incontinence in women. *Cochrane Database System Rev* 2001: CD001407.

8. Leach GE, Dmochowski RR, Appell RA *et al*. Female stress urinary incontinence. Clinical Guidelines Panel summary report on surgical management of female stress urinary incontinence. *J Urol* 1997; **158**: 875–880.

9. Agency for Health Care Policy and Research. *Urinary incontinence in adults: acute and chronic management*. Clinical Practice Guideline update no. 2. Rockville, MD: US Department of Health & Human Services Public Health Service, AHCPR, 1996.

10. Black N, Griffiths J, Pope C, Bowling A, Abel P. Impact of surgery for stress incontinence on morbidity: cohort study. *BMJ* 1997; **315**: 1493–1502.

11. Royal College of Obstetricians and Gynaecologists. *Clinical Standards: Advice on planning the service in obstetrics and gynaecology*. London: RCOG, 2002.

12. Black NA, Downs SH. The effectiveness of surgery for stress incontinence in women: a systematic review. *Br J Urol* 1996; **78**: 497–510.

13. Jarvis GJ. Surgery for genuine stress incontinence. *Br J Obstet Gynaecol* 1994; **101**: 371–374.

14. Bidmead J, Cardozo L. Sling techniques in the treatment of genuine stress incontinence. *Br J Obstet Gynaecol* 2000; **107**: 147–156.

15. Cardozo L, Hextall A, Bailey J, Boos K. Colposuspension after previous failed incontinence surgery: a prospective observational study. *Br J Obstet Gynaecol* 1999; **106**: 340–344.

16. Maher C, Dwyer P, Carey M, Gilmour D. The Burch colposuspension for recurrent urinary stress incontinence following retropubic continence surgery. *Br J Obstet Gynaecol* 1999; **106**: 719–724.

17. Colombo M, Zanetta G, Vitobello D, Milani R. The Burch colposuspension for women with and without detrusor overactivity. *Br J Obstet Gynaecol* 1996; **103**: 255–260.

18. Serels SR, Rackley RR, Appell RA. Surgical treatment for stress urinary incontinence associated with Valsalva induced detrusor instability. *J Urol* 2000; **163**: 884–887.

19. Ward KL, Hilton P, on behalf of the UK TVT Trial Group. Prospective multicentre randomised trial of tension-free vaginal tape and colposuspension as primary treatment for stress incontinence. *BMJ* 2002; **325**: 67–70.

20. Abrams P, Cardozo L, Fall M *et al*. Standardisation of terminology of lower urinary tract function: report from the Standardisation Sub-committee of the International Continence Society. *Neurourol Urodyn* 2002; **21**: 167–178.

21. Gorton E, Stanton S, Monga A, Wiskind AK, Lentz GM, Bland DR. Periurethral collagen injection: a long-term follow-up study. *Br J Urol Int* 1999; **84**: 966–971.

22. Lapitan MC, Cody DJ, Grant AM. Open retropubic colposuspension for urinary incontinence in women. *Cochrane Database System Rev* 2003: CD002912.

23. Moehrer B, Ellis G, Carey M, Wilson PD. Laparoscopic colposuspension for urinary incontinence in women. *Cochrane Database System Rev* 2000: CD002239.

24. Glazener CM, Cooper K. Bladder neck needle suspension for urinary incontinence in women. *Cochrane Database System Rev* 2004: CD003636.

25. Glazener CM, Cooper K. Anterior vaginal repair for urinary incontinence in women. *Cochrane Database System Rev* 2003: CD001755.

26. Bezerra CA, Bruschini H. Suburethral sling operations for urinary incontinence in women. *Cochrane Database System Rev* 2001: CD001754.

27. Pickard R, Reaper J, Wyness L, Cody DJ, McClinton S, N'Dow J. Periurethral injection therapy for urinary incontinence in women. *Cochrane Database System Rev* 2003: CD003881.

28. Alcalay M, Monga A, Stanton SL. Burch colposuspension: a 10–20 year follow up. *Br J Obstet Gynaecol* 1995; **102**: 740–745.

29. Moehrer B, Carey M, Wilson D. Laparoscopic colposuspension: a systematic review. *Br J Obstet Gynaecol* 2003; **110**: 230–235.

30. Mainprize TC, Drutz HP. The Marshall-Marchetti-Krantz procedure: a critical review. *Obstet Gynecol Surv* 1988; **43**: 724–729.

31. McDuffie Jr RW, Litin RB, Blundon KE. Urethrovesical suspension (Marshall-Marchetti-Krantz). Experience with 204 cases. *Am J Surg* 1981; **141**: 297–298.

32. Bergman A, Elia G. Three surgical procedures for genuine stress incontinence: five-year follow-up of a prospective randomized study. *Am J Obstet Gynecol* 1995; **173**: 66–71.

33. Davila GW, Ghoniem GM, Kapoor DS, Contreras-Ortiz O. Pelvic floor dysfunction management practice patterns: a survey of members of the International

Urogynecological Association. *Int Urogynecol J Pelvic Floor Dysfunct* 2002; **13**: 319–325.

34. Ward KL, Hilton P. A prospective multicenter randomized trial of tension-free vaginal tape and colposuspension for primary urodynamic stress incontinence: two-year follow-up. *Am J Obstet Gynecol* 2004; **190**. 324–331.

35. Paraiso MF, Walters MD, Karram MM, Barber MD. Laparoscopic Burch colposuspension versus tension-free vaginal tape: a randomized trial. *Obstet Gynecol* 2004; **104**: 1249–1258.

36. Nilsson CG, Falconer C, Rezapour M. Seven-year follow-up of the tension-free vaginal tape procedure for treatment of urinary incontinence. *Obstet Gynecol* 2004; **104**: 1259–1262.

37. deTayrac R, Deffieux X, Droupy S, Chauveaud-Lambling A, Calvanese-Benamour L, Fernandez H. A prospective randomized trial comparing tension-free vaginal tape and transobturator suburethral tape for surgical treatment of stress urinary incontinence. *Am J Obstet Gynecol* 2004; **190**: 602–608.

38. Morgan Jr TO, Westney OL, McGuire EJ. Pubovaginal sling: 4-year outcome analysis and quality of life assessment. *J Urol* 2000; **163**: 1845–1848.

39. Harriss DR, Iacovou JW, Lemberger RJ. Peri-urethral silicone microimplants (Macroplastique) for the treatment of genuine stress incontinence. *Br J Urol* 1996; **78**: 722–725.

40. Fulford SCV, Sutton C, Bales G, Hickling M, Stephenson TP. The fate of the 'modern' artificial urinary sphincter with a follow-up of more than 10 years. *Br J Urol* 1997; **79**: 713–716.

41. Blaives JG. The Emperor's New Clothes [Editorial]. *Neurourol Urodyn* 2003; **22**: 1

Adam H. Balen Martin R. Glass

11

What's new in polycystic ovary syndrome?

The condition we refer to as polycystic ovary syndrome (PCOS) is a many faceted heterogeneous problem and the commonest hormonal disturbance to affect women. There is a close association between disturbances of insulin metabolism and PCOS – indeed some believe that PCOS is the ovarian expression of the 'metabolic syndrome'. Whilst insulin resistance is seen in at least 40% of women with PCOS,[1] it is a variable finding and there are probably several routes to the pathophysiology of the syndrome. In recent years, there have been a number of developments in the understanding of the genetics and pathophysiology of PCOS which have provided a fruitful basis for the development of new strategies for its management. An understanding too of the long-term health consequences (type 2 diabetes, cardiovascular disease and endometrial cancer) provides an opportunity to develop strategies for the screening of at-risk women.

The classical symptoms of the 'Stein Leventhal syndrome' as it was eponymously known for many years – namely menstrual disturbance (amenorrhoea or oligomenorrhoea), hyperandrogenism and obesity – are now known to describe the extreme end of the spectrum of what is now recognised to be a very heterogeneous condition. The definition of the syndrome has been much debated. There are many extra-ovarian aspects to the pathophysiology of PCOS, yet ovarian dysfunction is central. At a joint consensus meeting of the American Society of Reproductive Medicine (ASRM) and the European Society of Human Reproduction and Embryology (ESHRE) held in Rotterdam, in May 2003, a refined definition of the PCOS was agreed. Namely the presence of two out of the following three criteria: (i) oligo- and/or anovulation; (ii) hyper-androgenism (clinical and/or biochemical); and (iii) polycystic ovaries, with

Adam H. Balen MD FRCOG (for correspondence)
Professor of Reproductive Medicine and Surgery, The General Infirmary, Leeds LS2 9NS, UK (E-mail: Adam.balen@leedsth.nhs.uk)

Martin R. Glass MD FRCOG
Consultant Obstetrician and Gynaecologist, The General Infirmary, Leeds LS2 9NS, UK

the exclusion of other aetiologies.[2] The morphology of the polycystic ovary has been redefined as an ovary with 12 or more follicles measuring 2–9 mm in diameter and/or increased ovarian volume (> 10 cm³).[3]

There is considerable heterogeneity of symptoms and signs amongst women with PCOS and, for an individual, these may change over time.[4] The PCOS is familial and various aspects of the syndrome may be differentially inherited. Polycystic ovaries can exist without clinical signs of the syndrome, which may then become expressed over time. There are a number of interlinking factors that affect expression of PCOS. A gain in weight is associated with a worsening of symptoms whilst weight loss will ameliorate the endocrine and metabolic profile and symptomatology.[5]

Elevated serum concentrations of insulin are more common in both lean and obese women with PCOS than weight-matched controls. Indeed, hyperinsulinaemia appears to be the key to the pathogenesis of the syndrome. Insulin stimulates androgen secretion by the ovarian stroma and appears to affect the normal development of ovarian follicles, both by the adverse effects of androgens on follicular growth and possibly also by suppressing apoptosis and permitting the survival of follicles otherwise destined to disappear.

WHAT IS POLYCYSTIC OVARY SYNDROME?

Polycystic ovaries are commonly detected by ultrasound or other forms of pelvic imaging, with estimates of the prevalence in the general population being in the order of 20–33%.[6,7] However, not all women with polycystic ovaries demonstrate the clinical and biochemical features which define the PCOS. The biochemical disturbance includes elevated serum concentrations of luteinizing hormone (LH), testosterone, androstenedione, and insulin.

THE POLYCYSTIC OVARY

Transabdominal and/or transvaginal ultrasound have become the most commonly used diagnostic methods for the identification of polycystic ovaries. Although the ultrasound criteria for the diagnosis of polycystic ovaries have never been universally agreed, the characteristic features are accepted as being an increase in the number of follicles and the amount of stroma as compared with normal ovaries. The transabdominal ultrasound criteria of Adams et al.[8] defined a polycystic ovary as one which contains, in one plane, at least 10 follicles (usually 2–8 mm in diameter) arranged peripherally around a dense core of ovarian stroma has been used for many years. However, at a recent joint ASRM/ESHRE consensus meeting, a refined definition of the PCOS was agreed, encompassing a description of the morphology of the polycystic ovary. According to the available literature, the criteria fulfilling sufficient specificity and sensitivity to define the polycystic ovary (PCO) are the presence of 12 or more follicles measuring 2–9 mm in diameter and/or increased ovarian volume (> 10 cm³).[3] If there is a follicle greater than 10 mm in diameter, the scan should be repeated at a time of ovarian quiescence in order to calculate volume and area. The presence of a single polycystic ovary is sufficient to provide the diagnosis. The distribution of the follicles and the description of the stroma are not required in the diagnosis. Increased stromal echogenicity and/or stromal volume are specific to PCO, but it has been shown that the measurement of the ovarian volume (or area) is a good surrogate for the quantification of the stroma in clinical practice. A woman having PCO in the absence of an ovulation disorder or hyperandrogenism ('asymptomatic PCO') should not be considered as having PCOS, although she may develop symptoms over time, for example if she gains weight.

DEFINING THE 'SYNDROME'

While it is now clear that ultrasound provides an excellent technique for the detection of polycystic ovarian morphology, identification of polycystic ovaries by ultrasound does not automatically confer a diagnosis of PCOS. Controversy still exists over a precise definition of the 'syndrome' and whether or not the diagnosis should require confirmation of polycystic ovarian morphology. The generally accepted view in Europe is that a spectrum exists, ranging from women with polycystic ovarian morphology and no overt abnormality at one end, to those with polycystic ovaries associated with severe clinical and biochemical disorders at the other end. Using a combination of clinical, ultrasonographic, and biochemical criteria, the diagnosis of PCOS is usually reserved for those women who exhibit an ultrasound picture of polycystic ovaries, and who display one or more of the clinical symptoms (menstrual cycle disturbances, hirsutism, obesity, hyperandrogenism), and/or one or more of the recognised biochemical disturbances (elevated LH, testosterone, androstenedione, or insulin).[4] At the joint ASRM/ESHRE consensus meeting in 2003, a refined definition of PCOS was agreed,[2] which, for the first time, included a description of the morphology of the polycystic ovary. The new definition requires the presence of two out of the following three criteria: (i) oligo- and/or anovulation; (ii) hyperandrogenism (clinical and/or biochemical); and (iii) polycystic ovaries, with the exclusion of other aetiologies.[2]

NATIONAL AND RACIAL DIFFERENCES

The highest reported prevalence of PCO has been 52% amongst South Asian immigrants in Britain, of whom 49.1% had menstrual irregularity.[9] Rodin et al.[9] demonstrated that South Asian women with PCO had a comparable degree of insulin resistance to controls with established type 2 diabetes mellitus. Generally, there has been a paucity of data on the prevalence of PCOS among women of South Asian origin, both among migrant and native groups. Type 2 diabetes and insulin resistance have a high prevalence among indigenous populations in South Asia, with a rising prevalence among women. Insulin resistance and hyperinsulinaemia are common antecedents of type 2 diabetes, with a high prevalence in South Asians. Type 2 diabetes also has a familial basis, inherited as a complex genetic trait that interacts with environmental factors, chiefly nutrition, commencing from fetal life. We have already found that South Asians with anovular PCOS have greater insulin resistance and more severe symptoms of the syndrome than anovular Caucasians with PCOS.[10] Furthermore, we have found that women from South Asia, living in the UK appear to express symptoms at an earlier age than their Caucasian British counterparts.

HEALTH CONSEQUENCES

Obesity and metabolic abnormalities are recognised risk factors for the development of ischaemic heart disease in the general population, and these are also recognised features of PCOS. The questions are whether women with PCOS are at an increased risk of ischaemic heart disease, and whether this will occur at an earlier age than women with normal ovaries? The basis for the idea that women with PCOS are at greater risk for cardiovascular disease is that these women are more insulin resistant than weight-matched controls and that the metabolic disturbances associated with insulin resistance are known to increase cardiovascular risk in other populations.

Insulin resistance is defined as a diminution in the biological responses to a given level of insulin. In the presence of an adequate pancreatic reserve, normal circulating glucose levels are maintained at higher serum insulin concentrations. In the general population, cardiovascular risk factors include insulin resistance, obesity, glucose intolerance, hypertension, and dyslipidaemia.

Hyperinsulinaemia has been demonstrated in both obese and non-obese women with PCOS, suggesting that a form of insulin resistance is specific to PCOS in addition to that caused by obesity. Obese women with PCOS have consistently been shown to be more insulin resistant than weight-matched controls. It appears that obesity and PCOS have an additive effect on the degree and severity of the insulin resistance and subsequent hyperinsulinaemia in this group of women.

Insulin sensitivity varies depending upon menstrual pattern. Women with PCOS who are oligomenorrhoeic are more likely to be insulin resistant than those with regular cycles – irrespective of their body mass index (BMI). Insulin resistance is restricted to the extra-splanchnic actions of insulin on glucose dispersal. The liver is not affected (hence the fall in SHBG and HDL), neither is the ovary (hence the menstrual problems and hypersecretion of androgens) nor the skin, hence the development of acanthosis nigricans. The insulin resistance causes compensatory hypersecretion of insulin, particularly in response to glucose, so euglycaemia is usually maintained at the expense of hyperinsulinaemia.

Central obesity

Simple obesity is associated with greater deposition of gluteo femoral fat while central obesity involves greater truncal abdominal fat distribution. Obesity is observed in 35–60% of women with PCOS. Hyperandrogenism is associated with a preponderance of fat localised to truncal abdominal sites. Women with PCOS have a greater truncal abdominal fat distribution as demonstrated by a higher waist:hip ratio. The central distribution of fat is independent of BMI and associated with higher plasma insulin and triglyceride concentrations, and reduced HDL cholesterol concentrations.

Impaired glucose tolerance and diabetes

Impaired glucose tolerance and diabetes are known risk factors for cardiovascular disease. It is reported that 18–20% of obese women with PCOS demonstrate impaired glucose tolerance. Dahlgren et al.[11] noted the prevalence of type 2 diabetes was 15% in women with PCOS compared with 2% in the controls. Most women with type 2 diabetes under the age of 45 years have

PCOS. Insulin resistance combined with abdominal obesity is thought to account for the higher prevalence of type 2 diabetes in PCOS. There is a concomitant increased risk of gestational diabetes.

Dyslipidaemia

Women with PCOS have high concentrations of serum triglycerides and suppressed high-density lipoprotein (HDL) levels, particularly a lower HDL_2 subfraction. High-density lipoproteins play an important role in lipid metabolism and are the most important lipid parameter in predicting cardiovascular risk in women. HDLs perform the task of 'reverse cholesterol transport'. That is, they remove excess lipids from the circulation and tissues to transport them to the liver for excretion, or transfer them to other lipoprotein particles. Cholesterol is only one component of HDL, a particle with constantly changing composition forming HDL_3 then HDL_2, as unesterified cholesterol is taken from tissue, esterified and exchanged for triglyceride with other lipoprotein species. Consequently, measurement of a single constituent in a particle involved in a dynamic process gives an incomplete picture.[12]

Thus, in summary, examining the surrogate risk factors for cardiovascular disease, there is evidence that insulin resistance, central obesity and hyperandrogenaemia are features of PCOS and have an adverse effect on lipid metabolism. Women with PCOS have been shown to have dyslipidaemia, with reduced HDL cholesterol and elevated serum triglyceride concentrations, along with elevated serum plasminogen activator inhibitor-I concentrations. The evidence is thus mounting that women with PCOS may have an increased risk of developing cardiovascular disease and diabetes later in life, which has important implications in their management.

However, in another study, Pierpoint et al.[13] reported the mortality rate in 1028 women diagnosed as having polycystic ovary syndrome between 1930 and 1979. All the women were older than 45 years and 770 women had been treated by wedge resection of the ovaries. A total of 786 women were traced; the mean age at diagnosis was 26.4 years and average duration of follow-up was 30 years. There were 59 deaths, of which 15 were from circulatory disease. Of these 15 deaths, 13 were from ischaemic heart disease. There were six deaths from diabetes as an underlying or contributory cause compared with the expected 1.7 deaths. The standard mortality rate both overall and for cardiovascular disease was not higher in the women with PCOS compared with the national mortality rates in women, although the observed proportion of women with diabetes as a contributory or underlying factor leading to death was significantly higher than expected (odds ratio 3.6; 95% CI 1.5–8.4). Thus despite surrogate markers for cardiovascular disease, in this study no increased rate of death from CVS disease could be demonstrated. A follow-up study of the same data-set, including 345 subjects with PCOS, found an odds ratio for coronary heart disease of 1.5 (95% CI 0.7–2.9) and for cerebrovascular disease of 2.8 (95% CI 1.1–7.1).

PCOS IN YOUNGER WOMEN

At what stage do the risk factors for cardiovascular disease become apparent in women with PCOS? The majority of studies which have identified the risk factors of obesity and insulin resistance in women with PCOS have investigated adult populations, commonly including women who have presented to specialist endocrine or reproductive clinics. However, PCOS has been identified in much younger populations,[7] in which women with increasing symptoms of PCOS were found to be more insulin resistant. These data emphasise the need for long-term prospective studies of young women with PCOS in order to clarify the natural history, and to determine which women will be at risk of diabetes and cardiovascular disease later in life. A study of women with PCOS and a mean age of 39 years followed over a period of 6 years, found that 9% of those with normal glucose tolerance developed impaired glucose tolerance and 8% developed NIDDM.[14] Of women with impaired glucose tolerance at the start of the study, 54% had NIDDM at follow-up. The risks of disease progression, not surprisingly, were greatest in those who were overweight.

A recent study to evaluate the cardiovascular risk was performed in 30 young (< 35 years) women matched against 30 age- and weight-matched controls.[15] Those with PCOS had higher fasting glucose and insulin levels (greater insulin resistance as assessed by HOMA), total cholesterol and LDL-cholesterol and lower HDL-cholesterol concentrations compared with controls. In addition, they had early signs of cardiovascular stress with increased left atrial size, left ventricular mass and lower left ventricular ejection fraction than controls, even though all were asymptomatic for cardiovascular disease.[15]

ENDOMETRIAL CANCER

Endometrial adenocarcinoma is the second most common female genital malignancy but only 4% of cases occur in women less than 40 years of age. The risk of developing endometrial cancer has been shown to be adversely influenced by a number of factors including obesity, long-term use of unopposed oestrogens, nulliparity and infertility. Women with endometrial carcinoma have had fewer births compared with controls and it has also been demonstrated that infertility *per se* gives a relative risk of 2. Hypertension and type 2 diabetes mellitus have long been linked to endometrial cancer, with relative risks of 2.1 and 2.8, respectively[16] – conditions that are now known also to be associated with PCOS. The true risk of endometrial carcinoma in women with PCOS, however, is difficult to ascertain.

Endometrial hyperplasia may be a precursor to adenocarcinoma, with cystic glandular hyperplasia progressing in perhaps 0.4% of cases and adenomatous hyperplasia in up to 18% of cases over 2–10 years. Precise estimation of rate of progression is impossible to determine. Some authors have reported conservative management of endometrial adenocarcinoma in women with PCOS with a combination of curettage and high-dose progestogens. The rationale is that cancer of the endometrium often presents at an early stage, is well differentiated, of low risk of metastasis and, therefore, is not perceived as being life-threatening, whilst poorly differentiated adenocarcinoma in a young woman has a worse prognosis and warrants hysterectomy. In general, however, the literature on women with PCOS and endometrial hyperplasia or adenocarcinoma suggests that this group of patients have a poor prognosis for fertility. This may be because of the factors that predisposed to the endometrial pathology – chronic anovulation combined often with severe obesity – or secondary to the endometrial pathology disrupting potential embryonic implantation. Thus a more traditional and radical surgical approach (*i.e.* hysterectomy) is suggested as the safest way to prevent progression of the cancer. Early stage disease may permit ovarian conservation and the possibility of pregnancy by surrogacy.

Although the degree of risk has not been clearly defined, it is generally accepted that for women with PCOS who experience amenorrhoea, or oligomenorrhoea, the induction of artificial withdrawal bleeds to prevent endometrial hyperplasia is prudent management. There are no data on the frequency with which women with PCOS should shed their endometrium. It seems prudent to induce a withdrawal bleed either monthly or at least every 3 months, not only to prevent endometrial hyperplasia but also to enable the bleed to be acceptable when it occurs – as progressive endometrial development may lead to a prolonged and heavy bleed when it does occur. For those with oligo-/amenorrhoea who do not wish to use cyclical hormone therapy, we recommend an ultrasound scan to measure endometrial thickness and morphology every 6–12 months (depending upon menstrual history). An endometrial thickness greater than 10 mm in an amenorrhoiec woman warrants an artificially induced bleed, which should be followed by a repeat ultrasound scan and endometrial biopsy if the endometrium has not been shed. Another option is to consider a progestogen secreting intrauterine system, such as the Mirena.

BREAST CANCER

Obesity, hyperandrogenism, and infertility occur frequently in PCOS, and are features known to be associated with the development of breast cancer. However, studies examining the relationship between PCOS and breast carcinoma have not always identified a significantly increased risk. The study by Coulam *et al.*[17] calculated a relative risk of 1.5 (95% CI 0.75–2.55) for breast cancer in their group of women with chronic anovulation which was not statistically significant. After stratification by age, however, the relative risk was found to be 3.6 (95% CI 1.2–8.3) in the postmenopausal age group. More recently, Pierpoint *et al.*[13] reported a series of 786 women with PCOS in the UK who were traced from hospital records after histological diagnosis of polycystic ovaries between 1930 and 1979. Mortality was assessed from the national registry of deaths and standardised mortality rates calculated for patients with PCOS compared with the normal population. The average follow-up period was 30 years. The standardised mortality rate for all neoplasms was 0.91 (95% CI 0.60–1.32) and for breast cancer 1.48 (95% CI 0.79–2.54). In fact, breast cancer was the leading cause of death in this cohort.

MANAGEMENT OF PCOS

The management of the PCOS is symptom orientated. Whilst obesity worsens the symptoms, the metabolic scenario conspires against weight loss. Diet and exercise are key to symptom control. Initial reports of the use of insulin-sensitising agents (*e.g.* Metformin) have been encouraging and suggest an improvement in biochemistry, symptoms and an increase in fertility. Ovulation induction has traditionally involved the use of clomiphene citrate and then gonadotrophin therapy or laparoscopic ovarian surgery in those who are clomiphene resistant. Patients with PCOS are not oestrogen deficient and those with amenorrhoea are at risk not of osteoporosis but rather of endometrial hyperplasia or adenocarcinoma. Cycle control and regular withdrawal bleeding is achieved with the oral contraceptive pill, which has the additional beneficial effect of suppressing serum testosterone concentrations and hence improving hirsutism and acne. Dianette and Yasmin, containing the anti-androgens cyproterone acetate and drosperinone, respectively, are usually recommended.

Women who are obese, and also many slim women with PCOS, will have insulin resistance and elevated serum concentrations of insulin (usually < 30 mU/l fasting). We suggest that a 75-g oral glucose tolerance test (GTT) be performed in women with PCOS and a BMI > 30 kg/m^2, with an assessment of the fasting and 2-h glucose concentration. It has been suggested that South Asian women should have an assessment of glucose tolerance if their BMI is greater than 25 kg/m^2 because of the greater risk of insulin resistance at a lower BMI than seen in the Caucasian population.

OBESITY

The clinical management of a women with PCOS should be focused on her individual problems. Obesity worsens both symptomatology and the endocrine profile and so obese women (BMI > 30 kg/m^2) should be encouraged to lose weight. Weight loss improves the endocrine profile, the likelihood of ovulation and a healthy pregnancy.

Much has been written about diet and PCOS. The right diet for an individual is one that is practical, sustainable and compatible with her life-style. It is sensible to keep carbohydrate content down and to avoid fatty foods. It is often helpful to refer to a dietician.

Anti-obesity drugs may help with weight loss. These can be prescribed by general practitioners and their use must be closely monitored. Metformin may improve with insulin resistance and may aid some women with weight loss, combined with a healthy diet and exercise programme. Metformin therapy is discussed below.

MENSTRUAL IRREGULARITY

The easiest way to control the menstrual cycle is the use of a low-dose combined oral contraceptive preparation. This will result in an artificial cycle and regular shedding of the endometrium. An alternative is a progestogen for 12 days every 1–3 months to induce a withdrawal bleed. It is also important, once again, to encourage weight loss.

In women with anovulatory cycles, the action of oestradiol on the endometrium is unopposed because of the lack of cyclical progesterone secretion. This may result in episodes of irregular uterine bleeding and, in the long-term, endometrial hyperplasia and even endometrial cancer (see above). An ultrasound assessment of endometrial thickness provides a bioassay for oestradiol production by the ovaries and conversion of androgens in the peripheral fat. If the endometrium is thicker than 15 mm, a withdrawal bleed should be induced; if the endometrium fails to shed, then endometrial sampling is required to exclude endometrial hyperplasia or malignancy.

INFERTILITY

First-line therapy in inducing ovulation remains the use of oral anti-oestrogens, such as clomiphene citrate, although there have been no prospective studies of clomiphene versus either gonadotrophins or laparoscopic ovarian diathermy in the first-line management of PCOS. There is also interest in the potential use of aromatase inhibitors and the *in vitro* maturation of oocytes collected from unstimulated polycystic ovaries – although these approaches remain very much in the confines of research protocols. Whilst clomiphene is successful in inducing ovulation in over 80% of women, pregnancy only occurs in about 40%. Clomiphene citrate should only be prescribed in a setting where ultrasound monitoring is available (and performed) in order to minimise the 10% risk of multiple pregnancy and to ensure that ovulation is taking place.[18] Once an ovulatory dose has been reached, the cumulative conception rate continues to increase for up to 10–12 cycles.[19]

The therapeutic options for patients with anovulatory infertility who are resistant to anti-oestrogens are either parenteral gonadotrophin therapy or laparoscopic ovarian diathermy. Because the polycystic ovary is very sensitive to stimulation by exogenous hormones, it is very important to start with very low doses of gonadotrophins and follicular development must be carefully monitored by ultrasound scans and treatment suspended if two or more mature follicles develop, to reduce the risk of multiple pregnancy.

Ovarian diathermy is free of the risks of multiple pregnancy and ovarian hyperstimulation and does not require intensive ultrasound monitoring. Laparoscopic ovarian diathermy has taken the place of wedge resection of the ovaries (which resulted in extensive peri-ovarian and tubal adhesions), and it appears to be as effective as routine gonadotrophin therapy in the treatment of clomiphene-insensitive PCOS.[20] The meta-analysis of laparoscopic ovarian diathermy includes data from the largest study to have been performed, in which a pragmatic approach was taken to the management of patients who failed to ovulate after ovarian surgery, by prescribing them first clomiphene citrate and then gonadotropins.[21] Gonadotrophin therapy was twice as successful as ovarian surgery at achieving a pregnancy after 6 months, although the cumulative conception rates were similar after 12 months.

INSULIN SENSITISING AGENTS AND METFORMIN

A number of pharmacological agents have been used to amplify the physiological effect of weight loss, notably Metformin. This biguanide inhibits the production of hepatic glucose and enhances the sensitivity of peripheral tissue to insulin, thereby decreasing insulin secretion. It has been shown that Metformin ameliorates hyperandrogenism and abnormalities of gonado-trophin secretion in women with PCOS and can restore menstrual cyclicity and fertility.[22] Metformin may also enhance the efficacy of clomiphene citrate and gonadotrophin therapy. The insulin-sensitising agent Troglitazone also appears to improve the metabolic and reproductive abnormalities in PCOS significantly, although this product has been withdrawn because of reports of deaths from hepatotoxicity. Newer thiazolinediones (rosiglitazone and pyoglitazone) are currently being evaluated.

Metformin is the most promising and safe sensitiser to insulin available in the UK at the present time and may have benefits for short- and long-term health, by improving hyperandrogenism, fertility, insulin sensitivity and lipid profile. There has been much publicity about its use and, as usual, inadequate scientifically sound data. Further research is required with adequately powered clinical studies. The current evidence suggests significant benefit of Metformin on reproductive function but not, despite earlier claims, on the ability to achieve weight loss.[22]

HYPERANDROGENISM AND HIRSUTISM

Hirsutism is characterised by terminal hair growth in a male pattern of distribution, including chin, upper lip, chest, upper and lower back, upper and lower abdomen, upper arm, thigh and buttocks. Treatment options include cosmetic and medical therapies. As drug therapies may take 6–9 months or longer before any improvement of hirsutism is perceived, physical treatments including electrolysis, waxing and bleaching may be helpful whilst waiting for medical treatments to work. For many years, the most 'permanent' physical treatment for unwanted hair has been electrolysis. There are many different types of laser in production and each requires evaluation of dose intensity, effectiveness and safety. The technique is promising, being faster and more effective than shaving, waxing or chemical depilation. Repeated treatments are required for a near-permanent effect because only hair follicles in the growing phase are obliterated at each treatment. At present, it is not widely available and is still an expensive option.

Medical regimens should stop further progression of hirsutism and decrease the rate of hair growth. Adequate contraception is important in women of reproductive age as transplacental passage of anti-androgens may disturb the genital development of a male fetus. The best pharmacological treatment of proven effectiveness is a combination of the synthetic progestogen cyproterone acetate (CPA, 50–100 mg) which is anti-gonadotrophic and anti-androgenic with ethinyl oestradiol (alone or as a combined contraceptive pill). Oestrogens lower circulating androgens by a combination of a slight inhibition of gonadotrophin secretion and gonadotrophin-sensitive ovarian steroid production and by an increase in hepatic production of sex hormone binding globulin resulting in lower free testosterone. The preparation Dianette contains ethinyl oestradiol in combination with cyproterone, although at a lower dose (2 mg).[23] The effect on acne and seborrhoea is usually evident within a couple of months. Cyproterone acetate can rarely cause liver damage and liver function should be checked regularly (after 6 months and then annually). It is generally advised that a switch should be made to a lower dose combined oral contraceptive pill once symptom control has been achieved – usually after 6–12 months of therapy with Dianette.

Spironolactone is a weak diuretic with anti-androgenic properties and may be used in women in whom the COCP is contra-indicated at a daily dose of 25–100 mg. Drosperinone is a derivative of spironolactone and contained in the new COCP, Yasmin, which appears to be well tolerated in women with PCOS.[24]

CONCLUSIONS

PCOS is a heterogeneous condition and the commonest cause of irregular menstrual cycles. Ovarian dysfunction leads to the main signs and symptoms and the ovary is influenced by external factors in particular the gonadotrophins, insulin and other growth factors, which are dependent upon both genetic and environmental influences. There are long-term risks of developing diabetes and possibly cardiovascular disease. Therapy, to date, has been symptomatic but by improved understanding of the pathogenesis treatment options are becoming available that strike more at the heart of the syndrome, such as the use of insulin sensitising agents.

Key points for clinical practice

- PCOS is the commonest endocrine disorder in women (prevalence 15–20%).
- PCOS is a heterogeneous condition. Diagnosis is made by the ultrasound detection of polycystic ovaries and one or more of a combination of symptoms and signs (hyperandrogenism [acne, hirsutism, alopecia], obesity, menstrual cycle disturbance [oligo/amenorrhoea]) and biochemical abnormalities (hypersecretion of testosterone, luteinizing hormone and insulin).
- Management is symptom orientated.
- If obese, weight loss improves symptoms and endocrinology and should be encouraged. A glucose tolerance test should be performed if the BMI is > 30 kg/m².
- Menstrual cycle control is achieved by cyclical oral contraceptives or progestogens.
- Ovulation induction may be difficult and require progression through various treatments which should be monitored carefully to prevent multiple pregnancy.
- Hyperandrogenism is usually managed with Dianette, containing ethinyl oestradiol in combination with cyproterone acetate. A new COCP, Yasmin, may also be of benefit. Alternatives include spironolactone. Flutamide and finasteride are not routinely prescribed because of potential adverse effects. Reliable contraception is required.
- Insulin sensitising agents (e.g. Metformin) are showing early promise but require further long-term evaluation and should only be prescribed by endocrinologists/reproductive endocrinologists.

Indications for referral to reproductive endocrinologist

- Serum testosterone > 5 nmol/l (to exclude other causes of androgen excess, e.g. tumours, late onset congenital adrenal hyperplasia, Cushing's syndrome).
- Infertility.
- Rapid onset hirsutism (to exclude androgen-secreting tumours).
- Glucose intolerance/diabetes.
- Amenorrhoea of more than 6 months – for pelvic ultrasound scan to exclude endometrial hyperplasia.
- Refractory symptoms.

References

1. Reaven GM. Role of insulin resistance in human disease (syndrome X): an expanded definition. *Annu Rev Med* 1993; **44**: 121–131.
2. Fauser B, Taratzis B, Chang J, Azziz R, Legro R, Dewailly D *et al.* 2003 ASRM/ESHRE consensus document. *Fertil Steril* 2004; **18**: 19–25.
3. Balen AH, Laven JSE, Tan SL, Dewailly D. The ultrasound assessment of the polycystic ovary: international consensus definitions. *Hum Reprod Update* 2003; 9: 505–514.
4. Balen AH, Conway GS, Kaltsas G *et al.* Polycystic ovary syndrome: the spectrum of the disorder in 1741 patients. *Hum Reprod* 1995; **10**: 2705–2712.
5. Clarke AM, Ledger W, Galletly C *et al.* Weight loss results in significant improvement in pregnancy and ovulation rates in anovulatory obese women. *Hum Reprod* 1995; **10**: 2705–2712.
6. Polson DW, Adams J, Wadsworth J, Franks S. Polycystic ovaries – a common finding in normal women. *Lancet* 1988; **1**: 870–872.
7. Michelmore KF, Balen AH, Dunger DB, Vessey MP. Polycystic ovaries and associated clinical and biochemical features in young women. *Clin Endocrinol (Oxford)* 1999; **51**: 779–786.
8. Adams J, Polson DW, Franks S. Prevalence of polycystic ovaries in women with anovulation and idiopathic hirsutism. *BMJ Clin Res Edn* 1986; **293**: 355–359.
9. Rodin DA, Bano G, Bland JM, Taylor K, Nussey SS. Polycystic ovaries and associated metabolic abnormalities in Indian subcontinent Asian women. *Clin Endocrinol* 1998; **49**: 91–99.
10. Wijeyaratne CN, Balen AH, Barth J, Belchetz PE. Clinical manifestations and insulin resistance (IR) in polycystic ovary syndrome (PCOS) among South Asians and Caucasians: is there a difference? *Clin Endocrinol* 2002; **57**: 343–350.
11. Dahlgren E, Johansson S, Lindstedt G *et al.* Women with polycystic ovary syndrome wedge resected in 1956 to 1965: a long term follow up focusing on natural history and circulating hormones. *Fertil Steril* 1992; **57**: 505–513.
12. Rajkowha M, Glass MR, Rutherford AJ, Michelmore K, Balen AH. Polycystic ovary syndrome: a risk factor for cardiovascular disease? *Br J Obstet Gynaecol* 2000; **107**: 11–18.
13. Pierpoint T, McKeigue PM, Isaacs AJ, Wild SH, Jacobs HS. Mortality of women with polycystic ovary syndrome at long-term follow-up. *J Clin Epidemiol* 1998; **51**: 581–586.
14. Norman RJ, Masters L, Milner CR, Wang JX, Davies MJ. Relative risk of conversion from normoglycaemia to impaired glucose tolerance or non-insulin dependent diabetes mellitus in polycystic ovary syndrome. *Hum Reprod* 2001; **16**: 1995–1998.
15. Orio F, Palomba S, Spinelli L *et al.* The cardiovascular risk of young women with polycystic ovary syndrome: an observational, analytical, prospective case-control study. *J Clin Endocrinol Metab* 2004; **89**: 3696–3701.
16. Elwood JM, Cole P, Rothman KJ *et al.* Epidemiology of endometrial cancer. *J Natl Cancer Inst* 1977; **59**: 1055–1060.
17. Coulam CB, Annegers JF, Kranz JS. Chronic anovulation syndrome and associated neoplasia. *Obstet Gynecol* 1983; **61**: 403–407.
18. National Institute for Clinical Excellence. *NICE Guidelines for the Investigation and Management of Infertility.* London: Department of Health, 2004.
19. Kousta E, White DM, Franks S. Modern use of clomiphene citrate in induction of ovulation. *Hum Reprod Update* 1997; **3**: 359–365.
20. Farquhar C, Vandekerckhove P, Lilford R. Laparoscopic 'drilling' by diathermy or laser for ovulation induction in anovulatory polycystic ovary syndrome (Cochrane Review). In: *The Cochrane Library*, Issue 4, 2002. Oxford: Update Software.
21. Bayram N, van Wely M, Kaajik EM, Bossuyt PMM, van der Veen F. Using an electrocautery strategy or recombinant follicle stimulating hormone to induce ovulation in polycystic ovary syndrome: randomized controlled trial. *BMJ* 2004; **328**: 192–195.
22. Lord J, Flight I, Norman R. Insulin-sensitising drugs: a meta-analysis. *Cochrane Review*, 2003.
23. Barth JH, Cherry CA, Wojnarowska F, Dawber RPR. Cyproterone acetate for severe hirsutism: results of a double-blind dose-ranging study. *Clin Endocrinol* 1991; **35**: 5–10.
24. Palep-Singh M, Mook K, Barth JH, Balen AH. An observational study of Yasmin in the management of polycystic ovary syndrome. *J Fam Plan Reprod Healthcare* 2004; **30**: 163–165.

Michael J. Gannon Peter O'Donovan

12

Update on endometrial ablation

THE FIRST GENERATION

The modern era of endometrial ablation commenced just over 20 years ago with the development of several methods of permanent endometrial destruction for women with menorrhagia. The procedures were carried out under hysteroscopic control by means of fine instruments introduced alongside the telescope. They varied in how endometrial destruction was achieved. Continuous fluid instillation was used to distend and irrigate the uterine cavity during surgery. Two hysteroscopic techniques were prominent in the early years.

NEODYMIUM YAG LASER

The neodymium YAG laser[1] delivered energy through an optical fibre via a specially adapted endoscope, which had a fluid inlet and outlet and a working channel. The activated fibre, 600 µm in diameter, was methodically drawn over the entire endometrial surface to achieve destruction down to the level of the superficial myometrium. Laser generators were big and expensive and required special training and handling. Use of this technique was confined to those centres with laser facilities and many of the operators doing laser endometrial ablation carried out large numbers of treatments.

ENDOMETRIAL RESECTION

Endometrial ablation became truly popular and wide-spread with the adaptation of the urological resectoscope for use in gynaecology. The

Michael J. Gannon MB PhD FRCSI FRCOG
Consultant Obstetrician and Gynaecologist, Midland Regional Hospital, Mullingar, Co. Westmeath, Ireland

Peter O'Donovan MB FRCS FRCOG
Professorof Obstetrics and Gynaecology, Bradford Royal Infirmary, Bradford, Yorkshire BD9 6RJ, UK

diathermy loop was used to shave off endometrium in strips up to 7-mm wide and 3–4-mm deep. This was commonly known as TCRE or transcervical resection of the endometrium from its urological origins. The uterus, unlike the bladder, does not act as a reservoir to store blood and debris. The resectoscope was modified for gynaecological use by the addition of a second fluid channel which allowed continuous replacement of bloodstained fluid with new distending medium, usually glycine. Endometrial resection[2] was easier to introduce than laser ablation because the instruments and diathermy were already in use in most hospitals. Camera stacks and modern light sources also became common-place with the advent of laparoscopic cholecystectomy at about this time. The technique of endometrial resection soon became popular for the surgical treatment of menorrhagia, but there were some concerns with respect to its safety and also its effectiveness. For instance, there were several reports of injuries to internal organs following uterine perforation with the diathermy loop.

Many observers felt that endometrial ablation was perhaps being performed for women with trivial symptoms and could not provide an alternative to hysterectomy. To answer these concerns, several clinical trials were set up, making endometrial ablation one of the most thoroughly studied of surgical procedures. The first trial[3] recruited from a cohort of women who were awaiting hysterectomy for menorrhagia. Half were randomly allocated to endometrial resection while the remainder underwent abdominal hysterectomy. The findings of the study were re-assuring. Women were happy to undergo endometrial ablation as a surgical alternative for menorrhagia, safety of the technique was demonstrated and, furthermore, there were striking benefits in shorter hospital stay and quicker recovery. Several further studies confirmed these findings. An interesting observation was that hysterectomy also carried a high level of satisfaction.

The initial enthusiasm for hysteroscopic endometrial ablation did not lead to its universal uptake. Reasons included the persistence of menses, albeit light, in many cases and the subsequent need for hysterectomy in up to a quarter of women. It was felt that this may have been due to inappropriate selection of candidates, higher failure rates being found in younger women and in those who had an abnormality such as fibroids. Those women with genuine menorrhagia, who had a measured menstrual blood loss of more than 80 ml, were more likely to have a good result.[4] With the benefit of experience, selection was more rigorous and counselling became more realistic. Women were generally advised not to anticipate total loss of bleeding, which occurred only in about 25% of cases. Most of those who had a successful procedure experienced light menstrual spotting, sometimes progressing to total amenorrhoea over several years.

ROLLERBALL ENDOMETRIAL ABLATION

Hysteroscopic surgery required a new skill which most gynaecologists did not have. Established consultants needed to receive instruction to become competent and not all undertook this. Minimally invasive surgery was taken on by a minority. In the late 1980s, rollerball endometrial ablation[5] was introduced as an easier to perform alternative to endometrial resection. The same basic equipment was used, the only difference being that the energy was delivered through a ball electrode rather than a loop, dispersing the current over a wider area. The ball was drawn methodically over the entire endometrial surface achieving destruction to a depth of 4–5 mm. The 3-mm diameter of the ball electrode enabled the procedure to be quicker than the laser or resection loop. The ball was also a good fit for the uterine cornua, making it potentially safer than the loop.

Rollerball ablation was enthusiastically taken up by American gynaecologists and became the preferred method in the US. The situation in the UK was different and loop resection kept its predominant place, perhaps because of its familiarity and versatility. Advantages claimed for the loop included the ability to deal with polyps or fibroids and its effectiveness for thicker, unprepared endometrium. The removed chips also provided a specimen for histological examination. A combined technique evolved in which the ball electrode was used for the fundus and cornua, and loop resection was carried out for the remainder of the endometrium

VERSAPOINT

The use of monopolar current required a non-electrolytic distending medium, usually glycine. Excess systemic absorption of glycine carried the risk of ammonia toxicity as in the TUR syndrome recognised by urologists. The Versapoint[6] system was developed using bipolar electrodes inserted through the 5f channel of a diagnostic hysteroscope or through a dedicated resectoscope. The main advantage was the use of saline as a distending medium thus avoiding possible glycine toxicity. Smaller electrodes were used for polyps and a bipolar loop resecting electrode and a vaporising electrode were developed for endometrial ablation. Clinical experience is limited.

THE SECOND GENERATION

Ten years ago, the Scottish Hysteroscopy Audit[7] and the MISTLETOE project[8] reported on endometrial ablation methods then in use. The Scottish figures were: loop, 65%; laser, 32%; and ball, 3%. The MISTLETOE figures for England and Wales were: combined (loop and ball), 40%; loop, 35%; laser, 17%; and ball, 6%. Complications described included uterine perforation, bleeding, and fluid overload due to absorption of the distending medium. In this audit, the resection loop was found to be associated with more complications than the other methods and the main recommendation was that use of the loop alone was not advised.

The learning curve and perceived level of complications led to a quest for an easier and safer method of endometrial ablation. Ideally, this could be performed under local anaesthesia as an ambulatory procedure. Attention was concentrated on producing a non-hysteroscopic method of achieving global endometrial destruction. This would generally involve the introduction of a device into the uterine cavity to destroy the endometrium permanently.

Most second generation methods rely on heat production. Uterine distension is usually produced by a balloon, and there is one method which uses free hot fluid. Some methods use an intra-uterine probe without distension which has the potential for better tolerability under local anaesthesia. Other variables which are important for ambulatory surgery are the diameter of the device and the length of time taken to perform the procedure. The ideal probe should be not more than 5 mm in diameter and procedure time not more than 2 min.

MOST WIDELY USED IN 2003

In September 2003, we sent 1410 questionnaires to UK and Irish consultant gynaecologists. Of 886 replies, 576 (66%) were performing endometrial ablation. The first choice procedures were in order: (i) thermal balloon; (ii) combined loop and ball; (iii) microwave endometrial ablation (MEA); (iv) loop; (v) ball; and (vi) laser. The thermal balloon was first choice of 75% of operators in Ireland and Wales, and of 37% in England and Scotland. MEA was first choice of 39% in Scotland, 14% in England and Wales, and was not used in Ireland. This survey confirmed that thermal balloon and MEA were the most popular second generation methods in use in the UK and Ireland during 2003.[9]

Uterine thermal balloon

The uterine thermal balloon[10] was developed just over 10 years ago and claimed to be as safe and effective as rollerball ablation in a randomised trial.[11] The device is simple and has the potential for use with local anaesthetic (Fig. 1). The drawbacks are that the balloon is only effective with a thin endometrium and might not reach the entire endometrial surface in an irregular cavity. Modifications were introduced, the most recent being ThermaChoice III which has an improved design to aid penetration at the cornua. Several competing balloons have been developed.[12] The Cavaterm plus balloon is made of flexible silicone and heat is produced centrally be a self-regulating element which is factory set to 80°C. An oscillating pump maintains a continuous flow of heated glycine around the system, producing a continuous temperature of 75°C for the treatment time of 15 min. The catheter has a unique feature which allows the balloon to be varied in length to fit the uterine cavity size. The Menotreat is the newest balloon, into which saline is circulated from the control unit at 85°C for 11 min. Two different sized disposable units are available for different

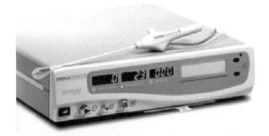 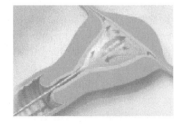

Fig. 1 Uterine thermal balloon (ThermaChoice). The apparatus consists of a distensible latex balloon at the tip of a catheter through which heated 5% dextrose in water is circulated at about 87°C for 8 min. The heating element is contained in the balloon. As a safety measure to confirm correct placement, a minimum pressure of 150 mmHg must be achieved to activate the device. There are pre-set limits for balloon pressure, temperature and duration of treatment.

sized uterine cavities. The simplicity of the thermal balloon technique is its great benefit and, despite the cost of this disposable device, many gynaecologists are now able to offer endometrial ablation for the first time. The ThermaChoice catheter has the smallest diameter of 5 mm making it more suited to office use. Against the use of local anaesthesia is the discomfort experienced during the pre-heating phase of balloon expansion and pressure stabilisation, and a treatment time of about 10 min. While there have been some reports of use in the office, most surgeons continue to use general anaesthesia in the operating theatre.

Microwave endometrial ablation

Microwave endometrial ablation (MEA)[13] was developed in Bath, UK at about the same time as the thermal balloon was being introduced (Fig. 2). Initial clinical results for MEA were very encouraging with active treatment times of less than 3 min and high satisfaction rates. A randomised trial comparing MEA and endometrial resection performed in Aberdeen showed an equivalent outcome with regard to satisfaction and health-related quality of life. Recent follow-up data favour MEA which has a 16% hysterectomy rate at 5 years compared to 25% following endometrial resection.[14] The technique involves more skill than use of the balloon and supervised training must be undertaken before performing MEA. Like the balloon methods, the procedure is blind. There is a continuous temperature display to help ensure that the operator is in correct position in the uterine cavity. Notwithstanding this feature, the US Food and Drug Administration (FDA) has recommended a number of safety checks including ultrasonic measurement of myometrial thickness, and

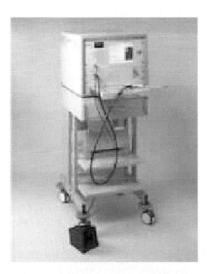
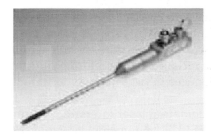

Fig. 2 Microwave endometrial ablation (MEA). The device is a metal tube containing a dielectric filling and radiating tip which propagates microwave energy at 9.2 GHz into the uterine cavity. The electromagnetic waves are generated in a magnetron to produce a hemispherical arc of heat between 70–80°C at the applicator tip. The operator sweeps the tip over and back while slowly withdrawing it from the uterine cavity. The temperature gradient is displayed and as a safety measure the device shuts off power at 90°C.

hysteroscopy to confirm uterine cavity integrity before use. Cervical dilation is required in almost all cases to allow introduction of the 8.5 mm diameter shaft, yet the short treatment time has enabled the Aberdeen group to employ local anaesthesia as a routine.

INNOVATIVE METHODS

There were several methods of endometrial ablation which had a limited time in clinical use. These were discontinued for a variety of reasons, having not fulfilled the criteria required for production and marketing of a successful endometrial ablation device or not having been developed to a sufficient extent for clinical use.

Radiofrequency induced endometrial ablation

One of the earliest second generation methods was radiofrequency induced endometrial ablation.[15] Hyperthermia was induced by a rapid oscillation of charged particles in tissue directly around an intra-uterine probe which was connected to a radiofrequency source. The slightly curved probe was rotated in a step-wise fashion within the uterine cavity to aid an even endometrial contact. A belt electrode around the patient's waist ensured a closed circuit by way of a return cable to the radiofrequency source. The technique fell out of favour largely because of safety concerns about inadvertent burns.

VestaBlate

The VestaBlate[16] consisted of a multi-electrode balloon which was inflated with air in the uterine cavity. Six foil electrodes on each side of the balloon made close contact with the endometrium. Thermistors on each electrode relayed to a computer module in the controller which was connected to a standard electrosurgical generator. On reaching a preset level between 65–75°C, the energy to an electrode was blocked and sent to another electrode where the temperature had dropped below its desired level. Active treatment lasted 4 min before automatic shut-off. Initial results with the Vesta system were promising but technical manufacturing difficulties meant that the system could not be produced in large quantity for clinical use.

Endometrial laser interstitial thermal therapy

The ELITT (endometrial laser interstitial thermal therapy)[17] device consisted of three laser fibres ending in cylindrical diffusers connected together by a Teflon bridge. Each lateral fibre folded alongside the central fibre for ease of access to the uterine cavity and, when pushed forward inside the cavity, gave the system an inverted triangular configuration without cavity distension. A pair of diode lasers was used to deliver power at 30 W for 5 min. Early clinical results were promising but the number of treatments was small. The system is not being actively marketed at the moment.

Photodynamic therapy

Photodynamic therapy (PDT) uses selective, drug-induced photosensitisation to target the endometrium for destruction by light of an appropriate wavelength. This technique has proved successful in targeting rapidly growing cancer tissues and is particularly effective for skin lesions. The use of PDT for endometrial ablation is still experimental, although promising results in photosensitising human endometrium have been achieved using 5-aminolaevulinic acid as a photosensitiser.[18] These results have not yet been translated into effective endometrial ablation using PDT in human studies.

NEWER METHODS

Several methods which employ a variety of energy sources are now being or are about to be marketed in the UK for clinical use. These have been developed and have undergone evaluation mainly in the US where there is a bigger drive for office-based endometrial ablation. Five systems have received FDA approval and are being marketed in the US. These are ThermaChoice and MEA as mentioned above, also Her Option, Hydro ThermAblator and NovaSure. Another method, Thermablate, is awaiting approval. The introduction of the latter four devices to the UK now provides a bigger than ever choice of technologies for endometrial ablation. It is difficult for a clinician to be familiar with all of the methods or even to assess the various techniques physically.

Her Option

Cryosurgery is the destruction of tissue through the application of extreme cold. Endometrial destruction with cryotherapy was first reported in the late 1960s with occasional reports since. The main problem was the establishment of an adequate temperature gradient and this was hindered by loss of contact between the probe and the endometrium and also by the presence of uterine perfusion. A modification using saline to form an ice ball did not have good results.[8] A new cryotherapy development known as Her Option[19] uses a tube containing a gas mixture as coolant which is circulated by a control unit in a closed system. Passage of the gas through a small diameter orifice at the tip of the probe causes a rapid expansion and drop in temperature of the coolant which is transferred to the tip of the surrounding disposable probe in contact with tissue. This produces a surface temperature of −115°C to −125°C at pressures of 300–350 psi. Under ultrasound guidance through a full bladder, the probe is inserted into one cornua and activated for 6 min to form a cryozone. After heating, removal and re-insertion, the second cornua is treated for 4–6 min. The ultrasound-detected cryozones are assessed to determine the need for a third freeze or a pull-back freeze in a large cavity. The technique compared favourably with rollerball ablation in a multicentre study.[20] Overall numbers are small and experience limited. Low surface temperatures are analgesic thus facilitating performance under local anaesthesia. The time required for treatment of from 12–15 min is longer than ideal and simultaneous ultrasound adds to the complexity.

Hydro ThermAblator

The Hydro ThermAblator (HTA)[21] uses heated saline which is circulated free in the uterine cavity to reach all parts of the endometrium, even in the presence of structural abnormalities. The device is an insulated sheath containing a 3 mm hysteroscope, which allows direct visualisation when introduced into the uterine cavity. The control unit circulates saline at room temperature and a loss of 10 ml from the system leads to shut-off. The saline is heated to 90°C and fed by gravity into the uterine cavity. The pressure attained, about 50–55 mmHg, is designed to prevent leakage through the tubes or cervix during the 10 min treatment cycle. At completion, the uterine cavity is flushed with room-temperature saline. A randomised trial comparing HTA and rollerball showed an equivalent outcome, although a thermal burn was reported in one HTA patient.[22]

Thermablate

Apart from cryotherapy, all of the second generation systems rely on heat production. The hot fluid systems produce a maximum temperature and pressure governed by the technical limitations of the system. Temperatures can not exceed the boiling point of dextrose in water or saline, and pressure in a free circulating system can not be higher than that which would open the tubes. The only variable which can increase treatment effect in the current hot fluid systems is a longer treatment time. Thermablate[23] is a new hot balloon system which uses a liquid which can be heated to 170°C. The liquid is supplied in a disposable treatment unit consisting of a prefilled cartridge connected to the balloon via an insulated catheter. The re-usable control unit is the size and shape of a hair dryer weighing only 700 g. The cartridge is locked onto the control unit with a bayonet connection and the liquid is heated. After insertion of the balloon into the endometrial cavity, an automatic check is performed prior to inflation with heated liquid. Treatment is carried out for 128 s and, at the conclusion, the fluid is returned to the cartridge before removal of the device. A 3-year follow-up has just been completed and a randomised trial is underway in the US and Canada.

NovaSure

NovaSure[24] is a global endometrial ablation system which does not distend the uterus (Fig. 3). An expanding bipolar electrode array is inserted through a 7.2 mm catheter and opened to fill the uterine cavity. No pretreatment is needed

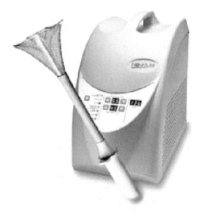
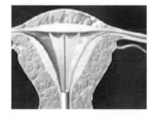

Fig. 3 NovaSure endometrial ablation. The device consists of a bipolar porous fabric mesh mounted on an expandable frame which is inserted into the uterine cavity through a sheath. Suction is continuously applied to bring the endometrium into contact with the electrode array. Power is delivered from the control unit according to uterine cavity measurements to a maximum of 180 W. A preliminary check for uterine perforation is carried out by inflation to 50 mmHg with carbon dioxide.

as suction is employed to draw the endometrium into the electrode mesh providing a good contact during treatment. Continuous suction removes hot gas, blood and debris from the uterine cavity. There is an automatic cut-off of power when tissue resistance reaches a preset level and the entire system shuts off at 2 min if treatment is continuing. The average time taken for active treatment is 90 s. Randomised trials showed 1-year outcomes equivalent to rollerball[25] and better than ThermaChoice.[26] There was a shorter treatment time for NovaSure patients than both other methods. NovaSure is more likely to be performed under local anaesthesia than rollerball and less likely than ThermaChoice. An observational study found that less than 3% of women had undergone hysterectomy at 3 years after NovaSure treatment.[27] The lack of uterine distension and short treatment time make this technique suitable for local anaesthesia, although the need for cervical dilation is a drawback.

Key points for clinical practice

- Fluid-distension, first generation methods are highly skill dependent. Rollerball ablation provides the best combination of ease and safety. Hydro ThermAblator (HTA) uses free hot fluid which may cause inadvertent burns.

- Balloon systems with enclosed distension fluid provide simpler, less versatile methods. The most widely used and preferred method for those with little hysteroscopic experience is ThermaChoice. The newer Thermablate is quicker and looks promising if clinical evaluation is satisfactory.

- A third group of methods uses various probes without distension media. Microwave endometrial ablation (MEA) has had good results in a randomised trial against loop resection. The NovaSure bipolar device which is suitable for office use has become a popular method of ablation in the US.

- The goal of the manufacturers is to produce safe, effective systems with smaller diameter catheters and quicker treatment times, which will help in the evolution of a truly ambulatory endometrial ablation method.

References

1. Goldrath MH, Fuller TA, Segal S. Laser photovaporization of the endometrium for the treatment of menorrhagia. *Am J Obstet Gynecol* 1981; **140**: 14–19.
2. DeCherney A, Polan ML. Hysteroscopic management of intrauterine lesions and intractable uterine bleeding. *Am J Obstet Gynecol* 1983; **61**: 392–397.
3. Gannon MJ, Holt EM, Fairbank J *et al.* A randomised trial comparing endometrial resection and abdominal hysterectomy for the treatment of menorrhagia. *BMJ* 1991; **303**: 1362–1364.
4. Gannon MJ, Day P, Hammadieh N, Johnson N. A new method for measuring menstrual blood loss and its use in screening women before endometrial ablation. *Br J Obstet Gynaecol* 1996; **103**: 1029–1033.
5. Vancaillie TG. Electrocoagulation of the endometrium with the ball-end resectoscope. *Obstet Gynecol* 1989; **74**: 425–427.

6. Vilos GA. Intrauterine surgery using a coaxial bipolar electrode in normal saline solution (Versapoint): a pilot study. *Fertil Steril* 1999; **72**: 740–743.
7. Scottish Hysteroscopy Audit Group. A Scottish audit of hysteroscopic surgery for menorrhagia: complications and follow up. *Br J Obstet Gynaecol* 1995; **102**: 249–254.
8. Overton C, Hargreaves J, Maresh M. A national survey of the complications of endometrial destruction for menstrual disorders: the MISTLETOE study. *Br J Obstet Gynaecol* 1997; **104**: 1351–1359.
9. Tahir A, Gannon MJ. Reaudit of endometrial ablation methods. In: *Proceedings of the Annual Scientific Meeting of the British Society for Gynaecological Endoscopy*, Dublin, Ireland 2004; 45.
10. Neuwirth RS, Duran A, Singer A, MacDonald R, Bolduc L. The endometrial ablator: a new instrument. *Obstet Gynecol* 1994; **83**: 792–796.
11. Meyer WR, Walsh BW, Grainger DA, Peacock LM, Loffer FD, Steege JF. Thermal balloon and rollerball ablation to treat menorrhagia: a multi-center comparison. *Obstet Gynecol* 1998; **92**: 98–103.
12. Friberg B, Wallsten H, Henriksson P *et al.* A new, simple, safe, and efficient device for the treatment of menorrhagia. *J Gynecol Techniques* 1996; **2**: 103–108.
13. Sharp NC, Cronin N, Feldberg I, Evans M, Hodgson D, Ellis S. Microwaves for menorrhagia: a new fast technique for endometrial ablation. *Lancet* 1995; **346**: 1003–1004.
14. Cooper KG, Bain C, Lawrie L, Parkin DE. A randomised comparison of microwave endometrial ablation with transcervical resection of the endometrium; follow up at a minimum of five years. *Br J Obstet Gynaecol* 2005; **112**: 470–475.
15. Phipps JH, Lewis BV, Roberts T *et al.* Treatment of functional menorrhagia by radio-frequency-induced thermal ablation. *Lancet* 1990: **335**: 374–376.
16. Dequesne JH, Gallinat A, Garza-Leal JG *et al.* Thermoregulated radiofrequency endometrial ablation. *Int J Fertil Women's Med* 1997; **42**: 311–318.
17. Donnez J, Polet R, Mathieu P-M, Konwitz E, Nisolle M, Casanas-Roux F. Endometrial laser interstitial hyperthermy: a potential modality for endometrial ablation. *Obstet Gynecol* 1996; **87**: 459–464.
18. Gannon MJ, Johnson N, Roberts DJH *et al.* Photosensitization of the endometrium with topical 5-aminolevulinic acid. *Am J Obstet Gynecol* 1995; **173**: 1826–1828.
19. Dobak JD, Ryba E, Kovalcheck S. A new closed-loop cryosurgical device for endometrial ablation. *J Am Assoc Gynecol Laparosc* 2000; **7**: 245–249.
20. Duleba AJ, Heppard MC, Soderstrom RM, Townsend DE. A randomized study comparing endometrial cryoablation and rollerball electroablation for treatment of dysfunctional uterine bleeding. *J Am Assoc Gynecol Laparosc* 2003; **10**: 17–26.
21. Baggish M, Paraiso M, Breznock EM, Griffey S. A computer-controlled, continuously circulating, hot irrigating system for endometrial ablation. *Am J Obstet Gynecol* 1995; **173**: 1842–1848.
22. Corson SL. A multicenter evaluation of endometrial ablation by Hydro ThermAblator and rollerball for the treatment of menorrhagia. *J Am Assoc Gynecol Laparosc* 2001; **8**: 359–367.
23. Mangeshikar P, Kapur A, Yackel DB. Endometrial ablation with a new thermal balloon system. *J Am Assoc Gynecol Laparosc* 2003; **10**: 27–32.
24. Laberge P. NovaSure technology overview. In: *Proceedings of the 2nd World Congress on Controversies in Obstetrics, Gynecology and Infertility, Vol. 1.* Paris, France 2001; 303–310.
25. Cooper J, Gimpelson R, Laberge P *et al.* A randomized, multicenter trial of safety and efficacy of the NovaSure system in the treatment of menorrhagia. *J Am Assoc Gynecol Laparosc* 2002; **9**: 418–428.
26. Bongers MY, Bourdrez P, Mol BWJ, Heintz APM, Brolmann HAM. Randomised controlled trial of bipolar radio-frequency endometrial ablation and balloon endometrial ablation. *Br J Obstet Gynaecol* 2004; **111**: 1095–1102.
27. Gallinat A. NovaSure impedance controlled system for endometrial ablation: Three-year follow-up on 107 patients. *Am J Obstet Gynecol* 2004; 191: 1585–1589.

Helga Gimbel

13

Total or subtotal hysterectomy – what is the evidence?

The first description of abdominal hysterectomy came from Charles Clay in 1843, who performed a subtotal abdominal hysterectomy.[16] The total abdominal hysterectomy was introduced in 1929 by the American surgeon, Richardson, to avoid serosanguinous discharge from the cervical stump and development of carcinoma of the cervix.[16] For these reasons, total abdominal hysterectomy became the predominant way of removing the uterus from the 1950s, whether it was done because of malignant or benign disease. The Papanicolau smear which could reduce the incidence rate of cervical cancer became available in the 1950s. However, it was not until the 1980s with the results of the cohort study performed by Kilkku *et al.*[13] and the discussion in 1991 of the laparoscopic approach of CASH (Classic Abdominal Semm Hysterectomy) that the case for subtotal hysterectomy was raised again.[12]

FACTORS INFLUENCING THE CHOICE OF HYSTERECTOMY AND HYSTERECTOMY METHOD

During the 1990s, several papers were published regarding factors influencing the choice of hysterectomy method. The attitudes of the gynaecologist might be important for the choice of method. A temporary correlation was found between the publication of results from the Finish[13] comparison of total and subtotal hysterectomy favouring subtotal hysterectomy and the change in preference of hysterectomy methods seen in some Scandinavian countries.[6] This suggests that the urinary and sexual outcomes reported to be superior after subtotal hysterectomy are more important to the gynaecologist than the risk of carcinoma of the cervical stump.[7] In the UK,[24] however, the majority of responding gynaecologists preferred a total hysterectomy to a subtotal

Helga Gimbel MD
Specialist Registrar, Department of Obstetrics and Gynaecology, Hillerød County Hospital, 3400 Hillerød, Denmark

hysterectomy although they thought that more urinary and sexual adverse effects were found after total than after subtotal hysterectomy.

Other, more subtle, reasons for the preference of one hysterectomy method over the other might also exist: in a Danish survey,[7] subtotal hysterectomy tended to be recommended more often by gynaecologists employed in the capital than in the provinces. Gynaecologists employed in public hospitals also recommended subtotal hysterectomy more often than their colleagues in private practice. The abdominal methods of hysterectomy were recommended more often than any other methods of hysterectomy and subtotal hysterectomy was the preferred hysterectomy method in 3 out of 7 cases. The recommendation to the patients and the preferred hysterectomy method for the gynaecologists or their wives were the same and corresponded well with the national figures in Denmark at that time.

An increasing level of information about the different treatment modalities among patients as well as an increasing level of information about patients' rights has emerged during the last decade. These factors are also known to influence the hysterectomy rate as well as method.[5,18]

INCIDENCE RATES

The actual rates of hysterectomy and hysterectomy methods have been described from several countries. The hysterectomy rates vary among industrialised countries, the US[3] and Finland[27] having the highest rates (560 and 414 per 100,000 women per year, respectively) and Sweden and Norway having the lowest rates (145 and 164 per 100,000 women per year, respectively). In many areas (*e.g.* Finland,[27] England, and New South Wales[28]), the hysterectomy rate has increased during the past decades. In the US[23] and Denmark,[6] however, a decrease was found.

A decrease in total hysterectomy and an increase in subtotal hysterectomy during the past 15 years was found in New York State as well as overall in the US,[23] and in Denmark,[6] while the rates were unchanged in Finland.[27]

All subtotal hysterectomy rates were much lower than those of total hysterectomy. The highest ratios between the rate of the two hysterectomy methods were found in Sweden (0.56), while the smallest ratios were found in the UK (0.04) and New York State (0.11). Although different in rates, all Scandinavian countries have high ratios (0.56 in Sweden, 0.39 in Denmark, 0.32 in Finland and 0.27 in Norway).

TOTAL VERSUS SUBTOTAL HYSTERECTOMY

Total and subtotal hysterectomy have been compared extensively in the literature since the 1930s. However, the indications were mixed in many of the studies. Patients with malignant as well as benign indications for hysterectomy were included. Many of the papers were merely experiences and little data were reported. Most papers were retrospective reviews of hospital files and for many of the studies there was a lack of strict methodology.

This review is based on observational studies[10,11,13,19–21] as well as randomised clinical trials[8,9,14,15,25,26,29] which include patients having hysterectomies for benign conditions and which are performed according to

Table 1 Results of urinary incontinence after total and subtotal hysterectomy

First author and country	Outcome measure	Outcome for TAH (n/total)	Outcome for SAH (n/total)	P-value
Kilkku, Finland[13]	Incontinence	30/104	24/107	0.29
Lalos, Sweden[14]	Incontinence	0/11	2/11	0.48
Thakar, UK[25]	Urge urinary incontinence	14/120	13/117	0.89
	Stress urinary incontinence	1.5 (± 0.9)	1.5 (± 0.9)	0.74
Learman, USA[15]	Stress incontinence	3/67	8/68	0.21
	Urge incontinence	2/67	4/68	0.68
Gimbel, Denmark[9]	Urinary incontinence	13/140	25/137	0.03
	Stress incontinence	3/140	8/137	0.13
	Urge incontinence	2/140	7/137	0.10
	Mixed incontinence	6/140	8/137	0.59
Gimbel, Denmark[10]	Urinary incontinence	10/65	9/91	0.33

TAH, total abdominal hysterectomy; SAH, subtotal abdominal hysterectomy.

[13]1981, observational study including 105 total hysterectomy patients and 107 subtotal hysterectomy patients. The data based on interviews 1 year after hysterectomy.

[14]1986, randomised clinical trial including 11 total hysterectomy patients and 11 subtotal hysterectomy patients. Data based on micturition study and cystometry 6 months after hysterectomy.

[25]2002, randomised clinical trial including 146 total hysterectomy patients and 133 subtotal hysterectomy patients. Data based on cystometrography, flowmetry and questionnaire 1 year after hysterectomy.

[15]2003, randomised clinical trial including 67 total hysterectomy patients and 68 subtotal hysterectomy patients. Data based on questionnaire 2 years after hysterectomy.

[9]In press, randomised clinical trial including 158 total hysterectomy patients and 161 subtotal hysterectomy patients. Data based on questionnaire 1 year after hysterectomy.

[10]2005, observational study including 80 total hysterectomy patients and 105 subtotal hysterectomy patients. Data based on questionnaire 1 year after hysterectomy.

strict methodology. Five of the studies are observational studies and, of these, four are prospective studies. Four are randomised clinical trials and the number of patients included varies from 22 to 319 with follow-up varying from 6 months to 2 years. The outcomes are almost exclusively measured through hospital charts and interviews/questionnaires, but two of the papers are based on objective examinations (gynaecological and urodynamic examinations).

OUTCOMES FAVOURING TOTAL HYSTERECTOMY

Urinary incontinence

The results of this outcome are variable (Table 1). In the largest trial,[9] more women were suffering from urinary incontinence after a subtotal hysterectomy than after a total hysterectomy. However, this difference is not reported in any of the other studies. The other studies report no difference between the two treatments although most of the randomised clinical trials tend to favour total hysterectomy.

The difference between the largest trial[9] and the other randomised clinical trials[14,15,25] is most likely due to difference in sample size. All the other randomised clinical trials are smaller in the numbers included and in the follow-up of patients than the largest randomised trial. Furthermore, the study by Thakar et al.[25] differs with respect to the race of the women included in the trial. As the incidence of urinary incontinence differs with race (the incidence is smaller for women of African origin than for Caucasian women), the sample size of a mixed race population should have been much larger in the Thakar et al.[25] study to demonstrate a difference.

Regarding evidence, the non-randomised clinical trials are either retrospective, prospective, or follow-up studies. It has previously been demonstrated that the results from observational and follow-up studies differ from the results of randomised clinical trials in an unpredictable way. Non-randomised studies tend to overestimate the treatment effect of a new treatment (i.e. subtotal hysterectomy), which also seems to be the case here.

So how could a possible difference between total and subtotal hysterectomy be explained? There is a general consensus that abnormal urethral support plays some role in the aetiology of stress urinary incontinence. As part of the abnormal urethral support, stress urinary incontinent women have increased bladder neck mobility. During the total hysterectomy procedure, many gynaecologists perform a suspension of the vaginal vault. A suspension of the cervical stump is not usually done in Denmark during the subtotal procedure. The suspension during the total hysterectomy might serve as a minor bladder neck suspension procedure thus decreasing/removing the problem of incontinence by decreasing bladder neck mobility.

A comparative study of 39 patients undergoing total abdominal hysterectomy and 30 controls has shown that the total hysterectomy procedure decreases bladder neck mobility. Procedures and devices often used to relieve urinary incontinence symptoms in general and stress urinary incontinence in particular (Burch's procedure and application of vaginal devices) also decrease the bladder neck mobility. Therefore, it is tempting to propose that the advantage of total hysterectomy over subtotal hysterectomy is the suspension. If the theory of suspension is correct, a suspension procedure of the cervical stump could be performed during subtotal hysterectomy in cases where it is impossible to undertake total hysterectomy.

All studies, however, report a relief of urinary incontinence symptoms in both treatment groups.

Cervical stump problems

All the studies found that some of the women who had a subtotal hysterectomy continued to have vaginal bleeding after the hysterectomy (Table 2). The rate of vaginal bleeding varied from 5–22%. Recent studies of laparoscopic supracervical hysterectomies[2,17] show that even after removing a cylinder of tissue including the endocervical canal and the transformation zone, 8–11% of women still experience vaginal bleeding.

In one study, most of the women who experienced vaginal bleeding after the subtotal procedure described the amount of bleeding as mild or very mild and that the bleeding did not interfere with their daily life. However, most of the women would have preferred to be without the bleeding.

Table 2 Results of cervical stump problems after subtotal hysterectomy

First author and country	Outcome measure	Number of patients (n/total)
Ruoss, UK[21]	Cervical stump bleeding	4/50
Thakar, UK[25]	Cervical stump bleeding	9/121
Learman, USA[15]	Cyclic vaginal bleeding	4/68
Gimbel, Denmark[8]	Cervical stump bleeding	27/137
Gimbel, Denmark[10]	Cervical stump bleeding	14/91
Okara, UK[17]	Vaginal bleeding	8/70
Ewies, UK[2]	Cyclic vaginal bleeding	12/150

[21]1995, follow-up study including 50 total hysterectomy patients and 50 subtotal hysterectomy patients. Data based on questionnaire 1 year after hysterectomy.

[25]2002, randomised clinical trial including 146 total hysterectomy patients and 133 subtotal hysterectomy patients. Data based on cystometrography, flowmetry and questionnaire 1 year after hysterectomy.

[15]2003, randomised clinical trial including 67 total hysterectomy patients and 68 subtotal hysterectomy patients. Data based on questionnaire 2 years after hysterectomy.

[8]2003, randomised clinical trial including 158 total hysterectomy patients and 161 subtotal hysterectomy patients. Data based on questionnaire 1 year after hysterectomy.

[10]2005, observational study including 80 total hysterectomy patients and 105 subtotal hysterectomy patients. Data based on questionnaire 1 year after hysterectomy.

[17]2001, follow-up study of 70 laparoscopic subtotal hysterectomy patients. Data based on interview 52 to 84 months after hysterectomy.

[2]2000, retrospective analysis of 150 subtotal hysterectomy patients. Data based on interview.

The most serious difference between total and subtotal hysterectomy is the risk of carcinoma of the cervical stump after subtotal hysterectomy. Although no studies included patients with former or present dysplasia or cancer of the cervix uteri, three studies reported one or more women having abnormal cytology in the follow-up period. In most of the other studies, this outcome was not reported.

OUTCOMES FAVOURING SUBTOTAL HYSTERECTOMY

Peri-operative blood loss, operation time and length of stay

Peri-operative blood loss and operation time were both in favour of subtotal hysterectomy (Table 3). However, the actual differences were not large and are unlikely to be of significant clinical importance except for difficult cases, in which a subtotal hysterectomy may be performed instead of a total hysterectomy.

Two studies found a difference regarding hospitalisation. One study favours total hysterectomy while the other favours subtotal hysterectomy. All other studies found no difference. In one study,[8] the difference between the treatments was explained by a difference in complication rates. The difference between the two studies could be explained by evidence grade. One of the studies was an observational study while the other was a randomised clinical trial. Another explanation could be tradition. Hospitalisation has been found to be very dependent on doctor's information and can be changed by change of attitude among the doctors.

Table 3 Results of duration of operation, intra-operative blood loss, and length of hospital stay after total and subtotal hysterectomy

First author and country	Outcome measure	Outcome for TAH	Outcome for SAH	P-value
Ruoss, UK[21]	Operating time (min – mean, range)	57 (35–88)	45 (23–57)	SAH less than TAH
	Length of hospital stay (days – mean, range)	5.5 (3–9)	4.7 (3–9)	Not reported
Roovers, The Netherlands[19]	Length of hospital stay (days – mean, SD)	8.3 (1.7)	9.2 (3.4)	SAH associated with longer hospital stay than TAH
Thakar, UK[25]	Duration of operation (min – mean ± SD)	71.1 ± 23.4	59.5 ± 20.6	< 0.001
	Blood loss (ml – mean ± SD)	422.6 ± 301.8	320.1 ± 271	0.004
	Length of hospital stay (days – mean ± SD)	6.0 (4.7)	5.2 (1.1)	0.04
Learman, USA[15]	Operation time (min – mean ± SD)	123 ± 46	113 ± 35	No significant difference
	Blood loss (ml – mean ± SD)	418 ± 306	382 ± 355	No significant difference
	Length of hospital stay (days – mean ± SD)	3.5 ± 1.2	3.3 ± 1.1	No significant difference
Gimbel, Denmark[8]	Operation time (min – median, range)	85 (35–255)	70 (34–165)	< 0.001
	Blood loss (ml – median, range)	400 (25–4500)	250 (10–2500)	<0.001
Gimbel, Denmark[10]	Operation time (min – median, range)	80 (35–210)	65 (30–150)	< 0.001
	Blood loss (ml – median, range)	350 (100–1300)	250 (25–1400)	< 0.001

TAH, total abdominal hysterectomy; SAH, subtotal abdominal hysterectomy.

[21]1995, follow-up study including 50 total hysterectomy patients and 50 subtotal hysterectomy patients. Data based on questionnaire 1 year after hysterectomy.

[19]2003, observational study including 164 total hysterectomy patients and 84 subtotal hysterectomy patients. Data based on questionnaire 6 months after hysterectomy.

[25]2002, randomised clinical trial including 146 total hysterectomy patients and 133 subtotal hysterectomy patients. Data based on cystometrography, flowmetry and questionnaire 1 year after hysterectomy.

[15]2003, randomised clinical trial including 67 total hysterectomy patients and 68 subtotal hysterectomy patients. Data based on questionnaire 2 years after hysterectomy.

[8]2003, randomised clinical trial including 158 total hysterectomy patients and 161 subtotal hysterectomy patients. Data based on questionnaire 1 year after hysterectomy.

[10]2005, observational study including 80 total hysterectomy patients and 105 subtotal hysterectomy patients. Data based on questionnaire 1 year after hysterectomy.

OUTCOMES NOT FAVOURING ANY OF THE HYSTERECTOMY METHODS

Lower urinary tract symptoms other than incontinence

No differences were found between total and subtotal hysterectomy regarding lower urinary tract symptoms other than incontinence in most studies. One study found a significant difference between the treatments regarding dysuria and sensation of residual urine. Both differences were in favour of subtotal hysterectomy. The study was, however, an observational study where the surgeon was supposed to decide the operation method. A suspicion of bias could be raised from the baseline parameters as most women with urinary tract symptoms before the operation had subtotal hysterectomy. As no studies had been able to repeat this finding whether performed as observational studies or randomised trials, the evidence seems to be that the operation methods do not differ regarding lower urinary tract symptoms apart from incontinence.

Peri- and postoperative complications

Many would assume that complications with hysterectomies would be less with subtotal hysterectomy as this procedure is less invasive than total hysterectomy. A general belief would be that more injuries to the bladder and ureter occur during total hysterectomy but studies showing this difference have not been identified. The reason might be that such complications are rare and the number of patients required in such studies would be large.

One UK study[25] found a difference between total and subtotal hysterectomy regarding postoperative complications (Table 4). Women having a total hysterectomy were more likely to have a postoperative complication than women having a subtotal hysterectomy. This finding was especially pronounced regarding pyrexia and use of antibiotics. Similar findings have not been reported by any of the other studies (Table 4). The other studies reported no difference between the operation methods although some had a tendency towards more complications in the subtotal hysterectomy group.

One explanation of this finding could be contamination of the abdominal cavity by the vaginal flora during total hysterectomy. Another explanation could be that the studies report fever differently. In most studies and trials, no definition is found as to postoperative fever. In two studies, fever was reported according to a more conservative rule than the study describing the difference between the two hysterectomy methods. This could affect the results. In any case, it is tempting to change the prophylactic antibiotics or to increase the dose if any difference between the hysterectomy methods is found regarding this complication.

Overall complication rates between 8% and 41% were found in the studies and trials. The reasons for the differences could be the length of follow-up, the data source, or the training of the surgeon.

Quality of life and psychiatric symptoms

Quality of life measured with the SF-36 questionnaire showed no difference between total and subtotal hysterectomy in three studies.[8,10,26] One study[26] showed a significant difference in one item (emotions) out of eight with a greater improvement in the subtotal hysterectomy group than in the total hysterectomy group. When this difference was examined further by looking at change in the General Health Questionnaire-28 subscales, there were no significant differences between total and subtotal hysterectomy women.

All of the studies, however, reported that quality of life was improved significantly after both hysterectomy methods. The postoperative scores in two studies were similar to those from an age-matched group from the same

Table 4 Results of peri- and postoperative complications after total and subtotal hysterectomy

First author and country	Outcome measure	Outcome for TAH (n/total)	Outcome for SAH (n/total)	P-value
Roover, The Netherlands[19]	Postoperative complications	15/109	4/50	0.43
Thakar, UK[25]	Re-admission	4/146	1/133	0.37
	Intra-operative complications	21/146	11/133	0.11
	Postoperative complications			
	Before discharge	40/146	13/133	< 0.001
	– Pyrexia	28/146	8/133	0.001
	– Retention of urine	2/146	0/133	0.50
	– Vault haematoma	1/146	0/133	1.00
	– Wound haematoma	4/146	3/133	1.00
	– Wound infection	3/146	2/133	1.00
	– Ileus	1/146	0/133	1.00
	– Vaginal bleeding	1/146	0/133	1.00
	After discharge	9/146	14/133	0.20
	– Bowel obstruction	2/146	0/133	0.50
Learman, USA[15]	All febrile morbidity	16/65	10/68	0.15
	Urinary tract injury	2/65	0/67	0.24
	Intra-operative haemorrhage or blood transfusion	3/65	4/67	1.00
	Delayed return of bladder function	3/65	1/67	0.36
	Total re-admissions	15	29	
	Total number of patients re-admitted	11/65	21/67	0.053
Gimbel, Denmark[8]	Total number of women having one or more complications	64/158	54/161	0.20
Gimbel, Denmark[10]	Total number of women having one or more complications	25/80	39/105	0.40

TAH, total abdominal hysterectomy; SAH, subtotal abdominal hysterectomy.

[19] 2003, observational study including 164 total hysterectomy patients and 84 subtotal hysterectomy patients. Data based on questionnaire 6 months after hysterectomy.

[25] 2002, randomised clinical trial including 146 total hysterectomy patients and 133 subtotal hysterectomy patients. Data based on cystometrography, flowmetry and questionnaire 1 year after hysterectomy.

[15] 2003, randomised clinical trial including 67 total hysterectomy patients and 68 subtotal hysterectomy patients. Data based on questionnaire 2 years after hysterectomy.

[8] 2003, randomised clinical trial including 158 total hysterectomy patients and 161 subtotal hysterectomy patients. Data based on questionnaire 1 year after hysterectomy.

[10] 2005, observational study including 80 total hysterectomy patients and 105 subtotal hysterectomy patients. Data based on questionnaire 1 year after hysterectomy.

country. Similarly, all women showed improvement in psychiatric and psychological symptoms.

Bowel function

No studies observed any difference between the total and the subtotal hysterectomy women regarding any bowel function. Constipation pre-operatively was a significant predictor for constipation after hysterectomy in a multivariate analysis.[8] Thus, constipation might be a problem unrelated to hysterectomy.

Prolapse

Older studies not included in this review were all in favour of subtotal hysterectomy regarding prolapse. More women were shown to have prolapse after subtotal than after total hysterectomy. Many of the studies were, however, retrospective or based on data from women admitted because of prolapse.

Although no significant difference was found in the recently performed studies regarding prolapse, trends of more women having prolapse after subtotal than after total hysterectomy were found (Table 5). The reason for the finding of no difference could be that the follow up time was too short and prolapse would be expected to occur late in life.

Although no significant difference was found between total and the subtotal hysterectomy, the trend of more women having prolapse after subtotal hysterectomy than after total hysterectomy supports the theoretical considerations for the difference between the two methods regarding incontinence. The difference between the operation methods regarding incontinence as well as prolapse could be explained by the suspension of the vaginal vault during the total hysterectomy procedure and the lack of such a suspension of the cervical stump in the subtotal hysterectomy procedure.

Table 5 Results of prolapse after total and subtotal hysterectomy

First author and country	Outcome measure	Outcome for TAH (n/total)	Outcome for SAH (n/total)	P-value
Thakar, UK[25]	Cervical prolapse	–	2/133	–
Learman, USA[13]	Prolapse	1/64	1/61	1.00
Gimbel, Denmark[8]	Prolapse	0/140	3/137	0.12
Gimbel, Denmark[10]	Prolapse	1/65	2/91	1.00

TAH, total abdominal hysterectomy; SAH, subtotal abdominal hysterectomy.

[25]2002, randomised clinical trial including 146 total hysterectomy patients and 133 subtotal hysterectomy patients. Data based on cystometrography, flowmetry and questionnaire 1 year after hysterectomy.

[13]2003, randomised clinical trial including 67 total hysterectomy patients and 68 subtotal hysterectomy patients. Data based on questionnaire 2 years after hysterectomy.

[8]2003, randomised clinical trial including 158 total hysterectomy patients and 161 subtotal hysterectomy patients. Data based on questionnaire 1 year after hysterectomy.

[10]2005, observational study including 80 total hysterectomy patients and 105 subtotal hysterectomy patients. Data based on questionnaire 1 year after hysterectomy.

Sexual life

The studies of Masters and Johnson from the 1960s suggested that, at least in some women, the uterus plays a role in the physiology of the female orgasm. Therefore, it was reasonable to predict that hysterectomy could have a detrimental effect on orgasm by eliminating the uterine contribution. A Finish study[13] suggested that subtotal hysterectomy was better regarding libido, dyspareunia and orgasmic coitus. The results were explained by the way the procedure preserved the nerves and ligaments and helped preserve normal postoperative sexual function better than the more invasive total hysterectomy procedure. Another explanation was that unconscious psychological reactions played an important role (Table 6).

Sexual life after total and subtotal hysterectomy has been examined in other studies regarding frequency of sexual desire, dyspareunia, frequency of intercourse, frequency of masturbation, frequency of orgasm, quality of orgasm, vaginal lubrication and satisfaction with sexual life. No significant difference was found between total and the subtotal hysterectomy in these studies whether performed as observational studies or randomised clinical trials. The reason for the findings in the Finish study could be bias between the two groups. More women in the subtotal hysterectomy group than in the total hysterectomy group had partners. The results from the recent studies and trials raise doubts about the Master and Johnson theory of orgasm.

Several studies reported that hysterectomy regardless of the operation method resulted in a relief of dyspareunia. This could be explained by removal of the tender and enlarged uterine body.

One study[29] found that satisfaction with sexual life before the operation, the relationship with the partner, and physical well-being were predictors of satisfaction with sexual life after the operation. This finding was supported by other studies on hysterectomy and sexuality. Thus, a good partner relationship seemed likely to be able to compensate for the problems arising from the new situation following hysterectomy. Consequently, women with a poor partner relationship or no relationship may be vulnerable to sexual problems after hysterectomy, and may perhaps require counselling.

Pelvic pain

No significant difference was found between total and subtotal hysterectomy regarding pelvic pain in any of the reports. However, a highly significant reduction in pelvic pain after hysterectomy regardless of operation method was found in many studies at 1-year follow-up. The reason for the resolution of pelvic pain following hysterectomy might be that most of the women having a hysterectomy for benign indications have painful fibroids. When they are removed, pelvic pain disappears.

CONCLUSIONS

Total hysterectomy differs from subtotal hysterectomy by less women suffering from urinary incontinence and prolapse and cervical stump problems after hysterectomy. However, subtotal hysterectomy is faster to perform, has less intra-operative bleeding, and seems to have less peri- and postoperative complications especially regarding infections. The latter

Table 6 Results of sexual life after total and subtotal hysterectomy

First author and country	Outcome measure	Outcome for TAH (n/total)	Outcome for SAH) (n/total)	P-value
Kilkku, Finland[13]	Coital frequency < once a week	45/98	37/107	0.10
	Dyspareunia	14/91	6/98	0.06
	Weak or absent libido	35/100	33/106	0.93
	Orgasm < one of four coituses	42/91	31/98	0.04
Ruoss, UK[21]	Increased sexual comfort and joy	19/50	32/50	0.01
	Decreased sexual comfort and joy	12/50	5/50	0.11
	Satisfactory orgasm as before	25/50	31/50	0.02
	Less satisfactory orgasm than before	9/50	7/50	0.79
Thakar, UK[25]	Orgasm	3.2 (± 0.9)	3.3 (± 0.9)	0.31
	Multiple orgasm	1.7 (± 1.0)	1.7 (± 1.0)	0.41
	Poor vaginal lubrication	22/84	25/90	0.81
	Superficial dyspareunia	9/85	15/91	0.28
	Deep dyspareunia	12/84	6/91	0.13
	Good relationship with partner	69/86	82/91	0.09
Gimbel, Denmark[29]	Sexual desire once a week or more	61/140	52/137	0.66
	Dyspareunia	9/140	13/137	0.38
	Intercourse once a week or more	53/140	45/137	0.38
	Masturbation once a week or more	13/140	7/137	0.25
	Orgasm always or often	110/140	106/137	0.81
	Quality of orgasm (excellent or good)	110/140	114/137	0.33
	Problems regarding vaginal lubrication	15/140	19/137	0.42
	Satisfaction with sexual life	95/140	86/137	0.37
Roovers, The Netherlands[20]	Problems with lubrication	22/145	12/76	0.90
	Problems with orgasm	18/145	11/76	0.67
	Problems with genital pain	18/145	5/76	0.25
	Problems with sensation in genitals	5/145	3/76	1.00
	Problems with arousal	23/145	14/76	0.63
	Any sexual problem	45/145	23/76	0.91
Gimbel, Denmark[29]	Sexual desire once a week or more	30/65	42/91	1.00
	Dyspareunia	5/65	10/91	0.59
	Intercourse once a week or more	25/65	36/91	0.89
	Masturbation once a week or more	2/65	5/91	0.70
	Orgasm always or often	53/65	70/91	0.49
	Quality of orgasm (excellent or good)	56/65	69/91	0.15
	Problems regarding vaginal lubrication	10/65	12/91	0.70
	Satisfaction with sexual life	44/65	59/91	0.71

TAH, total abdominal hysterectomy; SAH, subtotal abdominal hysterectomy.

[13]1981/1985, observational study including 105 total hysterectomy patients and 107 subtotal hysterectomy patients. The data are based on interviews 1 year after hysterectomy.

[21]1995, follow-up study including 50 total hysterectomy patients and 50 subtotal hysterectomy patients. Data based on questionnaire 1 year after hysterectomy.

[25]2002, randomised clinical trial including 146 total hysterectomy patients and 133 subtotal hysterectomy patients. Data based on cystometrography, flowmetry and questionnaire 1 year after hysterectomy.

[29]2004, randomised clinical trial including 158 total hysterectomy patients and 161 subtotal hysterectomy patients. Data based on questionnaire 1 year after hysterectomy.

[20]2003, observational study including 145 total hysterectomy patients, 76 subtotal hysterectomy patients and 89 vaginal hysterectomy patients. Data based on questionnaire 6 months after hysterectomy.

[29]2004, observational study including 80 total hysterectomy patients and 105 subtotal hysterectomy patients. Data based on questionnaire 1 year after hysterectomy.

problem should be solved by finding a suitable antibiotic regimen. Therefore, a total hysterectomy with appropriate antibiotic regimen is recommended. In difficult cases and in cases where a reduction in operation time is needed, subtotal hysterectomy could still be considered.

Key points for clinical practice

- More women seem to have urinary incontinence after subtotal hysterectomy than after total hysterectomy.

- Total hysterectomy takes longer to perform and has more intra-operative blood loss than subtotal hysterectomy.

- There is no difference between the hysterectomy methods regarding quality of life, bowel symptoms, lower urinary tract symptoms other than incontinence, pelvic pain and sexual life.

- A tendency towards more women with prolapse after subtotal hysterectomy and more women with urinary incontinence has generated the theory that the difference in the suspension during the operation procedures might be crucial.

- More postoperative complications, especially pyrexia and use of antibiotics, after total hysterectomy in one study suggests that the type and the dosage of intra-operative antibiotics are important.

- Of the women, 5–22% of the subtotally hysterectomised women have regular or irregular vaginal bleeding. Most women report that their daily activity is not influenced by the vaginal bleeding. However, they would have preferred to be without. Vaginal bleeding cannot be avoided by excision of the cervical canal.

- Although women have normal cervix cytology before subtotal hysterectomy, some develop abnormal cytology after subtotal hysterectomy. Thus, women having subtotal hysterectomy still require regular cervical cytology investigations postoperatively.

References

1. Drife J. Conserving the cervix at hysterectomy [Commentary]. *Br J Obstet Gynaecol* 1994; **101**: 563–564.
2. Ewies AAA, Olah KSJ. Subtotal abdominal hysterectomy: a surgical advance or a backward step? *Br J Obstet Gynaecol* 2000; **107**: 1376–1379.
3. Farquhar CM, Steiner CA. Hysterectomy rates in the United States 1990–1997. *Obstet Gynecol* 2002; **99**: 229–234.
4. Feridun M. The return of subtotal hysterectomy [Letter]. *Am J Obstet Gynecol* 2000; **182**: 1648–1649.
5. Geller SE, Burns LR, Brailer DJ. The impact of non-clinical factors on the practice variation: the case of hysterectomies. *Health Services Res* 1996; **30**: 729–750.
6. Gimbel H, Settnes A, Tabor A. Hysterectomy on benign indication in Denmark 1998. A register based trend analysis. *Acta Scand Gynecol Obstet* 2001; **80**: 267–272.

7. Gimbel H, Ottesen B, Tabor A. Danish gynecologists' opinion about hysterectomy on benign indication – results of a survey. *Acta Scand Gynecol Obstet* 2002; **81**: 1123–1131.
8. Gimbel H, Zobbe V, Andersen BM *et al.* Randomized controlled trial of total compared to subtotal hysterectomy with one-year follow up results. *Br J Obstet Gynaecol* 2003; **110**: 1088–1098.
9. Gimbel H, Zobbe V, Andersen BM *et al.* Lower urinary tract symptoms after total and subtotal hysterectomy. Results of a randomized controlled trial. *Int Urogyn J* 2005; In press.
10. Gimbel H, Zobbe V, Andersen BM *et al.* Total versus subtotal hysterectomy: an observational study with one-year follow up. *Aust NZ J Obstet Gynecol* 2005; **45**: 64–67.
11. Iosif CS, Bekassy Z, Rydhström H. Prevalence of urinary incontinence in middle-aged women. *Int J Gynaecol Obstet* 1988; **26**: 255.
12. Johns A. Supracervical versus total hysterectomy. *Clin Obstet Gynecol* 1997; **40**: 903–913.
13. Kilkku P. Abdominal hysterectomy versus supravaginal uterine amputation with reference to carcinoma of the cervical stump, urinary symptoms and sexual aspects. Academic dissertation, University of Turku, Finland 1982.
14. Lalos O, Bjerle P. Bladder, wall mechanics and micturition before and after subtotal and total hysterectomy. *Eur J Obstet Gynecol Reprod Biol* 1986; **21**: 143–150.
15. Learman LA, Summitt Jr RL, Varner E *et al.* for the Total or Supracervical Hysterectomy Research Group. A randomized comparison of total or supracervical hysterectomy: surgical complications and clinical outcomes. *Obstet Gynecol* 2003; **102**: 453–462.
16. Leonardo R-A. *History of Gynaecology*. New York: Foben, 1944.
17 Okara FO, Jones KD, Sutton C. Long term outcome following laparoscopic supracervical hysterectomy. *Br J Obstet Gynaecol* 2001; **108**: 1017–1020.
18. Roos NP. Hysterectomy: variations in rates across small areas and physicians' practices. *Am J Public Health* 1984; **74**: 327–335.
19. Roovers J-PWR, van der Bom JG, van der Vaart CH, Fousert DMM, Heintz PM. Does mode of hysterectomy influence micturition and defecation? *Acta Obstet Gynecol Scand* 2001; **80**: 945–951.
20. Roovers J-PWR, van der Bom JG, van der Vaart CH, Fousert DMM, Heintz PM. Hysterectomy and sexual well-being: prospective observational study of vaginal hysterectomy, subtotal abdominal hysterectomy and total abdominal hysterectomy. *BMJ* 2003; **327**: 774–778.
21. Ruoss CF. Supravaginal hysterectomy – a less invasive procedure. *J Obstet Gynecol* 1995; **15**: 406–409.
22. Scott JR, Sharp HT, Dodson MK, Norton PA, Warner HR. Subtotal hysterectomy in modern gynecology: a decision analysis. *Am J Obstet Gynecol* 1997; **176**: 1186–1192.
23. Sills ES, Saini J, Steiner CA, McGee 3rd M, Gretz 3rd HF. Abdominal hysterectomy practice patterns in the United States. *Int J Gynaecol Obstet* 1998; **63**: 277 283.
24. Thakar R, Manyonda I, Robinson G, Clarkson P, Stanton S. Total versus subtotal hysterectomy: a survey of current views and practice among British gynaecologists. *J Obstet Gynecol* 1998; **18**: 267–269.
25. Thakar R, Ayers S, Clarkson P, Stanton S, Manyonda I. Outcomes after total versus subtotal abdominal hysterectomy. *N Engl J Med* 2002; **347**: 1318–1325.
26. Thakar R, Ayers S, Georgakapolou A, Clarkson P, Stanton S, Manyonda I. Hysterectomy improves quality of life and decreases psychiatric symptoms: a prospective and randomised comparison of total versus subtotal hysterectomy. *Br J Obstet Gynaecol* 2004; **111**: 1115–1120.
27. Vuorma S, Teperi J, Hurskainen R, Keskimäki I, Kujansuu E. Hysterectomy trends in Finland in 1987–1995 – a register based analysis. *Acta Obstet Gynecol Scand* 1998; **77**: 770–776.
28. Yusuf F, Siedlecky S. Hysterectomy and endometrial ablation in New South Wales, 1981 to 1994–1995. *Aust NZ J Obstet Gynaecol* 1997; **37**: 210–216.
29. Zobbe V, Gimbel H, Andersen BM *et al.* Sexuality after total and subtotal hysterectomy. Results of a randomized clinical trial and a simultaneously performed observational study. *Acta Obstet Gynecol Scand* 2004; **83**: 191–196.

Gormlaith C. Hargaden Mary Keogan

14

Pelvic imaging of endometriosis

Endometriosis is defined as the presence of functioning endometrial tissue in a site outside the uterus. It is a common and debilitating condition occurring in up to 10% of women. Diagnosis has traditionally been by laparoscopy but recent advances in imaging technology have greatly improved non-operative diagnosis. Endometriomas in the ovary are usually relatively easily detected on ultrasound or MRI but the presence of small peritoneal deposits presents more of a challenge. This chapter will review the various imaging techniques available, describe the classic imaging findings in endometriosis and describe how endometriomas differ from other common pelvic pathology.

IMAGING MODALITIES

ULTRASOUND

Ultrasound is the first-line investigation of women suspected of having endometriosis due to its wide availability, good resolution, low cost and lack of ionising radiation. Three techniques are available – transabdominal, transvaginal and endorectal scanning. Transabdominal (TA) scanning is performed using a convex 3–5-MHz probe, and a full bladder is required to visualise the uterus and ovaries. Distension of the bladder helps to lift small bowel loops out of the field of view in addition to reducing the normal anteversion of the uterus. Transvaginal (TV) scanning is performed with a high resolution 6–10-MHz probe placed in the vagina; the procedure is well tolerated by most patients and many prefer this technique as a full bladder is

Gormlaith C. Hargaden MB MRCPI FFR(RCSI)
Specialist Registrar in Radiology, Department of Radiology, St James's Hospital, Dublin 8, Ireland

Mary Keogan MB MRCPI FRCR (for correspondence)
Consultant Radiologist, Department of Radiology, St James's Hospital, Dublin 8, Ireland and Senior Lecturer in Radiology, Trinity College Dublin, Ireland (E-mail: MKeogan@stjames.ie)

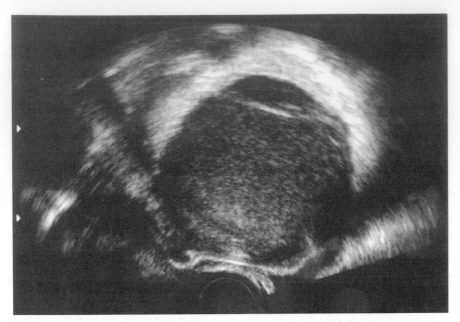

Fig. 1 Transvaginal ultrasound shows an enlarged right ovary with homogeneous echoes and cystic areas typical of endometriosis.

not required. Transvaginal scanning gives better resolution and image quality than the transabdominal technique. Transrectal scanning will be discussed later. Lesions on ultrasound are defined in terms of echogenicity with echogenic lesions appearing bright and hypo-echoic lesions appearing dark.

The main focus of TA and TV scanning is to visualise the ovaries and to characterise completely any cystic lesions in terms of internal echogenicity and wall morphology. Endometriomas have a wide variety of appearances on ultrasound but the more classical appearance is of a homogenous hypo-echoic mass within the ovary. The majority of lesions will have diffuse low-level internal echoes (Fig. 1) and only rarely is the lesion anechoic similar to a simple cyst. Lesions may be uni- or multilocular with either thin or thick septa; if nodularity of the wall is present, then a malignant lesion cannot be excluded on imaging alone.

Patel et al.,[1] in an extensive review of 252 adnexal masses seen on ultrasound, found that 95% of endometriomas display internal echoes and that a multiloculated mass with low-level echoes and no nodularity of the wall is 64 times more likely to be an endometrioma. Interestingly, 20% of the endometriomas displayed wall nodularity, a feature more usually associated with malignancy.

Wall nodularity should be differentiated from hyperechoic foci within the wall, as the latter, when identified in a lesion with low-level echoes and no malignant features, is very suggestive of an endometrioma. The pathological bases for these hyperechoic foci has not been clearly established but may relate to cholesterol deposits. Patel et al.[1] found that 35% of endometriomas had hyperechoic wall foci and this was the single highest predictor for endometrioma.

The differential diagnosis of an endometrioma includes dermoid cysts, haemorrhagic cysts and cystic neoplasms, all of which may look similar on ultrasound.[2] Dermoid cysts may contain fat (echogenic), fat-fluid levels or calcium (acoustic shadowing), which can help in the diagnosis. Differentiation between haemorrhagic cysts and endometriomas can prove more difficult; the former usually demonstrate high level internal echoes within a thin-walled cyst but, with time, may evolve and appear more complex. Fibrin formation may mimic thin septa but with interval scanning these lesions usually resolve. Patient history is also helpful in making the diagnosis of an acute haemorrhagic cyst as the symptoms are usually more acute. If a cyst has soft-tissue components, then a malignant lesion must be excluded.

Endorectal ultrasound is performed to look at the sigmoid for evidence of bowel infiltration by endometriosis. The technique involves: (i) placement of a 6–10-MHz probe within the rectum; (ii) the use of a flexible probe[3] which allows more distal placement in the sigmoid; and (iii) patient preparation requiring a rectal enema prior to the examination, but sedation is not required. The advantage of the endorectal position is that similar to the transvaginal technique the probe is close to the disease location, which increases the resolution and diagnostic accuracy. Unfortunately, the field of visualisation is quite restricted and only the distal bowel is imaged. Ultrasound of the bowel demonstrates five alternating hyper- and hypo-echoic layers and endometriotic deposits appear as rounded or triangular hypo-echoic deposits. Infiltration of the bowel wall can be seen as thickening of the muscularis propria.

A number of authors have looked at the use of endorectal ultrasound in patients with suspected endometriosis. Bazot et al.,[4] in a prospective study of 30 patients, reported sensitivity of 82%, with a specificity of 88% in the diagnosis of rectosigmoid endometriosis. More recently, Chapron et al.[3] reported sensitivity and specificity of 97% and 89%, respectively, with the use of endorectal ultrasound and they also found that it was superior to MRI for the diagnosis of rectal involvement in patients with endometriosis.

Endorectal ultrasound may also have a role in the diagnosis of rectovaginal endometriosis although the studies to date involve relatively small patient numbers. Fedele et al.[5] looked at 34 patients with deeply infiltrating endometriosis of the vagina and uterosacral ligaments and reported sensitivity and specificity of 80% and 97%, respectively. Further work is required but the initial results are promising.

In summary, ultrasound is an inexpensive and readily available technique for imaging the pelvis in patients with suspected endometriosis. Many of these patients are young and will undergo repeated investigations; ultrasound has the advantage of not only providing a quick and well-tolerated test but also avoiding the use of ionising radiation. The typical appearance of an endometrioma on ultrasound is that of a homogeneous hypo-echoic mass within the ovary with low-level internal echoes. Lesions may be uni- or multilocular and the presence of hyperechoic lesions within the wall is highly suggestive of an endometrioma. Transrectal scanning can be a useful technique to look for rectosigmoid deposits and possibly for assessing the rectovaginal area.

MAGNETIC RESONANCE IMAGING (MRI)

MRI is becoming more readily available and has the advantage of imaging the entire pelvis in multiple planes at a single examination. Images are obtained

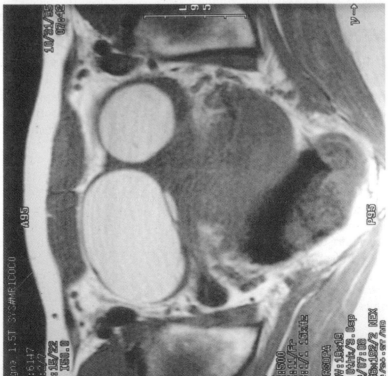

2A

2B

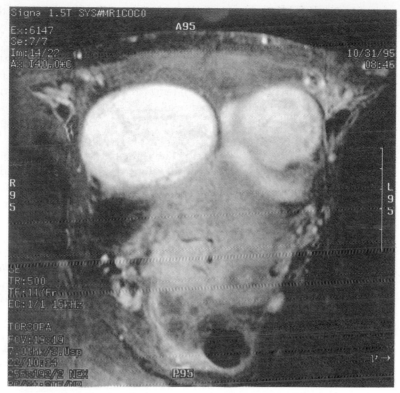

Fig. 2 (A) Small field of view axial MR image of the pelvis, T1 weighted, shows 2 well-defined bright masses consistent with dermoid cysts or endometriomas. (B) The same patient as in (A). T2-weighted image showing 'shading' effect of layering dark signal within masses typical of endometriomas. (C) Same patient as above. T1 weighted image to which fat saturation has been applied. Persistence of high signal within masses indicates blood products within endometriomas and excludes the possibility of dermoid cysts.

using a strong magnetic field in conjunction with various applied pulse sequences; where possible, a dedicated pelvic coil should be used. The use of the correct imaging sequences is critical to maximise diagnostic accuracy. Standard sequences include T1 (where water is dark and fat and fresh haemorrhage are bright) and T2 (where water is very bright and fat is also quite bright). Lesions that contain degenerated blood products, including methaemoglobin and concentrated protein, may appear bright on both T1- and T2-weighted sequences. The addition of a fat-suppressed T1 sequence (where the normally bright fat is now dark in signal) is critical, as this sequence is extremely useful in differentiating fat containing structures, such as dermoid cysts, from haemorrhagic lesions such as endometriomas. The use of contrast agents in endometriosis has not been shown to be helpful unless a malignant lesion is suspected. All sequences can be performed in multiple imaging plane – axial, sagital or coronal – with the sagital plane particularly useful for evaluating the cul-de-sac and rectum.

Endometriomas or 'chocolate cysts' of the ovary are mass lesions that contain blood products of various ages as a result of cyclical bleeding. They are usually seen on MR as hyperintense (bright) lesions on a T1-weighted sequence, and on T2 they are usually more hypo-intense (darker) with foci of hyperintensity, which gives the classical appearance of 'shading' (Fig. 2). Shading is due to the presence of blood products of various ages, and can range from very subtle layering to a complete signal void (black). The differentiation of endometriomas from haemorrhagic cysts can be difficult on MRI as both contain blood products; haemorrhagic cysts tend to be unilocular, do not demonstrate 'shading' and usually resolve on follow-up imaging. Diagnosing dermoid cysts is easier due to the presence of fat in these lesions, which on fat-suppressed sequences loses signal and becomes dark.

Endometrial deposits are typically found in the rectovaginal septum, the uterine ligaments and the muscular wall of the pelvis.[6] These solid nodules can be seen as a low-intermediate signal on T1 with punctate areas of high signal, and of uniform low signal on T2. The areas of high signal result from haemorrhage surrounded by fibrotic tissue. Unfortunately, the diagnosis of small deposits remains difficult with any combination of signal possible; although they can demonstrate enhancement post contrast, this is neither sensitive nor specific. Associated tubal abnormalities can be present in 30% of women with endometriosis. Dilated fallopian tubes from endometriosis may demonstrate high signal on T1 and also on T2, and their tubular nature can be readily apparent on multiplanar imaging helping to differentiate them from adnexal masses.

Involvement of the bowel is reported in 12–37% of patients. Direct visualisation of visceral deposits on MRI is possible. The commonest sites of involvement are the anterior and lateral rectal walls where low signal irregular thickening can be identified. Chapron et al.[3] reported sensitivity and specificity of 76% and 97%, respectively, using MR in the diagnosis of rectal endometriosis; although MR was more specific than endorectal ultrasound, the latter was more sensitive and had a higher negative predictive value. Endometriosis commonly results in the formation of adhesions, which may be diagnosed on MR as low-signal areas of stranding or suggested by the presence of a fixed retroverted uterus, angulated loops of bowel or displacement of the ovaries. However, the role of imaging in the diagnosis of adhesions is rather limited.

Although 20% of patients with endometriosis may have involvement of the genito-urinary system, they are usually asymptomatic except in the case of severe pelvic disease. The urinary bladder is most frequently involved with deposits usually on the serosal surface but occasionally infiltrating the muscle to appear as intraluminal masses. With MRI, the serosal deposits (typically at the dome of the bladder) as well as the infiltrating lesions can be clearly identified (Fig. 3). Characteristically, a hypo-intense mass with areas of hyperintensity is identified forming an obtuse angle with the bladder wall. Involvement of the ureters may result in stricture formation and secondary hydronephrosis which is well visualised on coronal imaging although the findings are non-specific.

Several authors have looked at the role of MRI in patients with endo-metriosis. Stratton et al.[7] looked at 48 women with suspected endometriosis and compared the findings at MRI with subsequent surgery and histopathology. They reported a sensitivity of 69% for detecting biopsy-proven endometriosis with a specificity of 75%. MRI detected most endometriomas (82%) and peritoneal defects (72%) visualised and excised at surgery. MRI

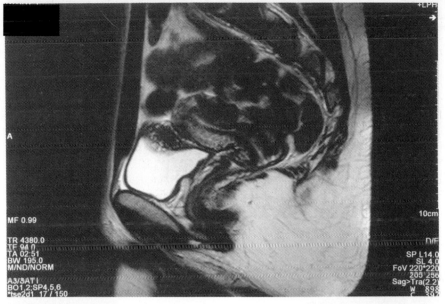

Fig. 3 Sagital T2-weighted image showing a mass involving the dome of the bladder. Note punctate areas of high signal (bright dots) indicate the presence of haemorrhage within a focus of endometriosis.

suggested the diagnosis in all patients with severe disease but overall identified fewer areas of endometriosis than surgery and was relatively insensitive in defining the extent of disease. These findings were similar to those of Tanaka *et al.*[8] who correctly identified 74% of cases and Ha *et al.*[9] who reported a sensitivity of 61% by fat-suppressed MRI, although the findings were less encouraging than those of Takahashi et al (10), who identified all lesions seen at surgery.

More recently, Bazot *et al.*[11] reported on 195 patients with suspected endometriosis and compared the MRI findings with surgery and histopathology. Overall, they reported a sensitivity of 90% with a specificity of 91%, and this rose to 98% and 87%, respectively, for the diagnosis of endometriomas. One of the reasons for their increased sensitivity may be attributable to the high prevalence of pelvic endometriosis and, specifically, of deep pelvic endometriosis in their study population.

In summary, in women with suspected endometriosis, MRI is sensitive for the diagnosis of endometriomas with the characteristic hyperintense lesion on T1 and 'shading' on T2. Although MRI may be helpful in diagnosis of endometrial deposits elsewhere within the pelvis, it is less sensitive than laparoscopy.

OTHER IMAGING TECHNIQUES

Ultrasound and MRI are the main imaging techniques in the diagnostic work-up of patients with endometriosis. However, some patients, in whom the diagnosis may not be suspected, undergo more traditional investigations such as barium enema or intravenous urography. The appearances of bowel deposits on double contrast barium enema can be varied. Typically, the deposits are serosal causing thickening and fibrosis of the muscularis propria,

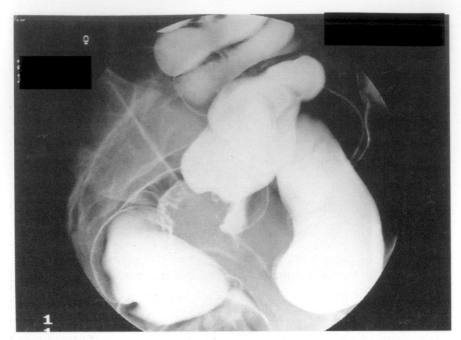

Fig. 4 Lateral view from a barium enema shows an eccentric impression on the wall of the sigmoid colon consistent with endometriosis in the cul-de-sac.

which is demonstrated as asymmetric narrowing with a crenulated or puckered appearance of the affected wall (Fig. 4). The differential diagnosis includes metastatic deposits and, if the lesion is more circumferential, it can be confused with an annular colon carcinoma, although this would be unusual.

On intravenous urography, serosal deposits may be seen at the dome of the bladder particularly if they have infiltrated the wall. On imaging, differentiation from a tumour is usually not possible and cystoscopy and biopsy are necessary. Involvement of the ureters is seen as a short- or medium-length tapering stricture, which may cause complete obstruction of the ureter with secondary hydronephrosis. The findings are non-specific and other causes of a ureteral stricture should be considered.

Computed tomography (CT) has not been particularly useful in this patient population. As in most pelvic conditions, the relative lack of resolution in visualisation of the ovaries and fallopian tubes with CT makes it less useful than MRI or ultrasound.

CONCLUSIONS

Ultimately, the diagnosis of endometriosis is based on histopathology; however, imaging is playing an increasingly important role in both diagnosis and follow-up. The major advantage of diagnostic imaging is that it is non-invasive and does not have the complications of laparoscopy. Ultrasound should be the first-line investigation with selected cases proceeding to MRI. Imaging can provide useful information but a significant number of patients with endometriosis may have normal findings.

Key points for clinical practice

- Endometriomas are often multiloculated lesions usually with low-level internal echoes on ultrasound.

- The presence of foci of high echogenicity within the wall on ultrasound is very suggestive of an endometrioma.

- Although up to 20% of endometriomas will demonstrate nodularity within the wall on ultrasound, any lesion that contains a soft tissue component should be regarded as malignant until proven otherwise.

- Haemorrhagic cysts can be confused with endometriomas on ultrasound but these are usually thin-walled cysts with high-level internal echoes that resolve with time.

- On MRI, endometriomas are classically hyperintense on T1 and hypointense with foci of hyperintensity on T2 known as 'shading'. This is due to the presence of degraded blood products.

- Fat-suppression sequences are useful in differentiating dermoid cysts from endometriomas on MRI.

- MRI can demonstrate peritoneal and deep pelvic deposits but is less sensitive than laparoscopy.

References

1. Patel MD, Feldstein VA, Chen DC, Lipson SD, Filly RA. Endometriomas: diagnostic performance of US. *Radiology* 1999; **210**: 739–745.
2. Woodward PJ, Sohaey R, Mezzetti Jr TP. Endometriosis: radiologic–pathologic correlation. *Radiographics* 2001; **21**: 193–216.
3. Chapron C, Vieira M, Chopin N et al. Accuracy of rectal endoscopic ultrasonography and magnetic resonance imaging in the diagnosis of rectal involvement for patients presenting with deeply infiltrating endometriosis. *Ultrasound Obstet Gynecol* 2004; **24**: 175–179.
4. Bazot M, Detchev R, Cortez A et al. Transvaginal sonography and rectal endoscopic sonography for the assessment of pelvic endometriosis; a preliminary comparison. *Hum Reprod* 2003; **18**: 1686–1692.
5. Fedele L, Bianchi S, Portuese A, Borruto F, Dorta M. Transrectal ultrasonography. I. The assessment of rectovaginal endometriosis. *Obstet Gynecol* 1998; **91**: 444–448.
6. Gougoutas CA, Siegelman ES, Hunt J, Outwater EK. Pelvic endometriosis: various manifestations and MR imaging findings. *Am J Roentgenol* 2000; **175**: 353–358.
7. Stratton P, Winkel C, Premkumar A et al. Diagnostic accuracy of laparoscopy, magnetic resonance imaging, and histopathologic examination for the detection of endometriosis. *Fertil Steril* 2003; **79**: 1078–1085.
8. Tanaka YO, Itai Y, Anno I et al. MR staging of pelvic endometriosis: role of fat-suppression T1-weighted images. *Radiat Med* 1996; **14**: 111–116.
9. Ha HK, Lim YT, Kim HS et al. Diagnosis of pelvic endometriosis: fat suppressed T1 weighted versus conventional MR. *Am J Roentgenol* 1994; **163**: 127–131.
10. Takahashi K, Okada M, Okada S et al. Studies on the detection of small endometrial implants by magnetic resonance imaging using a fat saturation technique. *Gynecol Obstet Invest* 1996; **41**: 203–206.
11. Bazot M, Darai E, Hourani R et al. Deep pelvic endometriosis: MR imaging for diagnosis and prediction of extension of disease. *Radiology* 2004; **232**: 379–389.

Enda McVeigh Philippe R. Koninckx

15

Surgery for advanced endometriosis

Endometriosis is characterised by the presence of glandular and stromal tissue in areas outside the uterus. It has been considered for decades as the result of the implantation of retrograde menstruated endometrial cells (Sampson's theory),[1] or as metaplasia[2,3] induced by menstrual debris or as lymphatic spread.[4,5] It occurs most frequently in the pelvic organs and peritoneum and is prevalent in 2.5–3.3% of women in the reproductive age. The evidence to support Sampson's theory seemed convincing: (i) transplantation of endometrium could induce endometriosis; (ii) retrograde menstruation occurred in almost all women;[6,7] menstrual fluid contained viable cells;[8] and (iv) endometrial cells can implant on the peritoneum.[9] The initial non-pigmented or subtle lesions were believed to progress to typical, cystic ovarian endometriosis and/or deep infiltrating endometriosis, and this was assumed to be the natural history of the disease (Fig. 1).[10–12] Endometriosis thus was considered as normal endometrial cells in an abnormal location and in an abnormal environment (*i.e.* the peritoneal fluid).[13]

This hypothesis of implantation/metaplasia and progression to more severe disease, however, has never been proved formally, and has been challenged by new concepts emphasising cellular differences (*e.g.* in the endometrial cells and in the endometriotic cells). From 'a normal cell in an abnormal location', endometriosis has become 'abnormal cells in an abnormal location'. This has led to the hypothesis that typical and severe endometriosis should be considered as a benign tumour, whereas subtle endometriosis could become a physiological condition occurring intermittently in all women. Only following cellular changes (*e.g.* a mutation), can these subtle lesions evolve into typical, deep

Enda McVeigh MB BCh BAO MPhil MRCOG (for correspondence)
Senior Fellow and Honorary Consultant, Nuffield Department of Obstetrics and Gynaecology, John Radcliffe Hospital, University of Oxford, Oxford OX3 9DU, UK
(E-mail: enda.mcveigh@obstetrics-gynaecology.oxford.ac.uk)

Philippe R. Koninckx MD PhD
Professor of Obstetrics and Gynaecology, University Hospital Gasthuisberg, Catholic University Leuven, B-3000 Leuven, Belgium (E-mail: philippe.koninckx@med.kuleuven.ac.be)

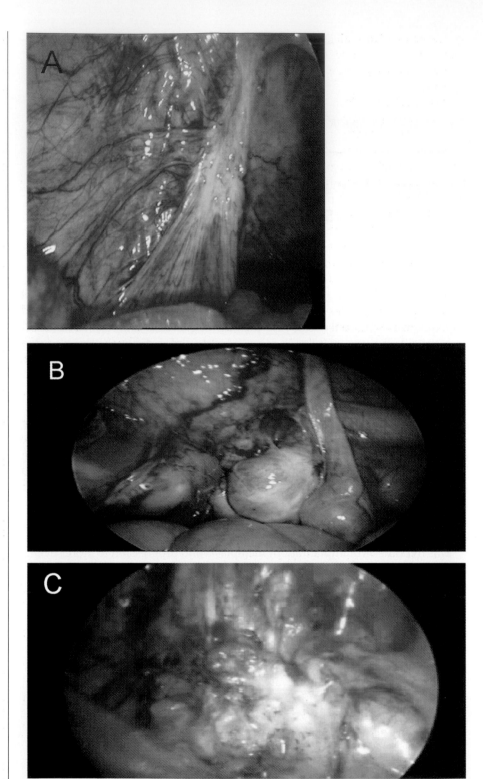

Fig. 1 Forms of endometriosis. (A) Peritoneal implant of endometriosis; (B) Bilateral cystic ovarian endometriosis; (C) Rectovaginal nodule of endometriosis.

or cystic ovarian endometriosis. To mark the difference between normal and abnormal cells, subtle endometriosis has been proposed as 'endometriosis', whereas the benign tumours (*i.e.* typical, cystic and deep) be called 'endometriotic disease'.[14]

Endometriosis is a surgical diagnosis. In hospital-based populations, however, the prevalence of endometriosis will vary depending on the type of the population being studied. For example, it is seen more frequently among women being investigated for infertility (21%) than among those undergoing sterilisation (6%). The incidence of endometriosis among those women being investigated for chronic abdominal pain is 15%, while among those undergoing abdominal hysterectomy, it can be as high as 25%.[15]

From a clinical history, the diagnosis of endometriosis may be assumed. The principal symptoms associated with endometriosis namely dysmenorrhoea, dyspareunia and pelvic pain are common. Establishing the diagnosis can be difficult because the presentation is so variable and considerable overlap can occur with other conditions such as irritable bowel syndrome and pelvic inflammatory disease. As a result, there is often delay between symptom onset and surgical diagnosis; this equates to about 3.5 years in adult women and over 10 years when onset occurs in adolescents.[16] The choice of treatment will depend upon the woman's age, her fertility plans, previous treatment, the nature and severity of the symptoms, and the location and severity of disease. Women with endometriosis-associated infertility and pain may have to decide which is the major priority as there is no evidence that hormonal therapy alone improves fertility.[17]

Medical management of endometriosis is a management strategy only in that it is not curative. For a cure of symptoms, the surgical removal of the ectopic endometrial glands is required. As the majority of women with endometriosis desire to maintain their fertility, the treatment modality that offers the least invasion and is also less expensive is desirable. The strategy for surgery is to remove the ectopic endometrial tissue and restore normal pelvic anatomy.

HISTORY OF SURGICAL TECHNIQUES

During the last 25 years, over 500 articles dealing directly with surgery in the title and over 1800 with surgery in the abstract were published. The vast majority of these articles have been observational studies or personal series with few randomised controlled trials (RCTs) in this area. This is especially true when dealing with severe endometriosis. The reason is probably that in the past 30 years there has been a rapid evolution in techniques and equipment, where the importance of training has clearly been shown. This set of circumstances has resulted in individual endometriosis surgeons and centres having progressively changed/improved their techniques with few, if any, of the individual surgeons claiming to be equally fluent with several techniques. Any RCT would thus risk being an evaluation of the surgeon rather than the technique. Some of the more notable RCTs[18] have thus been performed in one centre with one technique.

Up to the end of the 1970s, minimal and mild endometriosis was destroyed endoscopically by heat application (endothermia) and by unipolar or bipolar coagulation. Treatment of more severe endometriotic disease tended to result in radical surgery with hysterectomy, adnexectomies and anterior resections of the rectum often in young women.

In the late 1970s and the early 1980s, microsurgery was introduced, emphasising gentle tissue handling and careful destruction of superficial endometriosis by bipolar coagulation or resection and removal of cystic ovarian endometriosis followed by reconstruction of the ovary. The stripping technique for ovarian endometriosis was developed during this period and the 60% fertility results still can be considered as a key reference for non-destructive surgery.[19,20]

In the 1990s, deep endometriosis was recognised increasingly during laparoscopic surgery or by clinical examination. 'Resection of deep endometriosis' comprises techniques which vary from debulking, to complete discoid excision to resection–re-anastomosis of the rectum with large margins mimicking oncological surgery. These differences in technique are rarely stated clearly in the literature, thus making interpretation difficult. Another important and growing bias is the severity of deep endometriosis reported. In some series, deep endometriosis comprises mainly lesions larger than 1 cm^3; in other reports, lesions are limited to slightly deeper typical lesions. It is not surprising that in the former series deep lesions are generally unique, whereas in the latter series deep lesions are described as multifocal especially in the uterosacral ligaments.

TECHNIQUES OF SURGERY AND DIFFERENT ENERGY FORMS

Internationally, a number of centres of excellence exist for the surgery of advanced endometriosis. A variety of techniques are used in the approach to this difficult and challenging surgery. What is of importance, however, is that the results from these centres of excellence all seem to be equivalent. The majority of surgeons operating on advanced endometriosis will use some form of energy, the main two being electrical energy or CO_2-laser energy.

CO_2-laser surgery and electrosurgery differ in their energy characteristics and by the mode of application. The CO_2-laser energy is almost completely absorbed by water. The effect is thus a very superficial heating and, provided sufficient energy is used, instantaneously heating to temperatures inducing a vaporisation of tissue, with little thermal spread (*i.e.* less than 100 µm). To obtain this effect, the laser energy has to be focused on a small area. Theoretically, spot diameters of less than 0.5 mm can be achieved, but this requires a perfect lens and working at the exact focal distance. In addition, the CO_2 gas (from the pneumoperitoneum) in the laser channel of the laparoscope is heated by adsorption of the laser beam which results in widening of the spot diameter, an effect known as blooming. Therefore, cooling continuously the CO_2 of the laser channel (e.g. with an high flow insufflator or using a CO_2 isotope to generate the laser beam) is mandatory for a quality cut. The most important difference with electrosurgery is that the energy output is constant over time. The quality of cut, therefore, is constant whereas the depth varies with speed of movement of the beam over the tissue. The CO_2 laser has the advantage of coagulating smaller vessels thus providing a rather bloodless cut. Using a defocused beam offers the versatility of vaporising larger areas, or of

Fig. 2 The difference between laser and electrosurgery in the angle of access to the tissues.

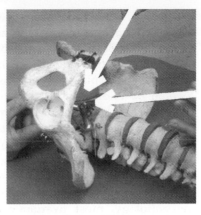

applying only superficial heat as in flowering a hydrosalpinx. The major drawback of CO_2-laser surgery is the cost of equipment, the smoke production during vaporisation and the blooming in the laparoscope.

Electrosurgery has the advantage of being more versatile, resulting in heating and coagulation below 200 V and in sparking with local heating of the air and the adjacent tissue and thus vaporisation above 200 V. Higher voltages, will, in addition, heat the tissue causing coagulation (*i.e.* damage). This was known in the past as blended current in electrosurgical units without voltage stabiliser. The quality of the cut is thus voltage dependent, and at exactly 200 V (*i.e.* with minimal sparking), the quality of a CO_2 laser and of an electrosurgical cut is comparable with similar limited tissue damage. The most important difference is that the energy output of electrosurgery is not constant since it essentially depends on the impedance of the tissues and on the area of contact between the electrode and the tissue. At higher output settings, the intensity of the current will be limited only by the impedance being smaller or higher according to the area of contact (*i.e.* the depth of cutting). Electrosurgery thus easily cuts to a constant depth notwithstanding an irregular surface. Limiting the energy output is not realistic, unless with a needle electrode in microsurgery, since any increase in contact area will result in a drop in voltage and thus will stop cutting and start coagulation.

Another difference between laser and electrosurgery is the angle of access to the tissues: the laser beam used through the laparoscope will have an almost horizontal access to the rectovaginal septum (Fig. 2). Energy used though the secondary ports will have a more vertical line of access, and this difference increases when secondary ports are introduced lower in the abdomen.

Finally, almost all laser surgery for endometriosis can be performed with two secondary ports only, placed low in the abdomen. For electrosurgery, generally three secondary ports are necessary, which for ergonomic reasons have to be placed higher in the abdomen.

CYSTIC OVARIAN ENDOMETRIOSIS

PHYSIOPATHOLOGY

The physiopathology of cystic endometriosis is not entirely understood. Many cystic ovarian endometriosis may originate from invagination of superficial implants.[21] When the ovary becomes adherent to the pelvic wall by endometriotic implants, it appears that a 'pseudocyst' is formed by the accumulation of old blood and debris, thus stretching the ovarian capsule over this cyst. This phenomenon of invagination and stretching of the ovarian capsule could explain why the inside of the cyst wall is not always entirely covered by endometriosis, which may be localised as focal endometriotic spots. It seems logical to suggest that only these endometriotic spots should be destroyed, and that removal of the cyst wall is equivalent to removing the ovarian surface. This mechanism of invagination and stretching of the ovarian capsule does not preclude that some cysts have a different origin. Careful histology of the cyst wall, moreover, reveals that endometriotic glands can be present in the 'so-called' cyst wall up to a depth of at least 5–6 mm. Whatever the aetiology, most ovarian cysts are clonal in origin, as repeatedly demonstrated.

SURGICAL MANAGEMENT AND THE SIZE OF THE OVARIAN CYST

From a surgical point of view, the size of the ovarian cyst is most important. For smaller cysts (< 5 cm), the cyst wall can generally be stripped easily from the ovary. This process seems to follow a natural plane of cleavage, confirmed indirectly by the lack of bleeding. For cysts larger than 5 cm diameter, the decision whether the cyst wall should be removed or destroyed, or whether a focal treatment will be sufficient is purely academic. Indeed, in those women with a large cyst, the remaining ovarian rim will be so thin that resection becomes either technically impossible or practically unrealistic since minimal or no ovarian tissue will be left. Also, the extensive vaporisation of these very large areas is unrealistic.

METHODS OF TREATMENT

Aspiration and rinsing of cystic ovarian endometriosis has been attempted but the recurrence rate is high. Ultrasound-guided aspiration will result in endometriotic fluid in the pelvis which, as reported during IVF, may result in pelvic infections and abscess formation. This fluid in the pelvis may also increase adhesion formation although chocolate fluid was shown not to induce adhesions when injected intraperitoneally in mice.

For smaller cysts (less than 5 cm diameter), the method of stripping the cyst from the ovary as initially described by the Clermont Ferrand group is our method of choice. It is rapid, technically easy, and results in a complete treatment especially when invading glands are present. Following adhesiolysis, drainage and rinsing, we incise with the CO_2 laser the ovarian capsule around the cyst opening. Once the plane of cleavage is found, the cyst wall is easily stripped from the ovary. The laser can assist cleavage in the right plane and prevent the ovarian capsule from been torn in the wrong direction. Closure of the ovary by tissue glue or a suture when the remaining ovarian flaps are unequal in size is suggested although not proven to be necessary.

Some concern has been reported that ovarian cystectomy may result in inadvertent removal or destruction of primordial follicles at the same time and thus reduce ovarian volume and reserve, and diminish fertility. To avoid this,

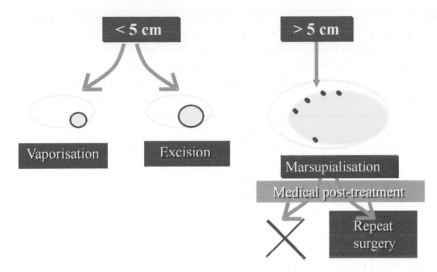

Fig. 3 Treatment of cystic ovarian endometriosis.

replacing cystectomy by fenestration and coagulation of the inner wall of the endometriotic ovarian cyst has been suggested. Some excellent results have been reported using this methodology but too superficial destruction resulted in inadequate treatment and deep destruction often caused bleeding. The third option besides wall excision and wall destruction is focal treatment, but this is overall equivalent to vaporisation.

For larger cysts, the pragmatism of size practically excludes excision and/or vaporisation. A two-stage procedure can be performed. At the first operation, a large window is made in the cyst wall, followed by rinsing, some focal treatment, no adhesiolysis and, postoperatively, 3 months of GnRH agonist treatment is given. If by ultrasound the cyst persists or reforms, this small cyst is treated during a second operation by excision. If no cyst is found, a second intervention may not be necessary in the absence of pain or infertility. This concept has the indirect advantage that the first operation can always be scheduled as a day case, without bowel preparation, whereas the necessity of a bowel preparation for the second intervention will be known in advance (Fig. 3).

RESULTS

In a case-control study,[22] cumulative clinical pregnancy rates and recurrence rates were comparable in women treated with cystectomy and with fenestration/coagulation after 36 months, but faster conception occurred in the fenestration/coagulation group. A more recent case-control study in 231 patients[23] reported a lower cumulative re-operation rate in the cyst excision group than in the fenestration/coagulation group after 18 (6% versus 22%) and 42 (24% versus 59%) months of follow-up. Furthermore, a randomised controlled trial[24] demonstrated that pain and subfertility caused by ovarian endometrioma were improved more by cystectomy than by fenestration/coagulation. A reduced recurrence of pain after 2 years (OR, 0.2; 95% CI, 0.05–0.77), an increased pain-free interval after operation (19 months versus 9.5 months) and an increased pregnancy rate (67%

Table 1 Removal versus ablation	
Recurrence after coagulation or laser	18.4%
Recurrence after cystectomy	6.4%

Data from a systematic review of four comparative trials (common odds ratio, 3.09; 95% CI, 1.78–5.36).[25]

versus 23%; OR, 2.83; 95% CI, 1.01–7.5) was found in the cystectomy group when compared to the fenestration/coagulation group. Systematic review of four comparative trials[25] looking at recurrence rates of endometrioma after coagualtion or laser compared to cystectomy showed an odds ratio of 3.09 (95% CI, 1.78–5.36) with a lower recurrence rate in the cystectomy group (Table 1). When ovarian function during IVF was considered in the two groups (vaporisation or cystectomy), neither appeared to compromise outcome.[26,27] Therefore, based on the current evidence, ovarian cystectomy seems to be the method of choice.

For larger cysts, no clear data are available favouring one or another technique. The size of the cyst, however, seems to dictate either an oophorectomy in women where fertility is not a factor or in a two-step surgery in women who want to preserve fertility.

DEEP ENDOMETRIOSIS

DIAGNOSIS, TYPES AND PREVALENCE

Endometriosis can infiltrate the surrounding tissues resulting in a sclerotic and inflammatory reaction which can translate clinically into nodularity, bowel stenosis and ureteral obstruction. The most severe forms such as rectovaginal endometriosis and endometriosis invading the rectum or the sigmoid have been known since the beginning of this century. These conditions, however, are relatively rare with an estimated prevalence of less than 1%.

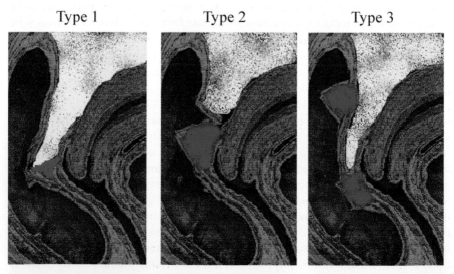

Fig. 4 Deep rectovaginal or sigmoidal endometriosis.

The endoscopic excision of endometriosis has revealed that endometriosis invading deeper than 5–6 mm is associated with pain and infertility. Three subtypes were described (Fig, 4).[28] Type I is characterised by a large pelvic area of typical and sometimes some subtle endometriotic lesions surrounded by white sclerotic tissue. Only during excision does it become obvious that the endometriotic lesion infiltrates deeper than 5 mm. Typically, the endometriotic area becomes progressively smaller as it grows deeper; the lesion is thus cone shaped.

Type II lesions are characterised by retraction of the bowel. Clinically, they are recognised by the obvious bowel retraction around a small typical lesion. In some women, however, no endometriosis can be seen through the laparoscope, and the bowel retraction is the only clinical sign. Diagnosis is generally not too difficult since during laparoscopy the retraction, under which an induration is felt, is obvious. In some women, however, the retraction is not seen and the induration can be hardly felt. Only during excision does the endometriotic nodule become apparent, emphasising the need for a pre-operative diagnosis and training in recognising these lesions.

Type III lesions are spherical endometriotic nodules in the rectovaginal septum. In their most typical form, these lesions are felt as painful nodularities in the rectovaginal septum. At laparoscopy, they generally present as a small typical lesion; in some women, a careful vaginal examination reveals some dark blue cysts (3–4 mm) in the posterior fornix. Type III lesions are the most severe lesions, and they often spread laterally up and around the uterine artery, sometimes causing sclerosis around the ureter. Sclerosing endometriosis invading the sigmoid is similar to the rectal endometriosis, but is situated 10 cm above the rectovaginal septum. This is another form of deep endometriosis, which is fortunately a rare condition and could be classified as type IV. By pathology, types II, III and IV are similar and present as adenomyosis externa (*i.e.* a glands and stroma in large areas of hyalinous muscular tissue). Since the pouch of Douglas is obliterated in women with deep endometriosis, it seems likely that these three lesions are pathophysiologically similar, type III being situated in the pouch of Douglas on the wall opposing the vaginal wall. Subsequently, the pouch is closed by retraction, giving the erroneous impression that these lesions are situated in the rectovaginal septum, which starts lower. These lesions are often vaginally visible since the distance between vaginal wall and peritoneal cavity is hardly 3–4 mm. The type II lesions are situated higher, generally between the back of the uterus and the rectosigmoid, whereas a lesion at the level of the sigmoid generally is not adherent to the surrounding structures, except occasionally to the ureter under the infundibulo pelvic ligament. These concepts seem to constitute another argument to differentiate between slightly larger and deeper typical lesions, the infiltrative type I deep endometriosis, and those with larger nodules, massive retraction and by pathology adenomyosis externa. The pathophysiology remains a subject of debate.

Diagnosis of deep endometriosis should be made before surgery. A retrospective analysis showed that by a routine clinical examination only 50% of the larger lesions are diagnosed. A menstrual clinical examination is the most powerful tool available to diagnose deep endometriosis types I, II and III. By clinical examination during menstruation,[29] painful nodularities are found in some 30% of women with pain or infertility. In the absence of cystic ovarian

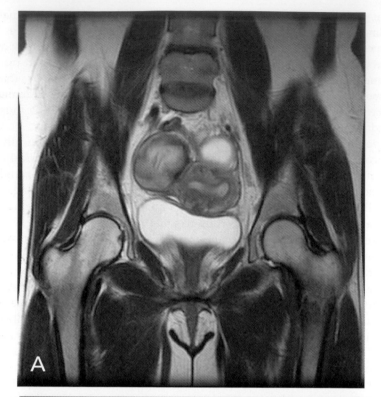

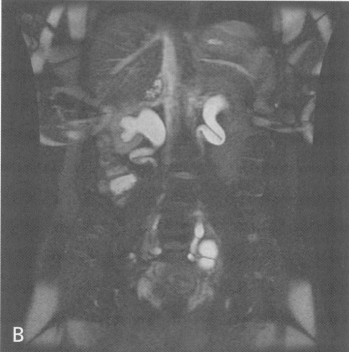

Fig. 5 Use of MRI in endometriosis. (A) MRI showing rectal involvement; (B) bilateral ureteric obstruction due to pelvic endometriosis.

endometriosis, these nodularities were in most of the women caused by deep endometriosis. Ultrasound and MRI can be used to diagnose deep endometriosis (Fig. 5), but their sensitivity is low especially for the smaller lesions. For type IV lesions, a contrast enema and/or a rectoscopy are necessary. Although hard data are not available, we presume that this diagnosis is easily missed, making prevalence higher than actually believed.

SURGICAL TREATMENT

Surgery for deep endometriosis is unpredictably difficult with the risk of severe complications. Therefore, a pre-operative ultrasound, contrast enema and intravenous pyelography are necessary in many cases, together with a full pre-operative bowel preparation. Surgery should be carefully planned. This planning comprises pre-operative ureter stenting if gross ureteric distortion or hydronephrosis is present together with the eventual collaboration of an urologist to perform ureter re-anastomosis or repair, bladder suturing, or ureter re-implantation. Pre operative planning often requires the collaboration of a colorectal surgeon, since surgery can unpredictably extend from a discoid excision with a muscularis defect, to a resection of the rectum or sigmoid wall necessitating suture, to a large transmural nodule requiring a resection anastomosis if the defect is too large. In the case of a combined rectal and sigmoid nodule which cannot be sutured, a pouch anastomosis requiring mobilisation of the left hemicolon will be required (Fig. 6). The type of lesion will also determine the position of the secondary trocars which have to be placed higher for a sigmoid lesion than for a rectum lesion.

The surgical excision of deep endometriosis relies upon a combination of visual inspection and tactile information. For the treatment of rectovaginal endometriosis up to the rectosigmoid, we prefer a CO_2 laser (80 W, Sharplan) with a high flow insufflator (Thermoflator, Storz AG)[30] which is mandatory for smoke evacuation and cooling the laser beam. Guided by visual inspection together with tactile information of the softness of the tissue, the peritoneum is incised below the lesion at the border between the normal soft tissue and the harder endometriosis. Endometriosis, moreover, glows yellowish in colour under the CO_2 laser beam. First, the lesion is circumscribed to mark the limits which are useful during later excision. Second, the lateral edges of the nodule are dissected to free the nodule if necessary from the ureter, the uterine artery, and from the sacrospinal ligament. This is technically the most difficult part of the surgery, since the lesion is often very deep and posterior and because of the presence of larger arteries and the nerve. If necessary, the lateral borders of the sigmoid have to be dissected and followed with identification of the ureters. Third, the pararectal spaces are identified. This marks the lateral edges of the nodule and, once identified, dissection is bluntly continued downwards. Finally, the posterior part of the nodule is dissected from the rectum. We feel it is important that, during this dissection, the nodule remains attached to the uterus and cervix or vagina thus elevating the nodule whereas the rectum progressively falls down by gravity. This dissection is continued as far as possible, at least until the rectum is completely freed from the rectovaginal septum. The need for a rectal probe is uncertain: it can be useful to identify

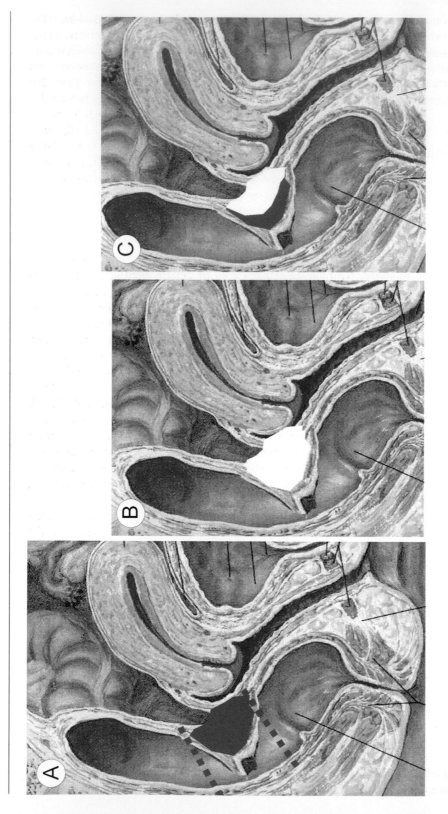

Fig. 6 Types of surgery. (A) Resection anastomosis; (B) complete excision; (C) debulking.

structures but it is not always helpful during dissection. Only after the completion of the dissection of the posterior part up to the vaginal wall, is the anterior side of the nodule dissected from the cervix and from the vagina. In about 20% of women, part of the vaginal fornix has to be removed because of endometriotic invasion whereas we estimate that in some 20% of women the rectum has to be opened to permit a complete resection.[31]

Three other techniques are used for the resection of deep endometriosis: (i) sharp dissection together with electrosurgery through the laparoscope; (ii) sharp dissection together with electrosurgery through the secondary ports; and (iii) a partial rectum resection followed by re-anastomosis usually with a circular stapler. It is obvious that each surgeon performs best using a preferred technique, and that few endoscopic surgeons are familiar with all techniques.

COMPLICATIONS, TREATMENT AND PREVENTION[32,33]

In the series of about 1000 cases in Louven and 200 in Oxford, complications of surgery have been: (i) the formation of 4 rectovaginal fistulas; (ii) the trans-section of the uterine artery necessitating clipping; (iii) a ureteric lesion in 2 women; and (iv) a late bowel perforation in 8 women. When part of the rectal wall has to be removed, or when the rectum is accidentally opened, the pelvis is rinsed with a 1% hibitane solution and the wall is sutured endoscopically with 2 layers of 3x0 Vicryl (Ethicon, USA). A defect in the posterior vaginal fornix is sutured either vaginally or endoscopically. In both cases of fistula formation in the Oxford series, the bowel was deemed not to have been perforated at the time of surgery (confirmed on review of surgical video). These lesions were thus the result of either a late perforation as a result of muscularis damage (surgical or thermal) or as a result of infection. Prevention of a late perforation by liberal prophylactic suturing of the rectum whenever a suspicion of lesion to the muscularis existed, and by careful pinpoint coagulation of the bowel wall when necessary, is mandatory. This rate of 1% is, however, similar to what might be expected at open surgery.

A lesion involving the ureter is a serious complication. In women with large nodules, a pre-operative intravenous pyelogram, a careful dissection of the ureter from its landmarks at the pelvic brim and a liberal preventive ureteric stenting, if necessary, are advocated. This is judged even more important, since it became evident that a ureter which is only half cut can be readily sutured endoscopically over a double J-stent.[34]

RESULTS

Preliminary analysis of our results in 200 women in Oxford in whom deep endometriosis has been excised with a CO_2-laser showed a cure rate of pelvic pain in 78% with a recurrence rate of less than 5% over a follow-up period of up to 5 years. These data should be interpreted carefully, since the completeness of excision has steadily increased. Recent results strongly suggest an almost complete cure rate without recurrences; this, however, may be an overoptimistic clinical impression, which will have to be proven by careful follow-up. In addition, medical treatment of pelvic pain is highly efficient, and the effect of treatment often persists after treatment has been stopped.[35]

Key points for clinical practice

- Surgery for advanced pelvic endometriosis requires extensive pre-operative investigation and planning, which may include IVPs, barium enemas and MRI.

- Surgery should involve a multidisciplinary team including a rectovaginal surgeon and a urologist. Referral to a specialist centre where this service exists may be required.

- As with all surgery, an on-going audit should occur to allow appropriate informed consent to take place.

- Ovarian endometriomas of less than 5 cm should have the cyst stripped from the ovarian capsule to avoid recurrence. Larger cysts may require a two-step procedure.

- Deep nodular endometriosis may require a partial rectal resection, which can be carried out laparoscopically.

References

1. Sampson JA. Peritoneal endometriosis due to the menstrual dissemination of endometrial tissue into the peritoneal cavity. *Am J Obstet Gynecol* 1927; **14**: 422–469.
2. El Mahgoub S, Yaseen S. A positive proof for the theory of coelomic metaplasia. *Am J Obstet Gynecol* 1980; **137**: 137–140.
3. Suginami H. A reappraisal of the coelomic metaplasia theory by reviewing endometriosis occurring in unusual sites and instances. *Am J Obstet Gynecol* 1991; **165**: 214–218.
4. Moore JG, Binstock MA, Growdon WA. The clinical implications of retroperitoneal endometriosis. *Am J Obstet Gynecol* 1988; **158**: 1291–1298.
5. Ueki M. Histologic study of endometriosis and examination of lymphatic drainage in and from the uterus. *Am J Obstet Gynecol* 1991; **165**: 201–209.
6. Koninckx PR, Ide P, Vandenbroucke W, Brosens IA. New aspects of the pathophysiology of endometriosis and associated infertility. *J Reprod Med* 1980; **24**: 257–260.
7. Halme J, Hammond MG, Hulka JF *et al.* Retrograde menstruation in healthy women and in patients with endometriosis. *Obstet Gynecol* 1984; **64**: 151–154.
8. Kruitwagen RF. Menstruation as the pelvic aggressor. *Baillière's Clin Obstet Gynaecol* 1993; **7**: 687–700.
9. van der Linden PQ, de Goeij AM, Dunselman GJ, Erkens HH, Evers JH. Amniotic membrane as an *in vitro* model for endometrium–extracellular matrix interactions. *Gynecol Obstet Invest* 1998; **45**: 7–11.
10. Redwine DB, Koninckx PR, D'Hooghe T, Oosterlynck D. Endometriosis: will the real natural history please stand up?. *Fertil Steril* 1991; **56**: 590–591.
11. Koninckx PR, Oosterlynck D, D'Hooghe T, Meuleman C. Deeply infiltrating endometriosis is a disease whereas mild endometriosis could be considered a non-disease. *Ann NY Acad Sci* 1994; **734**: 333–341.
12. Vercellini P, Bocciolone L, Crosignani PG. Is mild endometriosis always a disease? *Hum Reprod* 1992; **7**: 627–629.
13. Koninckx PR, Kennedy SH, Barlow DH. Pathogenesis of endometriosis: the role of peritoneal fluid. *Gynecol Obstet Invest* 1999; **47 (Suppl 1)**: 23–33.
14. Koninckx PR, Barlow D, Kennedy S. Implantation versus infiltration: the Sampson versus the endometriotic disease theory. *Gynecol Obstet Invest* 1999; **47 (Suppl 1)**: 3–9.
15. Mahmood TA, Templeton A. Prevalence and genesis of endometriosis. *Hum Reprod* 1991; **6**: 544–549.

16. Arruda MS, Petta CA, Abrao MS, Benetti-Pinto CL. Time elapsed from onset of symptoms to diagnosis of endometriosis in a cohort study of Brazilian women. *Hum Reprod* 2003; **18**: 756–759.
17. Hughes E, Fedorkow D, Collins J, Vandekerckhove P. Ovulation suppression for endometriosis. *Cochrane Database Syst Rev* 2000: CD000155.
18. Sutton CJ, Ewen SP, Whitelaw N, Haines P. Prospective, randomized, double-blind, controlled trial of laser laparoscopy in the treatment of pelvic pain associated with minimal, mild, and moderate endometriosis. *Fertil Steril* 1994; **62**: 696–700.
19. Gordts S, Boeckx W, Brosens I. Microsurgery of endometriosis in infertile patients. *Fertil Steril* 1984; **42**: 520–525.
20. Brosens I, Gordts S, Boeckx W, Koninckx PR. Surgical treatment of endometriosis in infertility. *Ir J Med Sci* 1983; **152 (Suppl 2)**: 18–21.
21. Donnez J, Nisolle M, Gillet N, Smets M, Bassil S, Casanas Roux F. Large ovarian endometriomas. *Hum Reprod* 1996; **11**: 641–646.
22. Hemmings R, Bissonnette F, Bouzayen R. Results of laparoscopic treatments of ovarian endometriomas: laparoscopic ovarian fenestration and coagulation. *Fertil Steril* 1998; **70**: 527–529.
23. Saleh A, Tulandi T. Reoperation after laparoscopic treatment of ovarian endometriomas by excision and by fenestration. *Fertil Steril* 1999; **72**: 322–324.
24. Beretta P, Franchi M, Ghezzi F, Busacca M, Zupi E, Bolis P. Randomized clinical trial of two laparoscopic treatments of endometriomas: cystectomy versus drainage and coagulation. *Fertil Steril* 1998; **70**: 1176–1180.
25. Vercellini P, Chapron C, De Giorgi O, Consonni D, Frontino G, Crosignani PG. Coagulation or excision of ovarian endometriomas? *Am J Obstet Gynecol* 2003; **188**: 606–610.
26. Donnez J, Wyns C, Nisolle M. Does ovarian surgery for endometriomas impair the ovarian response to gonadotropin? *Fertil Steril* 2001; **76**: 662–665.
27. Canis M, Pouly JL, Tamburro S, Mage G, Wattiez A, Bruhat MA. Ovarian response during IVF-embryo transfer cycles after laparoscopic ovarian cystectomy for endometriotic cysts of > 3 cm in diameter. *Hum Reprod* 2001; **16**: 2583–2586.
28. Koninckx PR, Martin DC. Deep endometriosis: a consequence of infiltration or retraction or possibly adenomyosis externa? *Fertil Steril* 1992; **58**: 924–928.
29. Koninckx PR, Timmermans B, Meuleman C, Penninckx F. Complications of CO_2-laser endoscopic excision of deep endometriosis. *Hum Reprod* 1996; **11**: 2263–2268.
30. Koninckx PR, Vandermeersch E. The persufflator: an insufflation device for laparoscopy and especially for CO_2-laser-endoscopic surgery. *Hum Reprod* 1991; **6**: 1288–1290.
31. Koninckx PR, Timmermans B, Meuleman C, Penninckx F. Complications of CO_2-laser endoscopic excision of deep endometriosis. *Hum Reprod* 1996; **11**: 2263–2268.
32. Van Rompaey B, Deprest JA, Koninckx PR. Enterocele as a consequence of laparoscopic resection of deeply infiltrating endometriosis. *J Am Assoc Gynecol Laparosc* 1996; **4**: 73–75.
33. Tate JJT, Kwok S, Dawson JW, Lau WY, Li AKC. Prospective comparison of laparoscopic and conventional anterior resection. *Br J Surg* 1993; **80**: 1396–1398.
34. Neven P, van Deursen H, Baert L, Koninckx PR. Ureteric injury at laparoscopic surgery: the endoscopic management. Case review. *Gynaecol Endosc* 1993; **2**: 45–46.
35. Shaw RW. Nafarelin in the treatment of pelvic pain caused by endometriosis. *Am J Obstet Gynecol* 1990; **162**: 574–576.

Deborah N. P. Haggai

16

Emergency contraception: a global overview among potential users

Emergency contraception is defined as the use of drugs or devices to prevent pregnancy within a few days of unprotected coitus.[1,2] It is sometimes referred to as 'Morning after' or postcoital contraception. Emergency contraception provides a safe and effective means of postcoital treatment and has been estimated to prevent at least 75% of expected pregnancies resulting from unprotected intercourse.[3]

Unintended pregnancy is a global problem, which affects women, their families and society at large. Abortion is a frequent consequence. There are about 50 million pregnancies terminated each year.[4] In the US, almost 50% of pregnancies are unwanted.[2] It has been calculated that the wide-spread use of emergency contraception in the US could prevent over a million abortions and 2 million unintended pregnancies that end in childbirth each year.[5] If emergency contraception was available to all women who have been raped, about 22,000 pregnancies per year could potentially be avoided in the US.[6]

There have been different approaches to this work. Some of the research was done among pregnant adolescents, some in the community, with others in institutions and colleges among teenagers. Studies done among pregnant women seeking abortion have been aimed at determining whether these women would have prevented the pregnancy if they had known about emergency contraception. Different approaches tend to start from basic assumptions about what the respondents will know and feel; for example, women attending family planning clinics might be expected to be more knowledgeable than women attending general practice. Similarly, a community-based survey will give information about the level of knowledge in the population at large and the general attitude towards use of emergency contraception. Institutional surveys, in schools and colleges, have been aimed

Deborah N. P. Haggai MBBCh FWACS MSc
Consultant/Lecturer, Department of Obstetrics and Gynaecology, Ahmadu Bello University Teaching Hospital, Zaria, Kaduna State, Nigeria. (E-mail: dhaggai@hotmail.com)

at identifying the knowledge and practice of emergency contraception in a population at particular risk of unintended pregnancy.

WHO MAY USE EMERGENCY CONTRACEPTION?

Almost every woman of reproductive age who is sexually active and fertile and wishes to prevent unintended pregnancy after unprotected intercourse can use emergency contraception.[7] As long as condoms continue to slip or break, diaphragms and cervical caps move out of place, pill-users forget to take their tablets regularly, there will be need for use of emergency contraception. Other potential users are women who engage in an unexpected sexual activity either by being forced (as in cases of rape) or coerced into having unplanned, unprotected intercourse. Emergency contraception is useful for women using withdrawal method in instances where withdrawal occurred too late or for women practising the rhythm or calendar method with any miscalculation of the 'safe' days for periodic abstinence. Emergency contraception is particularly suitable for adolescents because of their patterns of sexual behaviour and contraceptive use. They often do not plan their first intercourse or may have infrequent intercourse with no contraceptive protection.

METHODS OF EMERGENCY CONTRACEPTION

The Yuzpe regimen has been the most commonly used method of emergency contraception. It consists of two doses of a combination of 100 μg of ethinyl oestradiol and 500 μg of levonorgestrel, the first dose taken within 72 h of intercourse and the second dose 12 h later.[8] The common side-effects associated with this regimen are nausea and vomiting of which up to 50% and 20%, respectively, have been reported.[9]

During the 1960s and early 1970s, high doses of oestrogen were the standard regimen which was claimed to be as effective as the Yuzpe method but produced more side-effects and was thus not commonly used.

The levonorgestrel regimen consists of two doses of 0.75 mg levonorgestrel taken 12-h apart starting within 72 h of unprotected intercourse. A recent, randomised, controlled trial by the World Health Organization (WHO) has shown that this regimen was better tolerated and more effective than the Yuzpe regimen.[10]

The copper-bearing intra-uterine device is a highly effective postcoital contraceptive with failure rates of less than 1%.[3] It is used for up to 5 days after unprotected intercourse and is particularly appropriate for women who wish to use the device as a long-term method of contraception.

Mifepristone (RU486) is highly effective as emergency contraception and the regimen consists of a single dose of 600 mg given within 72 h of unprotected intercourse.[9] The WHO multicentre randomised trial to assess the safety and effectiveness of lower doses of mifepristone (50 mg and 10 mg) showed that reducing the dose did not decrease its efficacy and was associated with less disturbance of the menstrual cycle.[11] These lower doses might probably be more acceptable politically in countries where abortion is illegal compared with the high doses used as an abortifacient.

WHAT DO WOMEN KNOW ABOUT EMERGENCY CONTRACEPTION?

KNOWLEDGE, ATTITUDES AND PRACTICES AMONG POTENTIAL USERS IN INDUSTRIALISED COUNTRIES

One of the earliest studies done among pregnant women seeking abortion was by Johnston and colleagues in Dundee, Scotland.[12] The study was aimed at estimating the potential usage of postcoital contraception to prevent unwanted pregnancy. The findings showed that the knowledge of postcoital contraception was poor. However, after being told about it, 98% of women said they would have used it if they had known. Duncan et al.[13] also conducted a study among pregnant women undergoing termination of pregnancy in Oxford between September 1988 and March 1989. This was aimed at developing a strategy for prevention of unwanted pregnancy. The findings showed that 70.1% of pregnancies were potentially predictable by virtue of non-use of contraception or by recognition of method failure, but only 2.5% had used postcoital contraception. The findings from this survey also suggested that the increase in abortion rate was due to an increase in barrier method use with no back up method. Women should be advised on 'double contraception' to avoid contraceptive failure due to condom accidents. In another study by Bromham and Cartmill,[14] among pregnant women requesting termination of pregnancy, 93.4% of the patients would have preferred to use postcoital contraception than experience an unplanned pregnancy. Subsequent studies of women who are pregnant showed that poor knowledge of postcoital contraception was not a major factor in failure to use emergency contraception[15,16] but easy availability and accessibility were of most importance. The recommendation by some authors to deregulate emergency contraception should be considered more objectively by policy makers.[17,18] The study by Gordon et al.[16] also suggests that although women may be better informed about contraception (particularly emergency contraception), and more likely to use a method to try and prevent pregnancy, there is still an unaltered tendency not to relate unprotected intercourse or a failure of contraception with the risk of pregnancy.

The study of Danish women requesting termination of pregnancy by Perslev et al.[19] showed that the group of women with sufficient knowledge of emergency contraception are younger, more educated and more often use contraception. There is no evidence that a liberal attitude toward emergency contraception will have a negative effect on the use of contraception. This was shown in the study by Sorhaindo et al.[20] in which 55% of women adopted an on-going method following their first use of emergency contraceptive pills. Kozinszky et al.,[21] in Hungary, studied contraceptive behaviour of teenagers requesting abortion and showed that knowledge about emergency contraceptive pills was significantly poorer among teenagers compared to the older women requesting abortion.

Studies of women attending general practice and family planning clinics showed that the source of information also had some influence on the accuracy of knowledge of emergency contraception. Women attending a family planning clinic were more knowledgeable than women who received contraceptive advice in a general practice.[14] A study by George et al.[22] of women attending general practice showed that only 13.6% of respondents knew the correct 72-h time limit during which postcoital contraception could be used effectively. A similar study by Ziebland et al.[23] of women seeking emergency contraception showed that the knowledge of the correct time limit was 72%. The other striking finding among this group was that almost 43% of the respondents believed emergency contraception to be more risky to their health than regular use of combined oral contraceptive, which is an overestimation of the health risks. Emergency contraception has been proven to be quite safe and this should be emphasised. Educational messages must distinguish clearly between emergency contraception and abortifacient use as some of the women who had heard of RU486 were not sure of the difference between it and emergency contraception. In a study conducted by Cohall et al.[24] in the US among adolescents attending a general primary health clinic, 80% of those who had heard of RU486 were not sure whether emergency contraception was abortifacient or not. These concerns were also raised in another study by Bird et al.[25] among women attending family planning clinics. The study conducted by Hughes et al.[26] in a general practice in North Wales, noted that the source of information was mostly media and friends with a disappointing input from health care professionals.

Romo et al.[27] recently reported that in Latino women only 25% had heard of emergency contraception. Reasons for lack of use included poor knowledge of mechanism of action. A recent literature review by Croxatto et al.[28] on the mechanism of action of hormonal preparations used for emergency contraception concluded that further research was needed to determine fully the mode of action and provide a clear-cut answer to the mechanism by which emergency contraceptives prevent pregnancy.

Research can also be divided into that aimed at targeted populations and community studies. In a Scottish project,[29] the level of knowledge of emergency contraception among 14- and 15-year-olds in schools was investigated. This was a different setting, as previous studies were among adults or teenagers who were already pregnant and, therefore, sexually active. Of pupils who participated in the study, 93% had heard of emergency contraception and girls (98%) were more likely to have heard of it than boys (87%). Pupils attending schools above national average for academic attainment were more likely to have heard of emergency contraception compared to those attending schools below average. Pupils from less academic schools were more likely to have had sexual intercourse before the age of 16 years. The use of emergency contraception was encouraging with 31.4% of girls who admitted to sexual intercourse having used emergency contraception. Knowledge about the safety of emergency contraception may have affected the use of this method as only 13.5% of pupils thought that emergency contraception was safer than regular use of the oral contraceptive pill. Confidentiality is also a sensitive issue in this group, as most would not want their parents to be involved. This study also highlighted the fact that despite the high percentage of pupils, who had heard of emergency contraception, knowledge of the correct time limit was poor and was unrelated to the academic standard of the pupils' school. Only 26.4% of pupils gave the correct time-limit of 72 h and girls who had been sexually active were most likely to know the correct time-limit. Schools and magazines were the commonest sources of information about emergency contraception with health care providers contributing very little in disseminating information. It appears, therefore, that schools and media play an important role in educating the under sixteen age group since they rarely come into contact with health professionals. In a similar study conducted by Harper and Ellertson in the US among students at Princeton University,[30] the findings were similar to UK studies. Although the basic level of awareness was high, only few respondents had accurate detailed knowledge, and misconceptions existed in many areas. The survey also showed that students have a positive attitude towards emergency contraception with 80% saying it should be used and 76% would take it or recommend to a friend if needed.

A community-based study by Smith et al.[31] in 1996 in Scotland revealed that 94% of women knew about the existence of the postcoital pill. As with other studies, there was poor knowledge of the correct timing of effectiveness of the postcoital pill and intra-uterine contraceptive devices. Over 70% of women were in favour of increased advertising, which they believed would reduce the number of unwanted pregnancies. Of the respondents, 21% felt it should be sold over the counter, but only 14% had used emergency contraception. Gooder in England,[32] in a public survey of knowledge of emergency contraception amongst men and women, showed that 89% of women and 81% of men under 45 years had heard of emergency contraception while only 50% of men and women over 45 years had heard of emergency contraception. Knowledge of the correct time-limit after unprotected intercourse was poor in both men and women (8% and 13%, respectively). In the study by Crosier[33] among women aged between 16 and 49 years, 97% of respondents had heard of emergency contraception but only 24% knew the correct time-limit of 72 h after unprotected intercourse; only 12% of women reported having previously used the method. In other national surveys in industrialised countries, Delbanco et al.[34] in the US and Kosunen et al.[35] in Finland showed that only 1% and 4% (respectively) of women had ever used emergency contraception.

The study by Gould et al.[36] to assess knowledge and attitudes about the differences between emergency contraception and medical abortion among middle-class women and men of reproductive age in Mexico City showed that at least 50% of the participants regarded emergency contraception as a medical method of abortion rather than a method of contraception. Their attitudes towards emergency contraception, however, changed after receiving adequate information. All participants agreed that using emergency contraception is 'more responsible' than risking an abortion. Most participants supported its use and wanted to see greater dissemination of information about the method in Mexico.

Foster et al.[37] in California showed that there is still confusion between RU486 and emergency contraception; thus, clarifying the differences between emergency contraception and medical abortion may increase acceptability of emergency contraception.

KNOWLEDGE, ATTITUDES AND PRACTICES AMONG POTENTIAL USERS IN NON-INDUSTRIALISED COUNTRIES

The findings in less industrialised countries are even more disappointing. A survey conducted among nurses and nursing students in Nairobi, Kenya, by Gichangi et al. in 1998 (unpublished)[38] showed that almost half of the respondents considered emergency contraception as an abortifacient. Over 90% of respondents acknowledged their deficient knowledge and requested more information. It also showed that the overall ever-users of emergency contraception was 3.5%. The respondents also expressed concern about risky sexual behaviour if emergency contraception was easily available and accessible which is not proven by any study; on the contrary, it is improved.[39] The study conducted in Zaria, Nigeria by Bako[40] showed poor knowledge of postcoital contraception. The study also suggested that Nigerian women are interested in preventing unintended pregnancy as shown by the high percentage of respondents who resort to traditional methods of emergency contraception and by the report of those who had a termination of pregnancy that said they would have used emergency contraception if they had known about it. A national survey conducted in Nigeria by the Society for Family Health[41] in 1998 showed that less than 1% (0.7%) of women had ever used an effective method of emergency contraception.

The study conducted by Smit et al.[42] in South Africa among public sector primary healthcare clients showed that only 22.8% of clients had heard of emergency contraception and 9.1% of those who knew of emergency contraception had used it. Accurate knowledge was, however, lacking among those who knew of it. After correct information was given, most respondents were supportive of the method with 90.3% indicating that they would use it if need be in the future while 92.3% would recommend it to a friend. Concerns or worries about abuse, side-effects, spread of STI/HIV and promiscuity are issues that need to be addressed for competent implementation of wide-spread programmes.

The study by Baiden et al.[43] in Ghana to determine the perception of university students about emergency contraception showed that 43.2% of respondents had heard of modern emergency contraceptive methods but only 11.3% knew the correct time-limit. The use of concentrated sugar solutions, enema and douching were common traditional methods used, which is a clear indication that women are interested in preventing unintended pregnancy, but adequate knowledge of modern methods was lacking. Almost all (97.4%) the respondents wanted to learn more about emergency contraception.

Sorhaindo et al.[20] also conducted a survey among university students in Kingston, Jamaica which showed that general awareness of emergency contraceptive pills was high (84%) but many students were unaware of specific details such as the correct time-limit. Only 28% knew that a woman must take the first dose within 72 h of unprotected sex. Many (86%) participants said that they would recommend this method to a family member or friend. Roberts et al.[44] in Durban, South Africa reported that in students, 56.5% had heard of emergency contraception but only 11.8% knew the correct time-limit.

CONCLUSIONS

All of the studies among potential users of emergency contraception have shown that in places where the method is available, knowledge and use increase with time (as shown by the UK studies), even though detailed knowledge improved more slowly than knowledge of existence of the method. This is not surprising because of the conflicting messages from 'morning-after' pill, to within 72 h after unprotected intercourse, and most recently to 'the sooner the better'.

The new interest in emergency contraception should dispel the myths and misunderstandings. Providers will become better informed and may start, pro-actively, to inform their clients. The development of more effective and better tolerated methods (such as levonorgestrel) will inevitably lead to preparations becoming available without the need to see a doctor; this will further enhance awareness and knowledge which should result in greater use. Less developed countries will probably follow the example of industrialised countries and, by the year 2010, emergency contraception will be as well known and as well used as the oral contraceptive pill. Whether this will lead to a reduction in unwanted pregnancies and abortion rates, remains to be seen. More research is needed in this field.

Key points for clinical practice

- Knowledge improves with time after emergency contraception becomes available.

- Knowledge of existence of emergency contraception improves rapidly.

- Knowledge of the details, e.g. correct timing of 72 h after unprotected intercourse, improves more gradually.

- The degree of knowledge varies among different groups within the same country.

- Younger people appear to be better informed which is a good thing. They are usually involved in more risky sexual behaviour and their contraceptive use is also low. Most are in school and would not want to disrupt their studies because of an unintended pregnancy.

- Although the intention or desire to use emergency contraception is high, actual use is very low.

- Reasons for non-use or concerns among users are similar in different settings. These concerns can be corrected by proper education on the mode of action and the safety of the method.

- The mass media and schools have been identified as important sources of information about emergency contraception in most of the reported studies; thus, detailed and correct information must be given through these sources.

References

1. Glasier A. Emergency post coital contraception. *N Engl J Med* 1997; **337**: 1058–1064.
2. Westley E. Emergency contraception: a global overview. *J Am Med Women's Assoc* 1998; **53**: 215–218, 237.
3. Trussell J, Ellertson CE. Efficacy of emergency contraception. *Fertil Control Rev* 1995; **4**: 8–11.
4. Van Look PFA, von Hertzen H. Induced abortion: a global perspective. In: Baird DT,

Grimes DA, Van Look PFA. (eds) *Modern Methods of Inducing Abortion*. Oxford: Blackwell, 1995; 1–24.

5. Trussell J, Ellertson C, Stewart F. The effectiveness of the Yuzpe regimen of emergency contraception. *Fam Plan Perspect* 1996; **28**: 58–64.

6. Stewart FH, Trussell J. Prevention of pregnancy resulting from rape a neglected preventive health measure. *Am J Prev Med* 2000; **19**: 228–229.

7. Robinson ET, Metcalf-Whittaker M, Rivera R. Introducing emergency contraceptive services: communications strategies and the role of women's health advocates. *Fam Plan Perspect* 1996; **22**: 71–75, 80.

8. Trussell J, Ellertson C, Rodriguez G. The Yuzpe regimen of emergency contraception: how long after the morning after? *Obstet Gynecol* 1996; **88**: 150–154.

9. Glasier A, Thong KJ, Dewar M, Mackie M, Baird DT. Mifepristone (RU486) compared with high-dose estrogen and progestogen for emergency postcoital contraception. *N Engl J Med* 1992; **327**: 1041–1044.

10. Task Force on Postovulatory Methods of Fertility Regulation. Randomised controlled trial of levonorgestrel versus the Yuzpe regimen of combined oral contraceptives for emergency contraception. *Lancet* 1998; **352**: 428–432.

11. Task Force on Postovulatory Methods of Fertility Regulation. Comparison of three single doses of mifepristone as emergency contraception: a randomised trial. *Lancet* 1999; **353**: 697–702.

12. Johnston TA, Howie PW. Potential use of postcoital contraception to prevent unwanted pregnancy. *BMJ* 1985; **290**: 1040–1041.

13. Duncan G, Harper C, Ashwell E, Mant D, Buchan H, Jones I. Termination of pregnancy: lessons for prevention. *Br J Fam Plan* 1990; **15**: 112–117.

14. Bromham DR, Cartmill RSV. Knowledge and use of secondary contraception among patients requesting termination of pregnancy. *BMJ* 1993; **306**: 556–557.

15. Pearson VAH, Owen MR, Phillips DR, Pereira Gray DJ, Marshall MN. Pregnant teenagers' knowledge and use of emergency contraception. *BMJ* 1995; **310**: 1644.

16. Gordon AF, Owen P. Emergency contraception: change in knowledge of women attending for termination of pregnancy from 1984 to 1996. *Br J Fam Plan* 1999; **24**: 121–122.

17. Glasier A. Emergency contraception – time for de-regulation? *Br J Obstet Gynaecol* 1993; **100**: 611–612.

18. O'Drife JO. Deregulating emergency contraception. *BMJ* 1993; **307**: 695–696.

19. Perslev A, Rorbye C, Boesen HC, Norgaard M, Nilas L. Emergency contraception: knowledge and use among Danish women requesting termination of pregnancy. *Contraception* 2002; **66**: 427–431.

20. Sorhaindo A, Becker D, Fletcher H, Garcia SG. Emergency contraception among university students in Kingston, Jamaica: survey of knowledge, attitudes and practices. *Contraception* 2002; **66**: 261–268.

21. Kozinszky Z, Bartai G. Contraceptive behaviour of teenagers requesting abortion. *Eur J Obstet Gynecol Reprod Biol* 2004; **112**: 80–83.

22. George J, Turner J, Cooke E *et al*. Women's knowledge of emergency contraception. *Br J Gen Pract* 1994; **44**: 451–454.

23. Ziebland S, Maxwell K, Greenhall E. 'It's a mega dose of hormones, isn't it?' Why women may be reluctant to use emergency contraception. *Br J Fam Plan* 1996; **22**: 84–86.

24. Cohall AT, Dickerson D, Vaughan R, Cohall R. Inner-city adolescents' awareness of emergency contraception. *J Am Med Women's Assoc* 1998; **53**: 258–261.

25. Bird ST, Harvey SM, Beckman LJ. Emergency contraception pills: an exploratory study of knowledge and perceptions among Mexican women from both sides of the border. *J Am Med Women's Assoc* 1998; **53**: 262–265.

26. Hughes H, Myres P. Women's knowledge and preference about emergency contraception: a survey from a rural general practice. *Br J Fam Plan* 1996; **22**: 77–78.

27. Romo LF, Berenson AB, Wu ZH. The role of misconceptions on Latino women's acceptance of emergency contraceptive pills. *Contraception* 2004; **69**: 227–235.

28. Croxatto HB, Devoto L Durand M *et al*. Mechanism of action of hormonal preparations used for emergency contraception: a review of the literature. *Contraception* 2001; **63**: 111–121.

29. Graham A, Green L, Glasier AF. Teenagers' knowledge of emergency contraception: questionnaire survey in southeast Scotland. *BMJ* 1996; **312**: 1567–1569.
30. Harper CC, Ellertson CE. The emergency contraceptive pill : a survey of knowledge and attitudes among students at Princeton University. *Am J Obstet Gynecol* 1995; **173**: 1438–1445.
31. Smith BH, Gurney EM, Aboulela L, Templeton A. Emergency contraception : a survey of women's knowledge and attitudes. *Br J Obstet Gynaecol* 1996; **103**: 1109–1116.
32. Gooder P. Knowledge of emergency contraception amongst men and women in the general population and women seeking an abortion. *Br J Fam Plan* 1996; **22**: 81–84.
33. Crosier A. Women's knowledge and awareness of emergency contraception. *Br J Fam Plan* 1996; **22**: 87–90.
34. Delbanco SF, Mauldon J, Smith MD. Little knowledge and limited practice: emergency contraceptive pills, the public, and the obstetrician-gynecologist. *Obstet Gynecol* 1997; **89**: 1006–1011.
35. Kosunen E, Sihvo S, Hemminki E. Knowledge and use of hormonal emergency contraception in Finland. *Contraception* 1997; **55**: 153–157.
36. Gould H, Ellertson C, Corona G. Knowledge and attitudes about the differences between emergency contraception and medical abortion among middle-class women and men of reproductive age in Mexico city. *Contraception* 2002; **66**: 417–426.
37. Foster DG, Harper CC, Bley JJ *et al*. Knowledge of emergency contraception among women aged 18 to 44 in California. *Am J Obstet Gynecol* 2004; **191**: 150–156.
38. Gichangi PB *et al*. Knowledge, attitudes and practice about emergency contraception among nurses and nursing students in two hospitals in Nairobi, Kenya, 1998; Unpublished.
39. Glasier A, Baird D. The effects of self-administering emergency contraception. *N Engl J Med* 1998; **339**: 1–4.
40. Bako AU. Knowledge and use of emergency contraception amongst Nigerian undergraduates, *J Obstet Gynaecol* 1998; **18**: 151–153.
41. Society for Family Health. *Emergency Contraception in Nigeria*. Lagos: Society for Family Health, 1998.
42. Smit L, McFadyen L, Beksinska M *et al*. Emergency contraception in South Africa: knowledge, attitudes and use among public sector primary healthcare clients. *Contraception* 2001; **64**: 333–337.
43. Baiden F, Awini F, Clerk C. Perception of university students in Ghana about emergency contraception. *Contraception* 2002; **66**: 23–26.
44. Roberts C, Moodley J, Esterhuizen T. Emergency contraception: knowledge and practices of tertiary students in Durban, South Africa. *J Obstet Gynaecol* 2004; **24**: 441–445.

Alaa A. El-Ghobashy C. Simon Herrington

17

Diagnosis and management of pre-invasive cervical glandular neoplasia

Invasive and pre-invasive cervical glandular lesions are reported to be increasing in incidence particularly in young women. This could be attributed to improved detection by pathologists, the high prevalence of HPV 18 and possibly the increased use of combined oral contraceptive pills.[1]

Cervical smear, with or without colposcopically directed biopsies, will detect only 38–69% of endocervical neoplasia before cervical conisation. Diagnosis is increased to 85% with the addition of biopsy and endocervical curettage (ECC).[2]

The incidence of cervical adenocarcinoma has risen from 5% in the 1950s to 10–22% in the mid 1990s.[3,4] In a Swedish study, the incidence of cervical adenocarcinoma increased from 1.59/100,000 in the 1950s and 1960s to 2.36 in the early 1990s.[5] The corresponding figures for cervical adenocarcinoma *in situ* (AIS) were 0.04 and 1.37, reflecting an even greater increase.

Debate is ongoing regarding the management of cervical glandular intra-epithelial neoplasia (CGIN) and micro-invasive adenocarcinoma.[6] Different procedures, such as hysterectomy and cone excision of the cervix, have been used. However, residual disease following conisation with negative margins, and pelvic recurrence following radical hysterectomy, have been reported.

In this review, the pathology of preneoplastic and early invasive glandular lesions of the cervix will be discussed. The efficacy of different interventions to manage such lesions will be appraised in the light of currently available evidence.

Alaa A. El-Ghobashy MD MRCOG (for correspondence)
Specialist Registrar in Obstetrics and Gynaecology, Bradford Royal Infirmary, Bradford, West Yorkshire, UK

C. Simon Herrington MA DPhil FRCP FRCPath
Professor of Pathology, University of St Andrews, Bute Medical School, Westburn Lane, St Andrews, Fife KY16 9TS, UK

PATHOLOGY

CERVICAL GLANDULAR INTRA-EPITHELIAL NEOPLASIA (CGIN)

Friedell and McKay[7] first described adenocarcinoma *in situ* in 1953. However, the term CGIN was first introduced by Brown and Wells in 1986.[8] It was realised that the originally proposed 3-tier grading of CGIN (equivalent to CIN I–III) was poorly reproducible in biopsies and in Pap smears, and in 1995 it was substituted by grading into low- and high-grade CGIN, the latter being equivalent to AIS.[9]

CGIN is much less common than its squamous counterpart (CIN) but, as with CIN, most CGIN lesions occur in the region of the transformation zone. The ratio of AIS (CGIN) to CIN III lesions (severe dysplasia/carcinoma) is 1:50 or 2%.[10] The majority of AIS lesions (46–72%) contain a counterpart squamous component – termed 'mixed disease' – which is usually a CIN III lesion.[10]

In contrast to CIN, separate foci may be found higher in the endocervical canal (skip lesions) in about 10% of CGIN lesions.[11] Smears from CGIN are characterised by abundant groups of endocervical cells showing nuclear crowding, pseudostratification, feathering at the edges and rosette formation. Dyskaryosis may be subtle and vary from cell to cell. Features suggesting invasion include the presence of a malignant diathesis, macronucleoli and windowing of nuclear chromatin.[12]

CGIN is recognised histologically by a combination of architectural atypia and cellular abnormalities. Low-grade lesions encompass similar histological abnormalities to high-grade CGIN, but to a lesser degree (Table 1). In most cases, CGIN occurs close to the transformation zone (TZ). Both the surface epithelium and the underlying crypts may be involved.

Table 1 Histological differences between low- and high-grade CGIN[24]

	Low-grade CGIN	High-grade CGIN
Cellular abnormalities		
	Minimal pseudostratification	Marked pseudostratification
	Nuclear atypia (enlargement, hyperchromasia, fine-to-moderate granular chromatin)	Increased nuclear atypia with a moderate-to-coarse granular chromatin pattern
	Evidence of cellular turnover (apoptotic bodies) and/or occasional mitoses (less than one or two per glandular grouping)	Increased apoptosis and frequent, possibly abnormal mitoses (more than two per glandular grouping)
Architectural abnormalities		
	Glandular crowding with minor degree of branching and budding	Increased complexity: cribriform pattern with branching and budding
	Occasional intraluminal papillary projection	Intraluminal papillary projections

One of the difficulties in the diagnosis of glandular intra-epithelial neoplasia is to exclude invasion. Normal glands are limited to a maximum depth of 7.8 mm and intra-epithelial lesions only involve glandular profiles. The presence of atypical glands outside the normal glandular field should always raise the suspicion of invasion.

MICRO-INVASIVE ADENOCARCINOMA

Micro-invasive adenocarcinoma is defined as a glandular neoplasm in which the extent of stromal invasion is so minimal that the risk of local lymph node metastasis is negligible. Unlike its squamous counterpart, early invasive adenocarcinoma or micro-invasive carcinoma remains a controversial category.[13] The hallmark of early invasive carcinoma is stromal invasion. The first sign of stromal invasion is often abrupt morphological change within a high-grade CGIN lesion, the cells becoming enlarged with abundant eosinophilic, squamoid-like cytoplasm [14] This appearance corresponds to stage 1A1 of the 1986 International Federation of Gynaecology and Obstetrics (FIGO) definition.[15] The depth of invasion and the width of the tumour should be measured for clinical management. However, the microscopic identification of early invasive adenocarcinoma is often difficult. Early invasive adenocarcinoma may present as an obvious small adenocarcinoma but, in some cases, invasion manifests as an extremely complex glandular pattern or the presence of small buds of cells originating from high-grade CGIN. The presence of stromal oedema, desmoplasia or inflammation indicates a stromal reaction and is a useful clue to the presence of early invasion, as is the development of a more 'squamoid' phenotype by cells at the epithelial–stromal interface. The accurate measurement of depth of invasion is often problematic in early endocervical adenocarcinomas as the endocervical glands are often architecturally complex;[16] hence an estimate is usually provided. In some cases, it may not be possible to ascertain with certainty whether invasion is present. A variety of cut-off points have been used to define micro-invasion, namely 1, 2, 3, or 5 mm or less.[14,17-24] Sometimes, the depth has to be measured from the surface rather than the point of origin, which may be hard to establish. Therefore, tumour thickness rather than 'depth of invasion' is often measured. Lesions with a volume of less than 500 mm^3 have a negligible risk of local recurrence and lymph node metastases.[25] However, it is not practical to express invasion in three dimensions. Moreover, gynaecologists tend to be less conservative in their treatment of micro-invasive adenocarcinomas arising in the endocervix than micro-invasive squamous cervical carcinomas.

Full clinicopathological correlation is, therefore, essential in order to establish the best management for individual patients.

PATHOGENESIS OF CERVICAL GLANDULAR NEOPLASIA

Women with high-grade CGIN are 10–20 years younger than those with invasive disease and invasive adenocarcinoma and CGIN commonly co-exist in the same specimen. In one study, the mean age of women progressively increased from 39 years for low-grade CGIN, to 43 years for both high-grade

CGIN and micro-invasive adenocarcinoma, and 48 years for adenocarcinoma, a span of approximately 10 years.[24] The natural history of low-grade CGIN is even less clear. Brown and Wells[8] have found that progression from low- to high-grade lesion could take place in 1.5–3 years. It has also been suggested that women with low-grade CGIN are at increased risk of further pre-invasive glandular changes in the genital tract.

Human papillomavirus (HPV) infection has been implicated as a potential risk factor in cervical glandular carcinogenesis. HPV 16, HPV 18 and HPV 31 have been identified in 80% or more of adenocarcinomas and adenosquamous carcinomas using sensitive polymerase chain reaction techniques and dot blot hybridisation. Other HPV types identified included HPV 45, HPV 52, and HPV 35.[26] There is a strong link between cervical adenocarcinoma and HPV infection, particularly HPV 18, although the reasons for the latter are unclear.[27] Some rare histological variants of cervical adenocarcinoma, such as clear cell and serous carcinoma, appear unrelated to HPV infection.[26]

Studies have identified a 1.5–5-fold increase in odds ratio for oral contraceptive pill users when compared with non users.[3,28,29] Adjustment for HPV infection reduced this association, which was then confined to adenocarcinoma *in situ* (AIS) and not invasive carcinoma. There appears to be no relationship between parity or smoking and cervical adenocarcinoma.

MANAGEMENT OF ENDOCERVICAL NEOPLASIA

Although the cytological features of CGIN have been better described recently, the diagnostic sensitivity of the cervical smear for the detection of glandular lesions remains less than for the squamous counterpart. The predictive value of abnormal glandular cytology, for preneoplastic and neoplastic pathology, varies between 17% and 95.7%.[30–33]

No single colposcopic appearance characterises adenocarcinoma *in situ*. Villous fusion and acetowhite changes proximal to the squamo-columnar junction have been reported in some cases.[34] Colposcopy lacks sensitivity for the diagnosis of glandular lesions[35,36] and punch biopsy has little role in their diagnosis.[37,38]

Diagnostic hysteroscopy and endometrial biopsy are recommended for perimenopausal women to exclude endometrial pathology.

The management of invasive cervical cancer including adenocarcinoma has been discussed in a previous edition of *Recent Advances in Obstetrics and Gynaecology*.[39] This review will focus on the management of glandular intra-epithelial neoplasia.

CONSERVATIVE MANAGEMENT

Many patients with CGIN are of child-bearing age and desire preservation of fertility. While hysterectomy remains the definitive treatment, a more conservative approach to the management of patients with these lesions has been proposed, provided that the excision margins are clear. Pathologists favour techniques that avoid thermal artefact in order to improve the assessment of excision margins.[37]

Nicklin *et al.*[40] reviewed the topography and behaviour of AIS. The authors reported that women younger than 36 years have a mean lesion length of 5.6 mm, versus 10.8 mm for women over 36 years. Only 1 of 14 younger women from a series of 31 patients had a linear length of more than 10 mm. In contrast 9 of 17 women in the older group had lesion lengths of more than 10 mm, with a maximum of 25 mm.[40] Bertrand et al.[41] studied the highest focus of cervical involvement of AIS measured from the maximal convexity of the cervix in hysterectomy specimens. The highest focus did not exceed 19.9 mm in 78.9% of cases, the highest recorded focus being 29.9 mm.[41] By taking into account the distribution of lesions, such measurements could provide guidelines for determining the size of cylindrical excision specimens, particularly when the endocervical canal is involved.

Cold-knife conisation

Cold-knife conisation (CKC) has been the traditional procedure for diagnosis and treatment of cervical dysplasia and early cervical carcinoma and is ideally performed in a hospital setting with general or regional anaesthesia. The adequacy of cervical conisation as conservative management of AIS was investigated in one retrospective study. A total of 28 patients, with a diagnosis of AIS made by cone biopsy, were reviewed. Patients were subsequently managed by either hysterectomy ($n = 13$) or conservatively with repeat conisation of the cervix ($n = 6$)/close follow-up ($n = 9$). Of patients managed conservatively, 47% had a recurrent glandular lesion detected in subsequent conisation; two of these recurrences were invasive adenocarcinoma. Patients who underwent conservative management had been followed by endocervical curettage (ECC) in combination with routine smears. The ECC was positive in only 43% of patients with glandular lesions prior to subsequent conisation. This retrospective study raises questions about the safety of conisation as conservative management of patients with AIS and stresses the potential inadequacy of following these patients with smears and ECC.[42]

The primary treatment of CGIN by conisation was examined in a CRC multicentre prospective cohort study. Fifty-one women with CGIN diagnosed on a cervical cone specimen were managed by either follow-up (42 patients) using cytological and colposcopic examinations if the cervical cone margins were negative or by hysterectomy (9 patients) if the latter were involved. No apparent residual CGIN or invasive disease was present in 35 women (83%) after a median follow-up period of 12 months. The authors suggested that further surgery is unnecessary when a diagnosis of CGIN is made upon a cone biopsy and the margins of the cone specimen are free of disease,. They also recommended follow-up using cervical smear, including endocervical sampling, and colposcopy for these women.[36]

Kennedy et al.[43] suggested that cold-knife conisation was the preferred method of management for cervical AIS patients selecting conservative treatment. Despite initial conisation margins being uninvolved, such patients have an approximate risk of 10% for recurrent AIS.[43]

Large loop excision of the transformation zone (LLETZ)

The LLETZ (large loop excision of the transformation zone) procedure was described in 1989, by Prendiville and colleagues from Bristol, UK, as a new method of management for women with an abnormal cervical smear, which had the advantages of simultaneous conisation, local destruction and minimal tissue damage.[44]

A prospective trial in 616 patients assessed the efficacy and morbidity of LLETZ in the out-patient setting. Treatment was completed in a mean time of 3.47 min. There was minimal immediate morbidity and adequate histological specimens were obtained in over 90% of cases. It was possible to treat almost two-thirds of patients in their first visit and the overall failure rate on subsequent assessment, 6 months after treatment, was 4.4%.[45]

Less intra-operative blood loss and fewer immediate postoperative complications were noted after LLETZ[46] and the incidence of cervical stenosis after LLETZ was significantly lower than that following knife cone biopsy. No differences in fertility and menstrual symptoms were found, after 3 years, between women treated with LLETZ for abnormal cervical smears and control women with a history of negative smears.[47,48]

Maini et al.[49] followed patients with CGIN treated by LLETZ for a mean of 32.35 months. No invasive carcinomas were identified in the completely excised group. In this retrospective study, LLETZ was found to be an adequate primary management for CGIN, and the excision margin status of the LLETZ specimen did appear to be a prognostic factor for residual disease.[49]

However, it has been shown that LLETZ is associated with a 50% rate of positive margins compared with 33% for knife cone excision. Similarly, the disease recurrence rate is higher in patients treated with LLETZ (29%) than in those treated by cone excision (6%).[50] This differs from CIN lesions, where the loop excision procedure appears to be as effective as conisation.[51] Another randomised prospective study, including 180 women, failed to identify any objective differences between LLETZ and cold-knife conisation with regard to diagnostic and therapeutic results.[52]

Azodi et al.[53] reported that the endocervical margins were positive for glandular abnormalities in 24% of knife cones in comparison with 75% of loop cones. The ectocervical margins were positive for squamous and/or glandular abnormalities in 8% and 13% of knife and loop procedures, respectively. These authors concluded that women with AIS had residual disease in about one-third of cases with negative margins in cone biopsies and/or with negative endocervical curettage and in 56% of cases with positive endocervical margins.[53]

Conisation using either loop diathermy or cold knife is acceptable and is recommended as first-line treatment in most cases of CGIN.[6] The success of these treatments depends on the skill of the operator, which can vary significantly. The success of treatment will also depend upon the depth and quality of the biopsy. The rate of complete excision will be greater with a cylindrical biopsy or 'blunt' cone than with a sharply tapering one. Treatment should, however, be individualised to the particular patient and should take into account the size of the lesion, the age of the patient and wishes regarding future fertility.

Needle excision of the transformation zone (NETZ)

In the loop excision procedure, the amount of tissue and the shape of the sample are largely determined by the shape and size of the loop. The deep cutting edge of the loop is invisible during the procedure, so excision may be shallower than intended. As a result, loop diathermy may give poor results when dealing with disease inside the cervical canal. Large lesions are often removed in multiple fragments, making orientation of the specimen and assessment of completeness of excision impossible.[54]

In an attempt to combine the ease of loop excision with the surgical accuracy of cold-knife conisation, Sadek described the NETZ technique.[55] The needle electrode is a 150-mm long insulated electrode that fits standard diathermy pen handles. The exposed needle (tungsten wire) is 15–20 mm long and 0.5 mm in diameter and is angled 45° away from the axis.

One prospective study of 58 unselected women with histologically verified CIN who underwent conisation with the needle diathermy showed that NETZ is a simple and effective out-patient procedure that yields a one-piece cone specimen of high quality and carries a success rate of 94.8%.[55]

More recently, a randomised, controlled trial compared the use of LLETZ with NETZ in the treatment of CIN. Study subjects were recruited from women undergoing their first cervical treatment for CIN. Cone specimens were deeper in NETZ procedures (20 mm) compared with LLETZ procedures (14 mm; $P < 0.001$) and larger in volume (3143 mm^3) than LLETZ specimens (2404 mm^3; $P - 0.033$). Seventeen patients who underwent LLETZ (9.7%) had at least one involved margin in the surgical specimen compared with 5 (2.9%) in the NETZ group ($P - 0.031$). Histological diagnoses did not differ between groups.[56]

The use of NETZ in the management of CGIN has to be investigated further before conclusions about its efficacy can be made.

SIMPLE HYSTERECTOMY

Definitive treatment for cervical AIS is extrafascial hysterectomy and this has been previously recommended due to the possibility of multifocal pre-invasive disease and occult invasive adenocarcinoma.[57]

An overall incidence of 10.2% of residual disease after cervical conisation for AIS has been reported.[40] Moreover, residual high-grade CGIN was found in about 60% of hysterectomy specimens following cone excisions with involved margins.[58] Furthermore, occult invasive carcinoma has also been detected in such cases. Denehy et al.[59] found that negative endocervical curettings and uninvolved cone margins in patients with cervical adenocarcinoma in situ did not exclude the presence of residual endocervical glandular disease in subsequent surgical specimens. These findings have been used to support the use of hysterectomy for treatment of AIS. However, invasive disease is very uncommon following conisation treatment; therefore, if positive margins are found after conisation, repeat cone biopsy could be considered as an alternative to hysterectomy.

Consideration of hysterectomy has been recommended in the following situations:[60]

1   *There are positive cone margins after an adequate excision.*
2   *There is cervical stenosis following previous conisation.*
3   *There is recurrent high-grade cytological abnormality.*
4   *The patient has completed her family or fertility is not intended.*
5   *The patient is poorly compliant or unwilling to undergo conservative management.*
6   *The patient has associated gynaecological conditions.*

For those in whom a hysterectomy is the proposed 'definitive treatment', a second cone biopsy is usually required before hysterectomy to avoid inappropriate treatment of an occult invasive lesion.[61] Despite extrafascial hysterectomy for presumed high grade CGIN, a residual focus could remain and present later as invasive adenocarcinoma.[62]

MANAGEMENT OF CGIN DURING PREGNANCY

Pregnant patients with any type of abnormal cervical cytology are referred for colposcopy and, if needed, directed biopsies. Diagnostic conisation is recommended at 16–18 weeks' gestation if the cytology suggests invasion. Otherwise, women undergo colposcopy every 4–8 weeks and cervical smears are taken; they are then re-evaluated for treatment postpartum.[63] If indicated, it is not safe to extend the CKC to include skip lesions in pregnant women.

A recent study reported 11 patients, with a median age of 32 years, managed for AIS during pregnancy. Five patients in whom the diagnosis was made early in the second trimester underwent cold knife conisation between 14–19 weeks while the other 6 patients had post-partum conisation. All patients delivered through the normal vaginal route. One patient undergoing postpartum CKC required radical hysterectomy for stage IB1 cervical adenocarcinoma. Four subsequent pregnancies occurred among patients who had fertility-sparing surgery. The authors concluded that management of cervical AIS during pregnancy by early second trimester CKC is safe for mother and fetus.[64]

FOLLOW-UP

After treatment for CGIN, long-term follow-up using cytological and colposcopic assessment is essential to detect residual disease and early evidence of recurrence. Recurrent abnormalities have been reported after conisation as well as after hysterectomy for AIS.[42,50]

Abnormal smear after cervical cone biopsy is a sensitive indicator of residual disease.[36] Doubts have been expressed about the reliability of post-conisation cytology, especially in the presence of cervical stenosis.[2] The effectiveness of cytological follow-up has not been established by long-term prospective studies.

Cytology is relatively insensitive for the detection of glandular lesions after treatment but both Ayre's spatula and endocervical brush samples are required to ensure adequate sampling of the endocervical canal and maximise this sensitivity.

The length of follow-up period, and the interval between follow-up smears, in women treated for CGIN are unknown. One study proposed smears at 4-monthly intervals for 2 years and annually thereafter.[36] Others recommended cytology, colposcopy, and endocervical curettage every 4 months for 1 year and every 6 months thereafter.[50,65]

While there is a trend for managing patients with CGIN with negative margins more conservatively, further studies are needed with longer follow-up of patients. The risk of developing recurrent CGIN is 10% at the most.[43] Patients should be informed that recurrent CGIN, and rarely early invasive adenocarcinoma of the cervix, do occur over the long term and that regular follow-up with colposcopy, cytology, and ECC is necessary. The management of these patients after completion of child-bearing remains controversial. Most continue to advocate definitive treatment with simple hysterectomy.[66]

CONCLUSIONS

There is currently no standard treatment for pre-invasive glandular lesions of the cervix. Treatment of CGIN includes conservative therapy, conisation, or hysterectomy. Emphasis should be focused on confirming the diagnosis of CGIN, ruling out invasive adenocarcinoma, and examining the histopathological status of the endocervical margin, as a positive margin is predictive for residual *in situ* or possibly early invasive disease. The rates of residual CGIN after conisation are not guaranteed even with negative cone margins. Patients who choose to be followed conservatively should be counselled about the importance of compliance and the potential risks of undetected and recurrent glandular disease, despite negative follow-up findings.

Key points for clinical practice

- Malignant and premalignant endocervical glandular lesions are increasingly encountered in clinical and pathology practice.

- Women with high-grade cervical glandular intra-epithelial neoplasia (CGIN) are 10–20 years younger than those with invasive disease.

- Cervical cytology and colposcopy have limited ability to detect women with CGIN.

- Conservative management, including excision of the transformation zone, has replaced radical treatment for most cases of CGIN.

- A cylindrical biopsy or 'blunt' cone is associated with a higher rate of complete excision than a sharply tapering one.

- NETZ combines the ease of loop excision with the surgical accuracy of cold-knife conisation but, to date, data are inadequate to recommend this procedure as treatment for high-grade CGIN.

- Simple hysterectomy should be recommended for women who have completed their family or who have other gynaecological conditions.

- Treatment should be individualised for each patient, with particular reference to the size of the lesion and the age of the patient.

References

1. Bryson P, Stulberg R, Shepherd L, McLelland K, Jeffrey J. Is electrosurgical loop excision with negative margins sufficient treatment for cervical ACIS? *Gynecol Oncol* 2004; **93**: 465–468.
2. Muntz HG, Bell DA, Lage JM, Goff BA, Feldman S, Rice LW. Adenocarcinoma *in situ* of the uterine cervix. *Obstet Gynecol* 1992; **80**: 935–939.

3. Parazzini F, La Vecchia C. Epidemiology of adenocarcinoma of the cervix. *Gynecol Oncol* 1990; **39**: 40–46.

4. Stockton D, Cooper P, Lonsdale RN. Changing incidence of invasive adenocarcinoma of the uterine cervix in East Anglia. *J Med Screen* 1997; **4**: 40–43.

5. Hemminki K, Li X, Vaittinen P. Time trends in the incidence of cervical and other genital squamous cell carcinomas and adenocarcinomas in Sweden, 1958–1996. *Eur J Obstet Gynecol Reprod Biol* 2002; **101**: 64–69.

6. El-Ghobashy AA, Shaaban AM, Herod JJ, Herrington CS. The pathology and management of endocervical glandular neoplasia. *Int J Gynaecol Cancer* 2005; **15**: 583-592.

7. Friedell G, McKay D. Adenocarcinoma *in situ* of the endocervix. *Cancer* 1953; **6**: 887–897.

8. Brown LJ, Wells M. Cervical glandular atypia associated with squamous intraepithelial neoplasia: a premalignant lesion? *J Clin Pathol* 1986; **39**: 22–28.

9. Anderson MC. Glandular lesions of the cervix: diagnostic and therapeutic dilemmas. *Baillière's Clin Obstet Gynaecol* 1995; **9**: 105–119.

10. Colgan TJ, Lickrish GM. The topography and invasive potential of cervical adenocarcinoma *in situ*, with and without associated squamous dysplasia. *Gynecol Oncol* 1990; **36**: 246–249.

11. Ostor AG, Pagano R, Davoren RA, Fortune DW, Chanen W, Rome R. Adenocarcinoma *in situ* of the cervix. *Int J Gynecol Pathol* 1984; **3**: 179–190.

12. NHSCSP TRCoPat. *Achievable standards, benchmarks for reporting, and criteria for evaluating cervical cytopathology.* NHSCSP Publication No 1, 2000.

13. Ostor AG. Early invasive adenocarcinoma of the uterine cervix. *Int J Gynecol Pathol* 2000; **19**: 29–38.

14. Ostor A, Rome R, Quinn M. Microinvasive adenocarcinoma of the cervix: a clinicopathologic study of 77 women. *Obstet Gynecol* 1997; **89**: 88–93.

15. FIGO CCo. Staging announcement. *Gynecol Oncol* 1986; **25**: 383–385.

16. Fluhmann CF. Focal hyperplasia (tunnel clusters) of the cervix uteri. *Obstet Gynecol* 1961; **17**: 206–214.

17. Qizilbash AH. *In-situ* and microinvasive adenocarcinoma of the uterine cervix. A clinical, cytologic and histologic study of 14 cases. *Am J Clin Pathol* 1975; **64**: 155–170.

18. Teshima S, Shimosato Y, Kishi K, Kasamatsu T, Ohmi K, Uei Y. Early stage adenocarcinoma of the uterine cervix. Histopathologic analysis with consideration of histogenesis. *Cancer* 1985; **56**: 167–172.

19. Rollason TP, Cullimore J, Bradgate MG. A suggested columnar cell morphological equivalent of squamous carcinoma *in situ* with early stromal invasion. *Int J Gynecol Pathol* 1989; **8**: 230–236.

20. Matsukuma K, Tsukamoto N, Kaku T *et al.* Early adenocarcinoma of the uterine cervix – its histologic and immunohistologic study. *Gynecol Oncol* 1989; **35**: 38–43.

21. Kaku T, Kamura T, Sakai K *et al.* Early adenocarcinoma of the uterine cervix. *Gynecol Oncol* 1997; **65**: 281–285.

22. Nicklin JL, Perrin LC, Crandon AJ, Ward BG. Microinvasive adenocarcinoma of the cervix. *Aust NZ J Obstet Gynaecol* 1999; **39**: 411–413.

23. Schorge JO, Lee KR, Flynn CE, Goodman A, Sheets EE. Stage IA1 cervical adenocarcinoma: definition and treatment. *Obstet Gynecol* 1999; **93**: 219–222.

24. Kurian K, al-Nafussi A. Relation of cervical glandular intraepithelial neoplasia to microinvasive and invasive adenocarcinoma of the uterine cervix: a study of 121 cases. *J Clin Pathol* 1999; **52**: 112–117.

25. Kasper H, Dinh T, Mg D. Clinical implications of tumor volume measurement in stage 1 adenocarcinoma. *Obstet Gynecol* 1993; **81**: 296–300.

26. Pirog EC, Kleter B, Olgac S *et al.* Prevalence of human papillomavirus DNA in different histological subtypes of cervical adenocarcinoma. *Am J Pathol* 2000; **157**: 1055–1062.

27. Zaino RJ. Glandular lesions of the uterine cervix. *Mod Pathol* 2000; **13**: 261–274.

28. Brinton LA, Tashima KT, Lehman HF *et al.* Epidemiology of cervical cancer by cell type. *Cancer Res* 1987; **47**: 1706–1711.

29. Ursin G, Peters RK, Henderson BE, d'Ablaing 3rd G, Monroe KR, Pike MC. Oral contraceptive use and adenocarcinoma of cervix. *Lancet* 1994; **344**: 1390–1394.

30. Jackson SR, Hollingworth TA, Anderson MC, Johnson J, Hammond RH. Glandular lesions of the cervix – cytological and histological correlation. *Cytopathology* 1996; **7**: 10–16.

31. Leeson SC, Inglis TC, Salman WD. A study to determine the underlying reason for abnormal glandular cytology and the formulation of a management protocol. *Cytopathology* 1997; **8**: 20–26.

32. Waddell CA. Glandular abnormalities: dilemmas in cytological prediction and clinical management. *Cytopathology* 1997; **8**: 27–30.

33. Shin CH, Schorge JO, Lee KR, Sheets EE. Cytologic and biopsy findings leading to conization in adenocarcinoma *in situ* of the cervix. *Obstet Gynecol* 2002; **100**: 271–276.

34. Lickrish GM, Colgan TJ, Wright VC. Colposcopy of adenocarcinoma *in situ* and invasive adenocarcinoma of the cervix. *Obstet Gynecol Clin North Am* 1993; **20**: 111–122.

35. Luesley DM, Jordan JA, Woodman CB, Watson N, Williams DR, Waddell C. A retrospective review of adenocarcinoma-*in-situ* and glandular atypia of the uterine cervix. *Br J Obstet Gynaecol* 1987; **94**: 699–703.

36. Cullimore JE, Luesley DM, Rollason TP *et al*. A prospective study of conization of the cervix in the management of cervical intraepithelial glandular neoplasia (CIGN) – a preliminary report. *Br J Obstet Gynaecol* 1992; **99**: 314–318.

37. NHSCSP. *Histopathology reporting in cervical screening*. Sheffield: Working party of The Royal College of Pathologists and the NHS Cervical Screening Programme, 1999.

38. Ostor AG, Duncan A, Quinn M, Rome R. Adenocarcinoma *in situ* of the uterine cervix: an experience with 100 cases. *Gynecol Oncol* 2000; **79**: 207–210.

39. Hunter R, Brewster A. Recent advances in the treatment of advanced carcinoma of the cervix. In: Bonnar J. (ed) *Recent Advances in Obstetrics and Gynaecology*, vol 18. Edinburgh: Churchill Livingstone, 1994.

40. Nicklin JL, Wright RG, Bell JR, Samaratunga H, Cox NC, Ward BG. A clinicopathological study of adenocarcinoma *in situ* of the cervix. The influence of cervical HPV infection and other factors, and the role of conservative surgery. *Aust NZ J Obstet Gynaecol* 1991; **31**: 179–183.

41. Bertrand M, Lickrish GM, Colgan TJ. The anatomic distribution of cervical adenocarcinoma *in situ*: implications for treatment. *Am J Obstet Gynecol* 1987; **157**: 21–25.

42. Poynor EA, Barakat RR, Hoskins WJ. Management and follow-up of patients with adenocarcinoma *in situ* of the uterine cervix. *Gynecol Oncol* 1995; **57**: 158–164.

43. Kennedy AW, Biscotti CV. Further study of the management of cervical adenocarcinoma *in situ*. *Gynecol Oncol* 2002; **86**: 361–364.

44. Prendiville W, Cullimore J, Norman S. Large loop excision of the transformation zone (LLETZ). A new method of management for women with cervical intraepithelial neoplasia. *Br J Obstet Gynaecol* 1989; **96**: 1054–1060.

45. Luesley DM, Cullimore J, Redman CW *et al*. Loop diathermy excision of the cervical transformation zone in patients with abnormal cervical smears. *BMJ* 1990; **300**: 1690–1693.

46. Oyesanya OA, Amerasinghe C, Manning EA. A comparison between loop diathermy conization and cold-knife conization for management of cervical dysplasia associated with unsatisfactory colposcopy. *Gynecol Oncol* 1993; **50**: 84–88.

47. Bigrigg A, Haffenden DK, Sheehan AL, Codling BW, Read MD. Efficacy and safety of large-loop excision of the transformation zone. *Lancet* 1994; **343**: 32–34.

48. Cruickshank ME, Flannelly G, Campbell DM, Kitchener HC. Fertility and pregnancy outcome following large loop excision of the cervical transformation zone. *Br J Obstet Gynaecol* 1995; **102**: 467–470.

49. Maini M, Lavie O, Comerci G *et al*. The management and follow-up of patients with high-grade cervical glandular intraepithelial neoplasia. *Int J Gynecol Cancer* 1998; **8**: 287–291.

50. Widrich T, Kennedy AW, Myers TM, Hart WR, Wirth S. Adenocarcinoma *in situ* of the uterine cervix: management and outcome. *Gynecol Oncol* 1996; **61**: 304–308.

51. Gold M, Dunton C, Murray J. Loop electrocautery excisional procedure: therapeutic effectiveness as an ablation and a conization equivalent. *Gynecol Oncol* 1996; **61**: 241–244.

52. Duggan BD, Felix JC, Muderspach LI *et al*. Cold-knife conization versus conization by the loop electrosurgical excision procedure: a randomized, prospective study. *Am J Obstet Gynecol* 1999; **180**: 276–282.

53. Azodi M, Chambers SK, Rutherford TJ, Kohorn EI, Schwartz PE, Chambers JT. Adenocarcinoma *in situ* of the cervix: management and outcome. *Gynecol Oncol* 1999; **73**: 348–353.

54. Basu PS, D'Arcy T, McIndoe A, Soutter WP. Is needle diathermy excision of the transformation zone a better treatment for cervical intraepithelial neoplasia than large loop excision? *Lancet* 1999; **353**: 1852–1853.

55. Sadek AL. Needle excision of the transformation zone: a new method for treatment of cervical intraepithelial neoplasia. *Am J Obstet Gynecol* 2000; **182**: 866–871.

56. Panoskaltsis T, Ind TE, Perryman K, Dina R, Abrahams Y, Soutter WP. Needle versus loop diathermy excision of the transformation zone for the treatment of cervical intraepithelial neoplasia: a randomised controlled trial. *Br J Obstet Gynaecol* 2004; **111**: 748–753.

57. Buscema J, Woodruff JD. Significance of neoplastic atypicalities in endocervical epithelium. *Gynecol Oncol* 1984; **17**: 356–362.

58. Howard G, Muntz H. Can cervical adenocarcinoma in situ be safely managed by conization alone? *Gynecol Oncol* 1996; **61**: 301–303.

59. Denehy TR, Gregori CA, Breen JL. Endocervical curettage, cone margins, and residual adenocarcinoma *in situ* of the cervix. *Obstet Gynecol* 1997; **90**: 1–6.

60. NHSCSP. *Colposcopy and Programme Management*. Sheffield: NHS Cervical Screening Programme, 2004.

61. Soutter WP, Haidopoulos D, Gornall RJ *et al*. Is conservative treatment for adenocarcinoma *in situ* of the cervix safe? *Br J Obstet Gynaecol* 2001; **108**: 1184–1189.

62. Krivak TC, Retherford B, Voskuil S, Rose GS, Alagoz T. Recurrent invasive adenocarcinoma after hysterectomy for cervical adenocarcinoma *in situ*. *Gynecol Oncol* 2000; **77**: 334–335.

63. American College of Obstetricians and Gynecologists. *Diagnosis and Treatment of Cervical Carcinomas*. ACOG Practice Bulletin, Number 35. Washington, DC: American College of Obstetricians and Gynecologists, 2002.

64. Lacour RA, Garner EI, Molpus KL, Ashfaq R, Schorge JO. Management of cervical adenocarcinoma in situ during pregnancy. *Am J Obstet Gynecol* 2005; **192**: 1449–1451.

65. Kennedy AW, elTabbakh GH, Biscotti CV, Wirth S. Invasive adenocarcinoma of the cervix following LLETZ (large loop excision of the transformation zone) for adenocarcinoma *in situ*. *Gynecol Oncol* 1995; **58**: 274–277.

66. Andersen E, Nielsen K. Adenocarcinoma *in situ* of the cervix: a prospective study of conization as definitive treatment. *Gynecol Oncol* 2002; **86**: 365–369.

Michael Hannemann Jo Bailey John Murdoch

18

Recent advances in the surgical management of cervical cancer

Cancer of the uterine cervix is the world's commonest cause of gynaecological cancer death and responsible for about 300,000 deaths every year. Of these, around 1000 occur in the UK. Both the incidence of and mortality from cervical cancer have been reduced by systematic screening and treatment for premalignant cervical lesions. In the UK, the incidence of invasive cervical carcinoma has fallen by about 7% every year since 1988 when three changes to the screening programme were introduced. These were: (i) the setting of incentivised targets for general practitioners; (ii) a computerised recall system; and (iii) the use of comprehensive screening quality control. Despite these efforts, cervical cancer still occurs because the sensitivity of individual smears may be as low as 30%, and 15% of women (who are often at particularly increased risk) fail to attend for screening.

NATURAL HISTORY AND STAGING

Squamous carcinoma is responsible for 75% of cervix cancers. The major aetiological factor is persistent human papilloma virus infection, which induces premalignant changes in the cervical squamous epithelium. The latent phase prior to the development of invasive cancer lasts an average of 12 years,

Michael Hannemann MBBCh MRCOG PhD (for correspondence)
Specialist Registrar, Directorate of Obstetrics and Gynaecology and ENT, United Bristol Healthcare NHS Trust, St Michael's Hospital, Southwell Street, Bristol BS2 8EG, UK
(E-mail: mhannemann@blueyonder.co.uk)

Jo Bailey MRCS(Ed) MRCOG
Subspecialty Trainee in Gynaecological Oncology, Directorate of Obstetrics and Gynaecology and ENT, United Bristol Healthcare NHS Trust, St Michael's Hospital, Southwell Street, Bristol BS2 8EG, UK

John Murdoch MD FRCOG
Consultant, Directorate of Obstetrics and Gynaecology and ENT, United Bristol Healthcare NHS Trust, St Michael's Hospital, Southwell Street, Bristol BS2 8EG, UK

Table 1 FIGO staging of cervical cancer

Stage		Positive pelvic nodes	Survival
1a1	Micro-invasive ≤ 3 mm deep ≤ 7 mm wide	< 1%	> 95%
1a2	Micro-invasive 3–5 mm deep ≤ 7 mm wide	7%	93%
1b1	Confined to cervix ≤ 4 cm	15%	90%
1b2	Confined to cervix > 4 cm		80%
2a	Beyond cervix, but not parametrium or lower third of vagina	30%	75%
2b	Beyond cervix, with parametrial involvement but not the lower third of vagina		73%
3a	Involves the lower third of vagina	> 35%	50%
3b	Involves the pelvic side wall, or obstructive uropathy		45%
4a	Involvement of mucosa of adjacent organs such as bladder or rectum	> 50%	30%
4b	Beyond the true pelvis		22%

providing the opportunity for screening and prevention. Once invasion has occurred, spread is initially contiguous, within the cervix, and then laterally along the uterine support structures. Vertical spread into the vagina or uterine cavity occurs later. Lymphatic spread occurs into parametrial, then pelvic, and finally para-aortic lymph nodes. Haematogenous spread is less common.

Apart from the mortality, invasive cervical cancer and its treatment have significant morbidity: sexual dysfunction, loss of fertility, bladder dysfunction, pain from bony invasion, renal failure due to ureteric involvement, fistulae, and discharge.

Sexual dysfunction following treatment of cervical cancer has been studied,[1] and the incidence is both high and multifaceted. Patients have reduced autonomic responses such as engorgement, lubrication and orgasm, and significant dyspareunia arises due to vaginal shortening and stenosis. Bladder dysfunction, particularly voiding difficulty or urinary tract infection, is also very common.

Staging of cervical cancer is most commonly based on the FIGO classification, last modified in 1994 (Table 1). FIGO staging defines the extent of disease, guides treatment, allows prognostic information, and enables valid comparison of management approaches used around the world. Staging is based on clinical examination, a chest X-ray and an intravenous urogram; it does not include nodal status, tumour type or differentiation, or the presence of lymphovascular space invasion. Neither does it recognise modern imaging, which has a major impact on treatment planning. These factors affect prognosis. For example, the presence and number of positive lymph nodes reduces survival stage for stage. One study demonstrated 5-year, disease-free survival in 77% of women with negative nodes, 55% with one or two positive nodes, and 39% when more than two nodes were involved.[2] Furthermore, there is a poor correlation between true tumour size and invasion assessed pathologically compared to pre-operative staging.[3] FIGO staging, therefore, has deficiencies in both accurate prognostication and in determination of tumour resectability.

Modern pretreatment assessment attempts to take these aspects into account through imaging and staging surgery. Imaging methods such as CT, MRI and PET have been used to assist in delineating tumour volume and spread, and the presence of nodal disease. CT and MRI have greatly varying (25–80%) sensitivities and specificities in identifying nodal disease, depending on the size of nodal tumour.[4–6] Considerable evidence suggests that MRI has good sensitivity for the detection of both parametrial involvement, extracervical spread, and to a lesser extent, involvement of lymph nodes.[7] More recently, the use of PET has shown great promise in detecting nodal disease when the primary tumour is avid for 2-[^{18}F]-fluoro-2-deoxy-D-glucose,[8] with a sensitivity of 90%.

Laparoscopy to determine nodal status prior to radical surgery has increased in practice. Nodes can be examined for micrometastases which would be missed by pre-operative imaging for nodal status. Laparoscopic node dissection may be performed as an interval procedure prior to definitive surgery, or as the first part of a two-stage operation combined with frozen section for histopathological assessment. Node yields are comparable with open lymph node dissection (suggesting high sensitivity), and morbidity is low.[9,10] A less invasive means of assessing node status is the use of laparoscopic ultrasound to guide lymph node sampling.[11] Only suspicious nodes are removed, thus limiting the risk of lymphocoele or lymphoedema. This method has an attendant risk of missing microscopic metastases, and calls into question its value in preference to less invasive imaging techniques.

In keeping with recent developments in the management of other cancers (malignant melanoma, breast, vulva), identification of the sentinel lymph node has been proposed in women with early stage disease. This could avoid the removal of large numbers of normal lymph nodes with attendant morbidity. Using blue dye injected into the cervix, Dargent and Enria[12] were able to identify and remove the sentinel node(s) in 125 of 135 dissections and 19 sentinel nodes contained tumour. All cases in the series went on to have full pelvic lymph node dissections, and none were shown to have nodal disease elsewhere when the sentinel node was negative.[12] Plante et al.[13] suggest combining use of blue dye injection with pre-operative lymphoscintiography, and report detection of up to 93% sentinel nodes, although this success was related to experience. They also reported a 100% negative predictive value.

Other reports are less encouraging. Marchiole et al.,[14] in a series of 29 cases, noted 3 occurrences of false negative sentinel node when multilevel sectioning and immunohistochemical staining for cytokeratin were employed in addition to routine histopathological assessment, yielding a negative predictive value of 87%. Anaphylactic reaction to the blue dye can arise in 1–2%.

HISTORICAL MANAGEMENT

The primary aim of surgery for invasive cervical cancer is cure by complete resection of the tumour with clear margins of disease-free tissue and minimal morbidity. This is achieved by matching extent of radical surgery with extent of disease. Radical hysterectomy was described by Wertheim (abdominal) and Schauta (vaginal) in the early 1900s. This was designed to achieve clear margins of excision, even when the tumour had extended into the parametria or the upper vagina. Refinements followed, notably in the UK from Victor Bonney, and in 1945, radical hysterectomy was combined with pelvic lymphadenectomy for disease staging by Meigs. The presence of positive lymph nodes signified incomplete disease excision and, therefore, a need for adjuvant radiotherapy.

In the latter part of the 20th century, the amount of tissue removed was refined to suit the disease stage. This led to the Rutledge classification of hysterectomies for cervical cancer.[15] This classification had five categories of increasing radicality, starting with Class 1, a simple or extrafascial hysterectomy. Class 3 was the classical Wertheim operation which involves division of the uterine supports at their pelvic origin and, therefore, considerable dissection of the ureters. Morbidity, particularly urological, remained a particular concern, leading to the use in less advanced tumours of the Class 2, or modified radical hysterectomy. This involved removal of less parametrial tissue with division of the uterine arteries medial to the ureters which was less likely to cause morbidity. Class 5 denoted complete pelvic exenteration, an operation primarily reserved for local tumour recurrence after primary treatment.

PRINCIPLES OF MANAGEMENT

Survival in early stage disease is the same, whether primary treatment is surgical or with radiotherapy (with or without chemotherapy).[16] Other factors are, therefore, taken into account when selecting the most appropriate treatment modality. The most important of these are age, medical co-morbidity, fertility requirements, and the likely relative morbidities of the available treatments. Surgical morbidity is rarely severe and is usually short-lived, or at least stable and treatable. Mortality arises from complications such as venous thromboembolism (0.1–1%), haemorrhage and infection. Radiotherapy, in contrast, has a treatment-related mortality of virtually zero. Early and late morbidity, however, is common (5–15%), chronic, often poorly treatable, and progressive.[17] Notable problems include chronic diarrhoea, bladder irritation and vaginal stenosis. In a small number of cases, radiation damage causes fistulae or bowel obstruction requiring surgical intervention.[18] Another benefit of a surgical approach in preference to radiotherapy in young patients with squamous carcinomas (and more controversially, with potentially oestrogen-sensitive adenocarcinomas) is retention of ovarian function.

The least favourable outcome would be aggregation of morbidities by subjecting the patient to both treatment modalities, as there is no compensatory survival advantage. Therefore, surgery tends to be the primary treatment modality if complete resection with clear margins and negative lymph nodes are highly likely. Primary chemoradiation is reserved for more advanced tumours and patients with inordinately high surgical risk.

SURGICAL MANAGEMENT

STAGE IA1

This tumour is preclinical, and usually detected by screening, although it is sometimes found after a simple hysterectomy for an unrelated indication.

Loop excision, conisation or simple hysterectomy are usually adequate treatments. The choice depends on patient-specific factors, such as age, need for fertility, and the presence and amount of surrounding CIN. The risk of lymphatic spread is extremely low, and 5-year survival with optimal care is more than 95%.[19]

STAGE IA2

Treatment is more controversial. There is a very high chance of cure, and studies aiming to examine differences in outcome between the available surgical treatments would have to be very large. Options vary from local excision to Class 3 hysterectomy. All have excellent survival results, but varying morbidity. Universal use of Class 3 hysterectomy, with its high incidence of short-term morbidity arising from bladder denervation, would be overtreatment in the majority of cases, while limiting all to local excision would lead to a few deaths which would have been prevented by a more radical approach.

Risk of nodal disease at the time of surgery is low (7%). Pelvic lymphadenectomy has morbidity (vascular trauma, lymph collection and lymphoedema) but identifies the subgroup of patients who need adjuvant therapy.

Treatment may be individualised using other non-FIGO information to stratify patients with 1a2 tumours into high or low risk. This is based on histopathological features such as the presence or absence of lymphovascular space invasion, degree of differentiation, type of tumour (adeno- or squamous carcinoma), and on tumour volume (with high risk near the upper limits of the FIGO 1a2 stage). Low-risk cases may be treated more conservatively, with local excision or simple hysterectomy, while high-risk cases have more radical surgery, combined with lymph node dissection (Table 2). Laparoscopy is increasingly used for hysterectomy and pelvic node dissection.[20]

Table 2 Surgical management of cervical cancer

FIGO stage	Non-FIGO information	Treatment
1a1		Local excision (LLETZ, conisation) Simple hysterectomy (if other indications, e.g. fibroids)
1a2	Low risk	As for 1a1
	High risk	Conisation and node dissection Radical trachelectomy Radical hysterectomy (abdominal/vaginal/laparoscopic)
1b1	< 2 cm	Radical trachelectomy Laparoscopic radical hysterectomy Abdominal/vaginal radical hysterectomy
	> 2 cm and 'Node negative'	Abdominal/vaginal radical hysterectomy
1b2	'Node negative'	Abdominal/vaginal radical hysterectomy
	'Node positive'	Primary chemoradiation
2a/2b		As for 1b2
3/4		Primary chemoradiation

STAGE IB1–IIA (NON-BULKY)

Treatment of these patients is less controversial, in that most patients would be treated with a Class 3 hysterectomy and pelvic lymphadenopathy. If pelvic or para-aortic lymph nodes are clinically enlarged, a para-aortic lymph node dissection is also often undertaken. Adjuvant treatment with radiotherapy is indicated if any lymph nodes are found to be involved (15% of Ib, 30% of IIa), or the resection margins are not clear. Knowledge about para-aortic lymph node positivity may be helpful for planning appropriate radiation fields. Variations on this theme depend on availability of resources. One approach might be a preliminary laparoscopic lymphadenectomy with frozen section and abandonment of radical surgery in favour of primary chemoradiation if the nodes are positive.[20,21] This could reduce morbidity from multimodal therapy, while uterine conservation facilitates brachytherapy. More recently, the feasibility of adjuvant radiotherapy in node-negative stage 1b1 has been explored in cases where adverse pathological features such as tumour grade, lymphovascular space invasion and stromal invasion are apparent.[22] The findings were that the treatment is well tolerated, and may confer a survival benefit in these carefully selected cases.

The use of adjuvant Rutledge 1 hysterectomy after primary treatment with radiation in early stage disease has been suggested. With local recurrence rates of about 3% in tumours of less than 5 cm,[23] there is little to be gained from this approach in non-bulky tumours. In 1969, Durrance et al.[24] suggested that the 10% risk of recurrence of bulky stage 1b disease after primary radiotherapy is reduced by adjuvant hysterectomy, which led to its wide-spread adoption. More recently, however, a prospective GOG study suggested no clinically significant benefit from this approach.[25] Bearing in mind the increased morbidity of surgery performed after radiation,[26] adjuvant hysterectomy is now rarely indicated.

STAGE IIB AND BEYOND

This stage has at least clinical tumour involvement of the parametrium. Such patients are not suitable for surgery, because resection margins are often positive and there is a high node-positivity rate (30%). Adjuvant chemoradiation would frequently be needed, with its excess morbidity and no proven survival advantage. Thus, treatment is with primary chemoradiation. An alternative strategy is surgery after neo-adjuvant chemoradiation. The patients, with initially inoperable tumours, are first treated with chemotherapy and/or radiotherapy, and then subjected to surgery if they have responded to the extent that the tumour has become operable. The purpose of this intervention would be to prevent local recurrence. Studies conflict, with one suggesting a distinct survival advantage from neo-adjuvant chemotherapy before radical surgery,[27] while another failed to do so.[28] A second study showing benefit from neo-adjuvant chemotherapy[29] has been criticised for failure to use neo-adjuvant chemotherapy in the radiotherapy arm, and for using suboptimal doses of radiation. The results of an EORTC trial addressing this issue are awaited.

STAGE III AND BEYOND

These patients are treated with primary chemoradiation. Consideration may be given to laparoscopic or open para-aortic lymph node dissection (30% positive). The information thus gained is prognostic,[30] and may modify treatment such as planning of radiation fields in up to 40% of patients.[31] There may be some advantage in surgical debulking of enlarged para-aortic lymph nodes prior to extended field radiation therapy. Cosin *et al.*[32] suggested that this approach has similar survival and morbidity results compared with only microscopically positive nodes. Others, however, contend that only about 4% of patients subjected to the necessary staging surgery (with its morbidity) would gain from it.[33]

INNOVATIONS WHICH LIMIT MORBIDITY

FERTILITY-SPARING SURGERY

Beyond stage 1a1, all treatment modalities for Ca cervix have until recently rendered patients sterile. Bearing in mind the initial tendency of small cervical tumours to spread laterally into the parametria and lymph nodes rather than vertically into the uterus or vagina, it should theoretically be possible to resect the cervix, parametria and lymph nodes while preserving the vagina, uterus and ovaries. This operation, known as a radical trachelectomy, may be performed vaginally, abdominally or with laparoscopic assistance, in conjunction with laparoscopic or open lymph node dissection. In women with small volume disease showing no evidence of extracervical spread (stage 1a2 – small 1b1), survival results should be good. First described in 1994, variations on the radical trachelectomy concept have been studied by a small number of researchers. The most common procedure is the vaginal radical trachelectomy with laparoscopic extraperitoneal lymph node dissection. The cervical stump is permanently cerclaged, and future pregnancies necessarily delivered abdominally through a classical uterine incision. So far, survival data have compared well with the more traditional radical hysterectomy approach,[34] and many successful pregnancies have resulted. Bernardini and colleagues[35] described a series of 80 vaginal radical trachelectomy patients, from whom 39 attempted to conceive; 18 were successful, having 22 pregnancies between them. Eighteen live births occurred, of which 12 were at term.[35] Preterm, prelabour rupture of membranes appeared to be a common problem in this and other series. Shepherd *et al.*[36] described a series of 30 women subjected to trachelectomy, of whom 13 tried to conceive and 9 had live births. There were no tumour recurrences in this series. Some cases of recurrence have now been described, however.[34,37] It is clear, therefore, that many women even after choosing to have fertility sparing surgery, decide not to attempt pregnancy, and among those who do, there are considerable challenges to overcome. These points, and the uncertain long-term survival results, should form an important part of presurgery counselling. Women who achieve pregnancy after radical trachelectomy may benefit during their pregnancies from serial ultrasound assessment of the neo-cervix, as this may assist in identifying those likely to labour or rupture membranes prematurely.[38]

NERVE SPARING SURGERY

Much of the bladder, bowel-related[39] and sexual[1] morbidity after radical hysterectomy may be attributed to disruption of the autonomic nerve supply to the affected organs. The hypogastric (largely sympathetic) and pelvic splanchnic (largely parasympathetic) nerves forming the inferior hypogastric plexus contribute to bladder function, as well as the sexual arousal response and orgasm. These are consistently damaged by standard radical surgery. Nerve-sparing radical hysterectomy has recently been described, which reduces morbidity, while maintaining survival and preventing recurrence.[40] This technique has been in use in Japan for some time,[41] but is time consuming and may prove more difficult in Western European women, probably due to increased adiposity. So far, evidence is restricted to case series, and larger prospective studies are awaited.

SURGERY FOR RECURRENCE

In patients with central recurrence following primary radiotherapy, pelvic exenteration has a cure rate as high as 50%. However, it is a formidable procedure, involving removal of all the (previously irradiated) pelvic organs, and should only be embarked upon in carefully selected cases.

Patient selection and pre-operative care

Clinical detection in the irradiated pelvis can be difficult, so exenteration should only be considered when tumour recurrence or persistence has been histologically proven. Cure is only feasible if the tumour is resectable with disease-free margins, and there is no lymph node spread. Lymph node disease present at the time of exenteration is associated with a 5-year survival of less than 15%.[43] Thus, before definitive surgery is undertaken, examination under anaesthesia and CT or MRI may exclude unresectable pelvic tumours, or evidence of distant spread to liver or lungs. Patients should be fully counselled and aware of the likelihood of two stomas for urinary and faecal diversion. They should be admitted the day before operation and have full bowel preparation.

At laparotomy, the abdomen should be carefully assessed for evidence of extrapelvic disease, or of lymph node spread on frozen section. The resectability of the tumour is also re-assessed. The procedure is abandoned at this stage in 25% of cases.[44]

Surgery and reconstruction

After the initial confirmation of resectability, pelvic exenteration involves the removal of the uterus, adnexae, cervix, vagina, bladder and rectum. This necessitates diversion of both urinary and faecal systems. Exenteration may be limited to either anterior or posterior pelvis if either the rectum or bladder is not involved, and resection can be complete without their removal. This has the benefit of reducing the number of diversions and resultant stomas. The tumour is removed *en bloc*. When urinary diversion is indicated, the ureters are divided and anastomosed to a new urinary reservoir, usually made from an ileal segment to form a conduit, or from colon and terminal ileum to form a continent reservoir. Bowel diversion usually results in a terminal sigmoid colostomy, although in selected cases a low rectal re-anastomosis may be feasible in conjunction with a temporary diverting ileostomy.

Pelvic floor coverage may then be achieved by bringing down a 'J' flap of omentum separated from the greater curvature of the stomach. This provides a non-irradiated blood supply to the pelvis, partially fills the surgical defect (thus preventing empty pelvis syndrome), and in conjunction with suturing together the levator muscles in the midline, limits the risk of introital prolapse or evisceration. Several procedures have also been described to construct a neovagina after exenteration. These include the use of tubes made from omentum, rectus abdominis myocutaneous flaps, gracilis myocutaneous flaps, or segments of bowel. These have the potential to preserve sexual function, while providing a non-irradiated blood supply and filling the surgical defect in the pelvis.

Outcomes

Exenteration has significant mortality (8%) and considerable morbidity (30–50%).[43] Morbidity arises from the urinary or gastrointestinal diversions in the form of leak, obstruction or infection, while other morbidities such as haemorrhage and thromboembolism are also common. About 20% require re-operation.

Intra-operative radiotherapy (IORT)

Several reports have been published of case series where surgery for recurrence has been combined with radiotherapy intra-operatively. The purpose of this is to limit the risk of residual disease at the resection margins, or to treat areas of non-resectable disease in patients who would otherwise not have been suitable for surgery. Advantages include accurate location of treatment, and the ability to move away from the treatment field tissues susceptible to treatment-related morbidity, such as bowel. Survival, however, is strongly influenced by patient selection factors, and severe late treatment-related morbidity occurs in up to 35%.[45]

CONCLUSIONS

Excellent survival results are achievable in cervical cancer, when screening is combined with appropriate surgical management. Recent advances have reduced morbidity (including loss of fertility) while maintaining best survival rates. The use of laparoscopy for lymph node dissection and hysterectomy has allowed the surgeon to perform operations which better suit individual patients. Lack of information about disease spread has been a long-standing problem. Advances in sentinel node detection and in methods of imaging such as MRI and PET, should improve this, enabling more appropriate matching of disease with treatment.

Key points for clinical practice

- Survival rates of patients with early cervical cancer are the same, whether primary treatment is surgical or non-surgical.

- There are trends toward less radical surgery in early stage cervical cancer, as survival rates remain good, and there is less morbidity.

- Radical trachelectomy is a recent procedure, which may preserve fertility in carefully selected and counselled patients.

- Nerve-sparing radical hysterectomy may lessen urological and sexual morbidity.

- Sentinel lymph node mapping may assist in the further management of patients, often without the need for a full pelvic lymph node dissection.

References

1. Bergmark K, Avall-Lundqvist E, Dickman PW, Henningsohn L, Steineck G. Vaginal changes and sexuality in women with a history of cervical cancer. *N Engl J Med* 1999; **340**: 1383–1389.
2. Sevin BU, Nadji M, Lampe B *et al.* Prognostic factors of early stage cervical cancer treated by radical hysterectomy. *Cancer* 1995; **76**: 1978–1986.
3. Matsuyama T, Inoue I, Tsukamoto N *et al.* Stage Ib, IIa, and IIb cervix cancer, postsurgical staging, and prognosis. *Cancer* 1984; **54**: 3072–3077.
4. van Engelshoven JM, Versteege CW, Ruys JH, de Haan J, Sanches H. Computed tomography in staging untreated patients with cervical cancer. *Gynecol Obstet Invest* 1984; **18**: 289–295.
5. Vercamer R, Janssens J, Usewils R *et al.* Computed tomography and lymphography in the presurgical staging of early carcinoma of the uterine cervix. *Cancer* 1987; **60**: 1745–1750.
6. Togashi K, Nishimura K, Sagoh T *et al.* Carcinoma of the cervix: staging with MR imaging. *Radiology* 1989; **171**: 245–251.
7. Bipat S, Glas AS, van der Velden J, Zwinderman AH, Bossuyt PMM, Stoker J. Computed tomography and magnetic resonance imaging in staging of uterine cervical carcinoma: a systematic review. *Gynecol Oncol* 2003; **91**: 59–66.
8. Reinhardt MJ, Ehritt-Braun C, Vogelgesang D *et al.* Metastatic lymph nodes in patients with cervical cancer: detection with MR imaging and FDG PET. *Radiology* 2001; **218**: 776–782.
9. Childers JM, Hatch K, Surwit EA. The role of laparoscopic lymphadenectomy in the management of cervical carcinoma. *Gynecol Oncol* 1992; **47**: 38–43.
10. Vidaurreta J, Bermudez A, di Paola G, Sardi J. Laparoscopic staging in locally advanced cervical carcinoma: A new possible philosophy? *Gynecol Oncol* 1999; **75**: 366–371.
11. Cheung TH, Lo WK, Yu MY, Yang WT, Ho S. Extended experience in the use of laparoscopic ultrasound to detect pelvic nodal metastasis in patients with cervical carcinoma. *Gynecol Oncol* 2004; **92**: 784–788.
12. Dargent D, Enria R. Laparoscopic assessment of the sentinel lymph nodes in early cervical cancer. Technique, preliminary results and future developments. *Crit Rev Oncol Hematol* 2003; **48**: 305–310.
13. Plante M, Renaud M-C, Tetu B, Harel F, Roy M. Laparoscopic sentinel node mapping in early stage cervical cancer. *Gynecol Oncol* 2003; **91**: 494–503.
14. Marchiole P, Buenerd A, Scoazec J-Y, Dargent D, Mathevet P. Sentinel lymph node biopsy is not accurate in predicting lymph node status for patients with cervical carcinoma. *Cancer* 2004; **100**: 2154–2159.

15. Piver MS, Rutledge F, Smith JP. Five classes of extended hysterectomy for women with cervical cancer. *Obstet Gynecol* 1974; **44**: 265–272.

16. Landoni F, Maneo A, Colombo A *et al.* Randomised study of radical surgery versus radiotherapy for stage Ib IIa cervical cancer. *Lancet* 1997; **350**: 535–540.

17. Maduro JH, Pras E, Willemse PHB, de Vries EGE. Acute and long term toxicity following radiotherapy alone or in combination with chemotherapy for locally advanced cervical cancer. *Eur J Cancer* 2003; **29**: 471–488.

18. Creutzberg CL, van Putten WL, Koper PC *et al.* The morbidity of treatment for patients with Stage I endometrial cancer: results from a randomized trial. *Int J Radiat Oncol Biol Phys* 2001; **51**: 1246–1255.

19. Gadducci A, Sartori E, Maggino T *et al.* The clinical outcome of patients with stage Ia1 and Ia2 squamous cell carcinoma of the uterine cervix: a Cooperation Task Force (CTF) study. *Cancer J* 2003; **24**: 513–516.

20. Possover M, Krause N, Kuhne-Heid R, Schneider A. Value of laparoscopic evaluation of paraaortic and pelvic lymph nodes for treatment of cervical cancer. *Am J Obstet Gynecol* 1998; **178**: 806–810.

21. Scholz HS, Lax SF, Benedicic C, Tamussino K, Winter R. Accuracy of frozen section examination of pelvic lymph nodes in patients with FIGO stage IB1 to IIB cervical cancer. *Gynecol Oncol* 2003; **90**: 605–609.

22. Rushdan MN, Tay EH, Khoo-Tan HS *et al.* Tailoring the field and indication of adjuvant pelvic radiation for patients with FIGO stage Ib lymph nodes-negative cervical carcinoma following radical surgery based on the GOG score – a pilot study. *Ann Acad Med Singapore* 2004; **33**: 467–472.

23. Eifel PJ, Morris M, Wharton JT, Oswald MJ. The influence of tumor size and morphology on the outcome of patients with FIGO stage IB squamous cell carcinoma of the uterine cervix. *Int J Radiat Oncol Biol Phys* 1994; **29**: 9–16.

24. Durrance FY, Fletcher GH, Rutledge FN. Analysis of central recurrent disease in stages I and II squamous cell carcinomas of the cervix on intact uterus. *Am J Roentgenol* 1969; **106**: 831–838.

25. Keys HM, Bundy BN, Stehman FB *et al.* Radiation therapy with and without extrafascial hysterectomy for bulky stage IB cervical carcinoma: a randomized trial of the Gynecologic Oncology Group. *Gynecol Oncol* 2003; **89**: 343 353.

26. Mendenhall WM, McCarty PJ, Morgan LS, Chafe WE, Million RR. Stage IB or IIA-B carcinoma of the intact uterine cervix greater than or equal to 6 cm in diameter: is adjuvant extrafascial hysterectomy beneficial? *Int J Radiat Oncol Biol Phys* 1991; **21**: 899–904.

27. Sardi JE, Giaroli A, Sananes C *et al.* Long-term follow-up of the first randomized trial using neoadjuvant chemotherapy in stage Ib squamous carcinoma of the cervix: the final results. *Gynecol Oncol* 1997; **67**: 61–69.

28. Chang TC, Lai CH, Hong JH *et al.* Randomized trial of neoadjuvant cisplatin, vincristine, bleomycin, and radical hysterectomy versus radiation therapy for bulky stage IB and IIA cervical cancer. *J Clin Oncol* 2000; **18**: 1740–1747.

29. Benedetti-Panici P, Greggi S, Colombo A *et al.* Neoadjuvant chemotherapy and radical surgery versus exclusive radiotherapy in locally advanced squamous cell cervical cancer: results from the Italian multicenter randomized study. *J Clin Oncol* 2002; **20**: 179–188.

30. Stehman FB, Thomas GM. Prognostic factors in locally advanced carcinoma of the cervix treated with radiation therapy. *Semin Oncol* 1994; **21**: 25–29.

31. Goff BA, Muntz HG, Paley PJ, Tamimi HK, Koh WJ, Greer BE. Impact of surgical staging in women with locally advanced cervical cancer. *Gynecol Oncol* 1999; **74**: 436–442.

32. Cosin JA, Fowler JM, Chen MD, Paley PJ, Carson LF, Twiggs LB. Pretreatment surgical staging of patients with cervical carcinoma: the case for lymph node debulking. *Cancer* 1998; **82**: 2241–2248.

33. Kupets R, Thomas GM, Covens A. Is there a role for pelvic lymph node debulking in advanced cervical cancer? *Gynecol Oncol* 2002; **87**: 163–170.

34. Plante M, Renaud M-C, Francois H, Roy M. Vaginal radical trachelectomy: an oncologically safe fertility preserving surgery. An updated series of 72 cases and review of the literature. *Gynecol Oncol* 2004; **94**: 614–623.

35. Bernardini M, Barrett J, Seaward G, Covens A. Pregnancy outcomes in patients after radical trachelectomy. *Am J Obstet Gynecol* 2003; **189**: 1378–1382.
36. Shepherd JH, Mould T, Oram DH. Radical trachelectomy in early stage carcinoma of the cervix: outcome as judged by recurrence and fertility rates. *Br J Obstet Gynaecol* 2001; **108**: 882–885.
37. Morice P, Dargent D, Haie-Meder C, Duvillard P, Castaigne D. First case of a centropelvic recurrence after radical trachelectomy: literature review and implications for the preoperative selection of patients. *Gynecol Oncol* 2004; **92**: 1002–1005.
38. Petignat P, Stan C, Megevand E, Dargent D. Pregnancy after trachelectomy: a high risk condition of preterm delivery. Report of a case and review of the literature. *Gynecol Oncol* 2004; **94**: 575–577.
39. Prospective multicenter study on urologic complications after radical surgery with or without radiotherapy in the treatment of stage IB IIA cervical cancer. *Int J Gynecol Cancer* 2000; **10**: 59–66.
40. Maas CP, Trimbos JB, DeRuiter MC, van de Velde CJH, Kenter GG. Nerve sparing radical hysterectomy: latest developments and historical perspective. *Crit Rev Oncol Hematol* 2003; **48**: 271–279.
41. Kuwabara Y, Suzuki M, Hashimoto M, Furugen Y, Yoshida K, Mitsuhashi N. New method to prevent bladder dysfunction after radical hysterectomy for uterine cervical cancer. *J Obstet Gynaecol Res* 2000; **26**: 1–8.
42. Trimbos JB, Maas CP, Deruiter MC, Peters AA, Kenter GG. A nerve sparing radical hysterectomy: guidelines and feasibility in Western patients. *Int J Gynecol Cancer* 2001; **11**: 180–186.
43. Shingleton HM, Soong SJ, Gelder MS, Hatch KD, Baker VV, Austin JM Jr. Clinical and histopathologic factors predicting recurrence and survival after pelvic exenteration for cancer of the cervix. *Obstet Gynecol* 1989; **73**: 1027–1034.
44. Miller B, Morris M, Rutledge F *et al*. Aborted exenterative procedures in recurrent cervical cancer. *Gynecol Oncol* 1993; **50**: 94–99.
45. Mahe MA, Gerard JP, Dubois JB *et al*. Intraoperative radiation therapy in recurrent carcinoma of the uterine cervix: report of the French intraoperative group on 70 patients. *Int J Radiat Oncol Biol Phys* 1996; **34**: 21–26.

Adam Rosenthal Ian Jacobs

19

Overview of ovarian cancer screening

Ovarian cancer is the commonest and most lethal gynaecological malignancy in the UK (Table 1). Despite increases in our understanding of the molecular events underlying malignancy, improved surgical technique and novel chemotherapeutic agents, ovarian cancer remains a challenging condition to manage and survival rates have hardly improved over the last three decades.[1] The poor prognosis of ovarian cancer has been attributed to the frequency with which the disease presents at an advanced stage (Table 2). Consequently, detection of early stage disease may offer a real opportunity to reduce mortality. However, to date, no screening strategy for ovarian cancer has been

Table 1 The ten commonest female solid cancers in the UK in 2001[5]

Site	Average annual incidence 1999–2001	Mortality: incidence ratio
Breast	40,740	0.32
Lung	14,878	0.87
Colorectal	15,939	0.48
Ovary	6663	0.67
Uterine corpus	5490	0.18
Melanoma	3833	0.19
Pancreas	3637	0.99
Stomach	3454	0.75
Bladder	3302	0.55
Cervix	3045	0.39

Adam Rosenthal PhD MRCOG
Clinical Lecturer in Gynaecological Oncology, Institute of Women's Health, University College London, Elizabeth Garrett Anderson Hospital, Huntley Street, London WC1E 6DH, UK

Ian Jacobs MD FRCOG
Professor of Gynaecological Oncology and Director, Institute of Women's Health, University College London, Elizabeth Garrett Anderson Hospital, Huntley Street, London WC1E 6DH, UK

Table 2 Five-year survival rates by stage at presentation in 4004 women treated from 1996–1998[6]

FIGO stage	Proportion of cases (%)	5-year survival (%)
Ia	11.7	89.3
Ib	1.4	64.8
Ic	14.0	78.2
IIa	1.8	79.2
IIb	2.6	64.3
IIc	5.1	68.2
IIIa	3.0	49.2
IIIb	6.3	40.8
IIIc	41.3	28.9
IV	12.8	13.4

shown conclusively to achieve this goal. Nevertheless, developments in tumour marker and ultrasound technology, combined with more sophisticated approaches to interpretation have improved the sensitivity and specificity of the potential screening strategies to levels which may now impact on mortality. These detection strategies are being tested in two large randomised controlled trials of ovarian cancer screening currently underway – one in the UK[2] and one in the US[3] (see below), but the results are not expected until 2012.

The World Health Organization (WHO) criteria for a screening programme[4] have been fulfilled by cervical screening, and the mortality from cervical cancer is falling in systematically screened populations. In this overview, we apply the WHO screening criteria to ovarian cancer to assess the potential for a successful screening programme.

WHO SCREENING CRITERIA AND OVARIAN CANCER

THE CONDITION SOUGHT SHOULD BE AN IMPORTANT HEALTH PROBLEM

Ovarian cancer is the fourth commonest solid cancer in UK women and the average annual incidence between 1999–2001 was 6663.[5] It is also the most lethal gynaecological malignancy, having a mortality:incidence ratio of 0.67.[5] These figures confirm that ovarian cancer is a major health problem.

One explanation for ovarian cancer's high mortality:incidence ratio is the fact that more than 70% of cases present with extra-ovarian disease (Table 2). This may reflect the absence of symptoms in early stage disease, due to the pelvic location of the ovaries and little interference with surrounding structures or local irritation until ovarian enlargement is considerable, or metastatic disease supervenes. When symptoms do occur, they are often non-specific with frequent GP consultations before further investigation or gynaecological referral. However, the vast majority of stage Ia and Ib ovarian cancers have an extremely good prognosis following surgery alone. Thus early detection of the disease should reduce the mortality from ovarian cancer.

THERE SHOULD BE AN ACCEPTED TREATMENT FOR PATIENTS WITH RECOGNISED DISEASE

Whilst certain issues remain to be resolved (*e.g.* the role of interval debulking following suboptimal primary surgery), the management of women presenting with a suspected ovarian cancer is well established with international agreed guidelines for the management of the disease.[7]

FACILITIES FOR DIAGNOSIS AND TREATMENT SHOULD BE AVAILABLE

The two most extensively investigated diagnostic modalities (serum CA125 measurement and transvaginal ultrasound) are both now routinely available in the majority of hospitals throughout the industrialised world. Ultrasound machines are often available in gynaecology clinics, and used for ovarian assessment.[8] Colour flow Doppler ultrasound has also been extensively investigated (see below), but the relatively high cost limits wide-spread use. Surgery and chemotherapy for ovarian cancer are also available throughout the industrialised world.

THERE SHOULD BE A RECOGNISABLE OR EARLY SYMPTOMATIC STAGE

Whilst no premalignant ovarian lesion has been conclusively identified and symptoms cannot be relied upon to identify women with early disease, the fact remains that patients with adequately staged, clinically detected stage I disease have an excellent prognosis. Consequently, stage I disease may be considered a 'recognisable latent phase' for the purposes of ovarian cancer screening. If in the future a premalignant ovarian lesion is identified, then screening for such a lesion should have a greater impact on mortality than screening for stage I disease. The length of the latent phase is of critical importance to the screening interval. A long latent phase, such as that seen in progression from CIN to cervical cancer, allows ample opportunity for disease detection even with screening every 3 years. Unfortunately, the rate of progression from stage I to stage III ovarian cancer is almost certainly variable, with some tumours demonstrating an indolent course, whilst others display an aggressive phenotype. It is hoped that annual screening will be both adequate and practical in this setting, but this remains to be proven.

THERE SHOULD BE A SUITABLE TEST OR EXAMINATION

High sensitivity (the probability of the test being positive in individuals with the disease) and high specificity (the probability of the test being negative in individuals without the disease) are important requirements for any screening test. Unfortunately, increasing the sensitivity of a test (*e.g.* by lowering the cut-off used for a tumour marker) tends to result in a reduction in specificity, and *vice versa*. Specificity is of paramount importance in ovarian cancer screening, because the majority of women testing positive will require exploratory surgery. Consequently, neither patients nor clinicians will accept large numbers of false positive screening results. Even a test with 98% specificity would result in 50 surgical procedures for every case of ovarian cancer detected on screening the postmenopausal population. A screening test for this population requires 99.6% specificity to yield a positive predictive value (PPV) of 10% (*i.e.* 10 operations for each case of cancer detected).[9] Lower specificity may be acceptable in high-risk populations (*e.g.* those with a strong family history of ovarian cancer), because their incidence of ovarian cancer will be higher.

A variety of different modalities have been used to detect ovarian cancer in asymptomatic women. These will be considered individually and then in combination, in the context of multimodal screening.

Vaginal examination

Most investigators would agree that this modality lacks sufficient sensitivity and specificity for asymptomatic screening. Evidence for this includes the following. One study[10] found that 18 of 24 patients with benign ovarian cysts, two with borderline malignancies and one with ovarian cancer, had 'normal' vaginal examinations prior to ultrasound. Another study of 4000 postmenopausal women[11] found that vaginal examination had a specificity of 97.3% for ovarian cancer but a specificity of 99.6% is required to achieve a positive predictive value of 10% in postmenopausal women. Vaginal examination remains important in the assessment of women presenting with gynaecological symptoms, but cannot be recommended as a first-line screening tool.

Tumour markers

The ability to detect human malignancy via a simple blood test has long been an objective in medical screening. The advantages of such an easy-to-use, relatively non-invasive and operator-independent test are self-evident. A variety of ovarian tumour markers have been studied. The most extensively investigated is CA125. This antigen was first recognised in 1981, using a murine monoclonal antibody developed in response to immunological challenge with an ovarian cancer cell line.[12] CA125 levels were found to be elevated in 50% of stage I and 90% of stage II ovarian cancers,[13] and in retrospective analysis, 25% of 59 samples stored more than 5 years prior to diagnosis had elevated levels of CA125.[14] Sensitivity for stage I disease using a simple cut-off of 30 IU/ml was limited; however, CA125 was capable of preclinical detection of ovarian cancer. Using CA125 with a cut-off of 30 IU/ml also lacks specificity, as the marker can be elevated in a variety of other conditions, both benign and malignant (*e.g.* fibroids, endometriosis, menstruation, endometrial cancer, many non-ovarian malignancies, pancreatitis, colitis, pericarditis, diverticulitis, and SLE).[15] Any condition which results in inflammation of a mesothelium-derived surface (pleura, peritoneum, pericardium, *etc.*) can cause an elevated CA125 level. The measurement of CA125 in patients with ascites but no pelvic mass risks an erroneous diagnosis of ovarian cancer.[16] Despite these limitations, CA125 has been used in prospective ovarian cancer screening trials, either alone, or in combination with ultrasound (Table 3). The largest CA125-based trial so far published has suggested that even using a simple CA125 cut-off as a first-line test may improve survival in the screened population.[17]

Important progress has been made by a more sophisticated approach to interpretation of CA125 results, using an algorithm incorporating age and rate

Table 3 Prospective ovarian cancer screening studies in the general population

Study	Population	Screening strategy	No. screened	No. of invasive EOC detected[a]	No. of positive screens	No. of oper./cancers detected
		CA125 alone				
Einhorn et al. 1992[31]	Age ≥ 40 years	CA125	5550	6; 2 stage I	175[b]	29[b]
		Multimodal approach – CA125 (level 1 screen), then USS (level II screen)				
Menon et al. 2003[32]	Age ≥ 50 years, postmenopausal	CA125, ROCA TVS if ROC↑	6532	3 (1); 2 stage I	16	5.3
Jacobs et al. 1999[17]	Age ≥ 45 years, postmenopausal	RCT, CA125, TAS/TVS if CA125↑	10,958; 3 annual screens	6; 3 stage I	29	4.8
Jacobs et al. 1996[33]	Age ≥ 45 years, postmenopausal	CA125, TAS if CA125↑	22,000	11; 4 stage I	41	3.7
Adonakis et al. 1996[34]	Age ≥ 45 years	CA125, TVS if CA125↑	2000	1(1); 1 stage I	15	15
Grover et al. 1995[35]	Age ≥ 40 years or family history (3%)	CA125, TAS/TVS if CA125↑	2550	1; 0 stage I	16	16
		USS-only approach – USS (level 1 screen), then repeat USS (level II screen)				
van Nagell et al. 2000[36]	Age ≥ 50 years and postmenopausal or ≥ 30 with family history	TVS; annual screens; mean 4 screens/woman	14,469	11 (6); 5 stage I	180	16.3
Sato et al. 2000[37]	Part of general screening programme	TVS; TVS + markers at level II	51,550	22; 17 stage I	324	14.7
Hayashi et al. 1999[38]	Age ≥ 50 years	TVS	23,451	3 (3); 2 stage I	258	13.6[c]
Tabor et al. 1994[39]	Aged 46–65 years	TVS	435	0	9	–
Campbell et al. 1989[26]	Age ≥ 45 years or with family history (4%)	TAS; 3 screens at 18 monthly intervals	5479	2 (3); 2 stage I	326	163
Millo et al. 1989[40]	Age ≥ 45 years or postmenopausal (mean 54)	USS (mode not specified)	500	0	11	–
Goswamy et al. 1983[41]	Age 39–78 years postmenopausal	TAS	1084	1; 1 stage I	–	–
		USS and CD (level I screen)				
Kurjak et al. 1995[42]	Aged 40–71 years	TVS and CD	5013	4; 4 stage I	38	9.5
Vuento et al. 1995[43]	Aged 56–61 years	TVS and CD	1364	(1)	5	–
		USS (level 1) and other test (level II screen)				
Parkes et al. 1994[44]	Aged 50–64 years	TVS then CD if TVS positive	2953	1; 1 stage I	14[d]	9
Holbert et al. 1994[8]	Postmenopausal, aged 30–89 years	TVS then CA125 if TVS positive	478	1; 1 stage I	33[e]	11

Some of these studies have previously been reported in earlier publications. To avoid data duplication, these have not been included in this table. EOC, epithelial ovarian cancer; RCT, randomised controlled trial; ROCA, risk of ovarian cancer algorithm; TAS, transabdominal ultrasound; TVS, transvaginal ultrasound; USS, ultrasound; CD, colour Doppler; oper., operations. [a]Primary invasive epithelial ovarian cancers. The borderline/granulosa tumours detected are shown in parenthesis. [b]Not all of these women underwent surgical investigation as the study design involved intensive surveillance rather than surgical intervention. [c]Only 95 women consented to surgery and there are no follow-up details on the remaining. [d]86 women had abnormal USS prior to CD. [e]Only 11 of these women underwent surgery.

of change of CA125 as well as absolute level.[18] This algorithm is based on the observation that women with ovarian cancer have rising levels of CA125 and women without ovarian cancer have static or falling levels, even if the levels remain above 30 IU/ml. This algorithm yielded a sensitivity of 83%, a specificity of 99.7% and a positive predictive value of 16% for predicting a woman's risk of developing ovarian cancer in the year following her last screen. Because this algorithm analyses rate of change of CA125 values, rather than a simple cut-off level, women with ovarian cancer can be recalled for an ultrasound scan before their CA125 level has reached 30 IU/ml, thus increasing sensitivity and facilitating earlier intervention. This 'risk of ovarian cancer' (ROC) algorithm is an important component of the UKCTOCS randomised controlled trial of ovarian cancer screening (see below).

The use of a combination of markers to increase sensitivity and specificity has been extensively investigated and some of the most promising include CA72-4 (TAG 72), M-CSF, OVX1, LPA, prostacin, osteopontin, inhibin and kallikrein.[19] Many of these exhibit complementarity to CA125 (*e.g.* mucinous tumours, which tend not to produce CA125, do produce some of these markers). The use of a panel of markers as a first-line test in ovarian screening is an attractive concept. The power of this strategy depends on interpretation of the pattern of different marker levels in relationship to each other, rather than the absolute levels of each marker. This can lead to observations which would be missed by less sophisticated analysis; for example, a fall in the level of marker A in relation to marker B may be associated with an increased risk of having a disease, whereas a rise in marker A may reduce the risk. Developments in bioinformatics may facilitate this strategy using either new markers or markers which have already been identified.

Recently, the use of surface-enhanced laser desorption ionisation time of flight (SELDI-TOF) mass spectrometry (MS) to analyse the serum proteome has been suggested as a possible means of screening asymptomatic women for ovarian cancer.[20] This technique involves using a laser to ionise the thousands of proteins contained in serum samples (the serum 'proteome') and separating them according to their molecular weight using the principle that heavier ions take longer to travel a set distance than lighter ions. Preliminary data[20] have demonstrated the ability of SELDI-TOF MS to differentiate women with ovarian cancer from healthy controls on the basis of the pattern of different proteins detected in their serum. These data have subsequently been criticised for the following reasons. First, the technique of protein pattern analysis used is a 'black box' technology, *i.e.* the complex statistical algorithm used to discriminate between cancer cases and controls is not transparent, and re-analysis of the raw MS data by other groups, using their own algorithms has suggested that the differences identified may have been an artefact.[21] Second, no specific proteins were identified as discriminating cancer cases from controls.[22] Third, the particular MS technique (SELDI) used in the study is not considered to be the most sensitive for the detection of subtle changes in the serum proteome, and matrix-assisted laser desorption ionisation time of flight (MALDI-TOF) MS may be a more appropriate technique.[23] Nevertheless, other groups have also used SELDI-based techniques to identify specific serum proteins in ovarian cancer.[24,25] In addition, MALDI-TOF has already been used successfully to gain prognostic information from biopsies in lung cancer.[26] The use of proteomic technology in screening for a variety of diseases is under investigation but has not been validated for use in a prospective ovarian cancer screening trial. The use of the CA125-based ROC algorithm has already enabled the implementation of single marker serum screening into a randomised controlled trial and we do not need to wait for the emergence of novel techniques before embarking on large-scale studies.

Ultrasound

Various different methods of ultrasonic assessment of the ovaries have been investigated. The first of these was standard transabdominal pelvic ultrasound.[27] This technique lacked sufficient specificity as over 50 women underwent surgical investigation for each case of cancer detected. The lack of specificity was due to the relatively poor resolution of the older ultrasound equipment used, in addition to the difficulties of imaging the pelvic organs through the abdominal wall. This problem has been successfully addressed by the development of transvaginal scanning, which offers greater resolution by virtue of closer proximity of the probe to the ovaries and improved morphological assessment. There have been attempts to quantify this information in the form of a morphological index, so that ovaries can be scored for their risk of malignancy.[28] This type of analysis has established a very low risk of ovarian cancer in simple cysts < 10 cm in diameter.[29] Specificity has been further enhanced by colour flow Doppler imaging; the neovasculature which arises in malignancies contains less smooth muscle than its benign counterpart and, therefore, offers less resistance to blood flow. This can be measured as the pulsatility index of the vessel. This technique has been used in a scoring system,[30] which incorporates the distribution of the vessels.

Other modalities

Other methods used to image ovarian cancer include 3 D ultrasound, computerised tomography, magnetic resonance imaging and radioimmuno-scintigraphy. None of these can currently be advocated as a first-line test for population screening due to cost, availability, patient acceptability and/or radiation exposure. These modalities may have a role in ovarian cancer screening when first-line tests (tumour markers and/or ultrasound) demonstrate that a patient is at a significantly increased risk of having an ovarian malignancy and so reduce the number of patients without cancer being referred for surgery.

Multimodal screening

The results of screening the general population with tumour markers and ultrasound individually, in combination, and sequentially are shown in Table 3. These data would suggest that the highest PPV can be achieved with multimodal screening, using CA125 as a first-line test, followed by ultrasound if CA125 is abnormal. However, the sensitivity of ultrasound as a first-line test for early stage ovarian cancer may be greater than that of CA125.

The use of multimodal screening to detect early ovarian cancer has three main advantages over strategies incorporating a single modality. First, using serum screening as a first-line test reduces cost. Second, reserving ultrasound as a secondary test reduces the number of women undergoing transvaginal assessment. Finally, combining different modalities can achieve sensitivity and specificity comparable to that of the most sophisticated protocols utilising colour flow Doppler ultrasound and morphological indices. Nevertheless, it remains to be proven that CA125, even if used with the ROC algorithm, has adequate sensitivity for early stage disease and consequently the use of ultrasound as a first-line test is also being investigated in the UKCTOCS trial (see below).

Two randomised controlled trials incorporating multimodal screening are currently underway. The first of these, the US NIH PLCO study,[3] will randomise 74,000 women over 60 years old to a control group or screening with clinical examination, ultrasound and CA125. Any abnormal tests will result in referral to a gynaecological oncologist for further investigation. The study duration to achieve 80% power for a 30% reduction in mortality is 16 years. The other study is UKCTOCS,[2] which aims to recruit 200,000 postmenopausal women aged 50–74 years old (Fig. 1). This trial opened in 2001 and has so far recruited over 150,000 women. These volunteers are being randomised to a control group or annual screening with CA125 or transvaginal ultrasound scanning (TVS). On the basis of the pattern of CA125 results analysed by the ROC algorithm, volunteers will be allocated to a low-risk group (annual CA125), intermediate-risk group (repeat CA125 sooner) or an elevated-risk group (TVS). An abnormal scan will trigger referral for surgery. This study has 80% power to detect a 30% reduction in mortality and should report in 2012. In a recently completed pilot study of 6532 women screened using the ROC algorithm,[32] a specificity of 99.8% and PPV 23.1% were achieved. This suggests that the ROC algorithm is suitable for assessment in the UKCTOCS trial.

On present evidence, some form of multimodal screening will probably provide the most cost-effective and acceptable strategy for the detection of early ovarian cancer in the general population.

THE TEST SHOULD BE ACCEPTABLE TO THE POPULATION

The successes of breast and cervical screening programmes have demonstrated that large numbers of women are willing to undergo uncomfortable and intimate examination at regular intervals in order to reduce their risk of dying from cancer. Few studies of the acceptability of ovarian cancer screening are available and socio-economic and demographic factors may influence acceptability.[45] Lower uptake rates in low socio-economic groups have provided cause for concern in breast and cervical screening programs as the incidence of these cancers is inversely related to social class. Ovarian cancer is more prevalent in professional classes[46] and employment was significantly associated with screening by ultrasound in women with a family history of ovarian cancer.[47] In the latter study, use of CA125 was associated with both an increasing number of affected family members and cancer worries, which increased ultrasound usage in women with one affected relative. These data suggest that women's fear of cancer exceeds their fear of screening, particularly when they have personal experience of malignancy, and that screening may be more acceptable to a population at higher risk.

A study of the acceptability of TVS in an English inner-city population[48] found that 76% of respondents were willing to be screened, but that women over 65 years were significantly less likely to accept screening compared to younger women, as were Caucasians compared to other ethnic groups. The

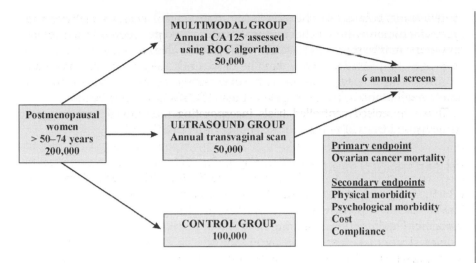

Fig. 1 UKCTOCS trial design. All women will be followed up for 7 years via 'flagging' through the Office of National Statistics and via postal questionnaires.

overall uptake of ultrasound screening in this study was 43% and, as expected, women who reported that they were less frightened of vaginal examination were more willing to undergo screening. Further evidence of test acceptability comes from a large pilot randomised trial of multimodal screening,[17] in which compliance with annual screening only fell marginally from 80% at the first screen to 77% at the third screen. More recently, our group performed a pilot study of test acceptability comparing venepuncture, cervical smears, mammography and transvaginal scanning amongst 100 randomly selected women aged 50–80 years, who had taken part in our pilot ovarian screening trial and had experienced all four screening techniques (U. Menon, personal communication). Over 80% of the 91 women returning the questionnaire rated venepuncture as their preferred screening method and transvaginal scanning had a similar level of acceptability to cervical cytology and mammography. A similar study of 54 women in an ovarian screening trial found TVS significantly less uncomfortable than smears or mammograms.[49] Recent evidence[50] from a more intensive screening protocol found that compliance with 6-monthly screening in 292 average to intermediate risk women fell from 97% of to 64% over 18 months, and compliance with TVS was worse than that with CA125. We conclude that the methods currently employed in annual ovarian screening are largely acceptable to the majority of women, but if a reduced screening interval is required, compliance may fall.

NATURAL HISTORY OF THE CONDITION, INCLUDING DEVELOPMENT FROM LATENT TO DECLARED DISEASE, SHOULD BE ADEQUATELY UNDERSTOOD

This is the requirement for screening least fulfilled by our knowledge of ovarian cancer. Although many of the molecular events in ovarian carcinogenesis have been identified, proof of the existence of a precursor lesion is still absent. At the present time, we must consider stage I as the 'latent disease'. However, this is problematic because of the possibility that stage I disease represents an indolent tumour whose behaviour is very different from more advanced stage tumours; maybe stage I disease never progresses and the patient succumbs to old age, completely unaware that she harbours a malignancy. Conversely, if transition from stage I to stage II occurs rapidly, then unless very short screening intervals are used, even the most sensitive and specific test is unlikely to reduce mortality. These issues are being addressed by the ongoing randomised trials of population screening described above.

THERE SHOULD BE AN AGREED POLICY ON WHOM TO SCREEN

As the incidence of a disease increases, the specificity required to achieve a given positive predictive value decreases. Thus a test which lacks the specificity required for screening the general population may be suitable in a high-risk population.

The 'high-risk' population

The results of screening studies in high-risk populations are summarised in Table 4. These data suggest that screening the high-risk population with established techniques has an acceptable PPV. However, annual screening does not detect all cancers at an early stage, interval cancers can occur and ovaries removed prophylactically can contain unsuspected malignancy. A recent meta-analysis[51] has suggested that screen-detected ovarian cancers in familial cases are not usually the high-grade serous carcinomas, which carry a poor prognosis, but rather tumours with better prognosis. This implies that screening this population using previous strategies may not reduce mortality, and consequently prophylactic oophorectomy on completion of child-bearing may be a safer option. Nevertheless, there remains a need to offer screening to women unwilling or not ready to undergo such surgery. Because an optimal screening strategy has yet to be defined, Cancer Research UK and the US NCI are supporting the UK Familial Ovarian Cancer Screening Study (UKFOCSS) to establish the optimum screening regimen in women with a > 10% life-time risk of ovarian cancer (Fig. 2). As it is considered unethical to randomise such a high-risk group to a non-screening arm, all volunteers are having annual CA125 and TVS at local centres. They are also providing 4-monthly serum samples for storage and retrospective analysis for novel tumour markers. A familial risk of ovarian cancer index will be calculated retrospectively, based on marker levels and scan results, combined with the knowledge of whether or not an individual developed ovarian cancer in the year following each screen. It is hoped that this strategy will facilitate the introduction of a validated screening programme for the high-risk population.

The general population

The two randomised controlled trials of screening in the general population described above both involve postmenopausal women only. The reasons for choosing the postmenopausal population are 3-fold. First, the incidence of epithelial ovarian cancer increases rapidly after the age of 50 years, such that the rate more than doubles in the 60–64 year age group as compared to the 45–49 year group.[5] Less than 15% of ovarian cancers occur in women under 50

Table 4 Prospective ovarian cancer screening studies in women with family history of ovarian or breast cancer or personal history of breast cancer

Study	Population	No. screened (% premeno.)	Screening protocol	No. referred for diag. tests (%)[a]	No. of invasive EOC detected (borderline tumours)	Cancers in screen –ve women
Weiner et al. 1993[52]	PMH of BC	600	TVS and CD	12 (3)	3; 1 Stage I	Not stated
Muto et al. 1993[53]	Aged > 25 yrs; FH of OC	384 (85)	TVS and CA125	15 (4)	0	Not stated
Belinson et al. 1995[54]	Aged > 23 yrs (mean 43 yrs); FH of OC	137	TVS and CD and CA125	5 (2)	1	Not stated
Menkiszak et al. 1998[55]	Aged > 20 yrs; FH of BC/OC	124	TVS and CA125 (6 monthly)	Not available	1 (3)	Not available
Karlan et al. 1993[56]	Aged >35 yrs; FH of OC, BC endometrial or colon cancer, PMH of BC	597[b] (75)	TVS and CD and CA125 6 monthly until 1995 then annually	10 (2)	0 (1)	Not stated
Karlan et al. 1999[57]		1261		Not stated	1 EOC (2), 3 PP, 1 Stage 1	4 PP (5, 6, 15, 16 months)
Dorum et al. 1996[58]	Aged > 25 yrs (mean <3 yrs); Strict criteria for FH of BC/OC	180[b]	TVS and CA125	16 (9)	4 (3)	2[c]
Dorum et al. 1999[59]		803		Not stated	16 (4)	Not stated
van Nagell et al. 2000[36]	FH of OC	3299	TVS then CD and CA125	Not stated	3 (1); 2 stage 1	2 (12, 14 months)
Taylor & Schwartz 2001[60]	Aged > 30 yrs; FH of OC	252 (83)	TVS and CD and CA125	3 (1)		1 (12 months)
Scheuer et al. 2002[61]	Aged > 35 yrs; BRCA1/2 mutation carriers	62	TVS and CA125 (6 monthly)	22 (36); 10 had surgery	4 EOC, 1 PP; 3 stage I	0[d]
Laframboise et al. 2002[62]	Aged > 22 yrs (mean 47 yrs); Strict criteria for FH of BC/OC	311	TVS and CA125 (6 monthly)	9 (3)	1 stage 1	Not stated
Tailor et al. 2003[63]	Aged > 17 yrs (mean 47 yrs); FH of OC	2500 (65)	TVS then CD	104 (3)	6 (4); 4 stage I	2 PP (20–40months); 7 EOC (9–46 months)
Fries et al. 2004[64]	Aged >28 yrs (mean 53 yrs); FH of OC/BC	53	TVS and CA125 (6 monthly)	3[e] (6)	0	Not stated

Some of these studies have previously been reported in earlier publications. To avoid data duplication, these have not been included in this table.
PMH, personal history; FH, family history; OC, ovarian cancer; BC, breast cancer; EOC, epithelial ovarian cancer; PP, primary peritoneal cancer; TVS, transvaginal ultrasound; CD, colour flow Doppler; premeno, premenopausal; diag. test, diagnostic tests; –ve, negative.
[a]Following positive secondary screens. [b]Incorporated in reference below. [c]Further 13 women underwent oophorectomy for BC, 2 had EOC not detected by TVS. [d]2 women who opted for oophorectomy with normal scans and CA125 had stage 1 EOC. [e]All three had surgery.

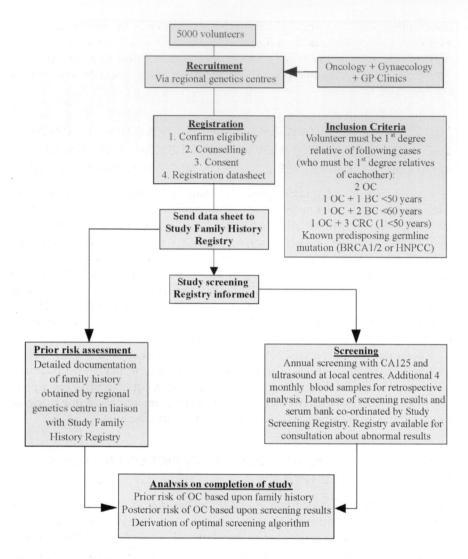

Fig. 2 Summary of the design and inclusion criteria of the UK Familial Ovarian Cancer Screening Study (UKFOCSS). OC, ovarian cancer; BC, breast cancer; CRC, colorectal cancer; HNPCC, hereditary non-polyposis colorectal cancer.

years and many of the malignancies in the younger age groups are non-epithelial and, therefore, either not amenable to screening by CA125 or have an excellent prognosis anyway. Consequently, screening younger age groups with a low incidence of ovarian cancer will reduce the specificity and hence the PPV of screening. Second, many of the physiological and benign pathological conditions associated with raised CA125 (*e.g.* menstruation, endometriosis and fibroids) occur either exclusively or more commonly in premenopausal women. Third, if premenopausal women were to be scanned, a variety of physiological and benign pathophysiological conditions of the ovary (*e.g.* functional cysts, endometriomas, *etc.*) would result in a greater number of 'abnormal' ultrasound scans and possibly higher rates of unnecessary surgical intervention in an age-group with a lower incidence of cancer. Use of a morphological index has its difficulties in the post-menopausal population, not least because of the reluctance of many patients and gynaecologists to ignore persistent abnormalities, despite some of these being at low risk of ovarian cancer.[29]

THE COST OF CASE-FINDING (INCLUDING DIAGNOSIS AND TREATMENT OF PATIENTS DIAGNOSED) SHOULD BE ECONOMICALLY BALANCED IN RELATION TO POSSIBLE EXPENDITURE ON MEDICAL CARE AS A WHOLE

In the absence of adequately powered trials of ovarian cancer screening, computer modelling has been used to estimate the cost per year of life saved.[65] Accepting the limitations with such techniques, it was concluded that even if the variance of rate of disease progression was higher than that used in the initial model, the cost of ultrasound was lower, or only 80% of tumours produced CA125 (instead of the 95% used in the initial analysis) then a multimodal approach was still the most cost-effective method of mass screening. A cost of less than $100,000 per year of life saved was achieved using annual CA125 screening as a first-line test, prompting TVS only if the value doubled since the previous screen or was > 35 IU/ml.

More information on cost will be available following completion of the UKCTOCS and PLCO trials. These data are extremely important to convince governments and health insurers that ovarian screening is worth funding. At the present time, UK health insurance companies are not recommending or funding ovarian screening as it has yet to be proven effective.

CASE-FINDING SHOULD BE A CONTINUING PROCESS AND NOT A 'ONCE AND FOR ALL' PROJECT

Clearly, if a disease can develop at any time over many years, then very little effect on mortality can be achieved if women are screened only once. The difficulty with ovarian cancer is to know how often to screen. Little is known of the natural history of the disease, in particular the rate at which it progresses. Even if this were known, the frequency of screening is often a compromise between what is felt to be the optimum screen interval, the test's cost and how often the population is willing to be tested. This complex interaction generally results in an evolving screening programme, which unfortunately is often controlled by health budgets rather than rigorous scientific analysis.

CONCLUSIONS

Ovarian cancer screening remains an enormous challenge. Following advances in tumour marker and ultrasound technology, combined with appropriate statistical design, the results of two large adequately powered randomised controlled trials of screening are eagerly awaited. In the meantime, further efforts should be concentrated on the discovery of even more sensitive and specific techniques for population screening. Serum proteomics appears to hold great promise, but requires rigorous validation before it can be incorporated into a randomised trial.

Key points for clinical practice

- Vaginal examination of asymptomatic women is neither sensitive nor specific enough to be used to screen for ovarian cancer.

- Many physiological, benign and malignant conditions can cause a high CA125, but rising levels of CA125 (even within the 'normal range') should raise the suspicion of an occult ovarian or primary peritoneal cancer. Conversely, measuring CA125 in patients presenting with ascites but no pelvic mass is unhelpful and may prompt unnecessary surgery.

- Screening with transvaginal ultrasound has high sensitivity for ovarian cancer, but may result in the detection of benign lesions, prompting unnecessary surgery.

- Ovarian cancer screening has the potential to cause psychological and physical morbidity and is currently of unproven benefit. Consequently, general population screening in the UK should not be performed outside of the context of the UKCTOCS randomised controlled trial.

- Women at high-risk of ovarian cancer due to a strong family history or documented germline mutation can be offered screening if they wish to avoid prophylactic oophorectomy. They should not undergo screening without being informed of its limitations. If they opt for screening, they should be offered participation in the UKFOCSS study to facilitate systematic screening data collection for retrospective analysis.

- Large randomised controlled trials in the general population are underway and should provide definitive evidence about the efficacy of ovarian cancer screening. Prospective studies of screening in the high-risk population are also in progress and should provide data on optimal screening strategies in this group.

Acknowledgement

We thank Usha Menon for providing Tables 3 and 4, which we have updated for this review.

References

1. Barnholtz-Sloan JS, Schwartz AG, Qureshi F, Jacques S, Malone J, Munkarah AR. Ovarian cancer: changes in patterns at diagnosis and relative survival over the last three decades. *Am J Obstet Gynecol* 2003; **189**: 1120–1127.
2. <http://www.ukctocs.org.uk/>.
3. Prorok PC, Andriole GL, Bresalier RS *et al.*, Prostate, Lung, Colorectal and Ovarian

Cancer Screening Trial Project Team. Design of the Prostate, Lung, Colorectal and Ovarian (PLCO) Cancer Screening Trial. *Control Clin Trials* 2000; **21 (6 Suppl)**: 273S–309S.

4. Wilson J, Jungner G. *WHO Principles and Practise of Screening for Disease.* Geneva: WHO, 1968; 66–67.

5. Office of National Statistics. *Cancer statistics registrations 2001.* Series MB1, No. 32. London: HMSO, <http://www.statistics.gov.uk/downloads/theme_health/MB1_32/MB1_32.pdf>.

6. FIGO (International Federation of Gynecology and Obstetrics) annual report on the results of treatment in gynecological cancer. *Int J Gynecol Obstet* 2003; **83 (Suppl 1)**: ix–xxii, 1–229.

7. Benedet JL, Hacker NF, Ngan HYS *et al.* Staging classifications and clinical practice guidelines of gynaecologic cancers. <http://www.figo.org/content/PDF/staging-booklet.pdf>.

8. Holbert TR. Screening transvaginal ultrasonography of postmenopausal women in a private office setting. *Am J Obstet Gynecol* 1994; **170**: 1699–1703.

9. Jacobs I, Oram D. Screening for ovarian cancer. *Biomed Pharmacother* 1988; **42**: 589–596.

10. Andolf E, Svalenius E, Astedt B. Ultrasonography for early detection of ovarian carcinoma. *Br J Obstet Gynaecol* 1986; **93**: 1286–1289.

11. Jacobs IJ, Oram DH. Potential screening tests for ovarian cancer. In: Sharp F, Mason WP, Leake RE. (eds) *Ovarian Cancer.* London: Chapman and Hall, 1990; 197–205.

12. Bast Jr RC, Feeney M, Lazarus H, Nadler LM, Colvin RB, Knapp RC. Reactivity of a monoclonal antibody with human ovarian carcinoma. *J Clin Invest* 1981; **68**: 1331–1337.

13. Zurawski Jr VR, Knapp RC, Einhorn N *et al.* An initial analysis of preoperative serum CA 125 levels in patients with early stage ovarian carcinoma. *Gynecol Oncol* 1988; **30**: 7–14

14. Zurawski Jr VR, Orjaseter H, Andersen A, Jellum E. Elevated serum CA 125 levels prior to diagnosis of ovarian neoplasia; relevance for early detection of ovarian cancer. *Int J Cancer* 1988; **42**: 677–680.

15. Jacobs I, Bast Jr RC. The CA 125 tumour-associated antigen: a review of the literature. *Hum Reprod* 1989; **4**: 1–12.

16. Silberstein LB, Rosenthal AN, Coppack SW, Noonan K, Jacobs IJ. Ascites and a raised serum CA 125 – confusing combination. *J R Soc Med* 2001; **94**: 581–582.

17. Jacobs IJ, Skates SJ, MacDonald N *et al.* Screening for ovarian cancer: a pilot randomised controlled trial. *Lancet.* 1999; **353**: 1207–1210.

18. Skates SJ, Menon U, MacDonald N *et al.* Calculation of the risk of ovarian cancer from serial CA-125 values for preclinical detection in postmenopausal women. *J Clin Oncol* 2003; **21 (10 Suppl)**: 206–210.

19. Menon U, Jacobs IJ. Tumour markers and screening. In: Berek JS, Hacker NF. (eds) *Practical Gynecologic Oncology,* 4th edn. Philadelphia, PA: Lippincott, Williams and Wilkins, 2005; 43–66.

20. Petricoin EF, Ardekani AM, Hitt BA *et al.* Use of proteomic patterns in serum to identify ovarian cancer. *Lancet.* 2002; **359**: 572–577.

21. Sorace JM, Zhan M. A data review and re-assessment of ovarian cancer serum proteomic profiling. *BMC Bioinformatics* 2003; **4**: 24.

22. Diamandis EP. Mass spectrometry as a diagnostic and a cancer biomarker discovery tool: opportunities and potential limitations. *Mol Cell Proteomics* 2004; **3**: 367–378.

23. Villanueva J, Philip J, Entenberg D *et al.* Serum peptide profiling by magnetic particle-assisted, automated sample processing and MALDI-TOF mass spectrometry. *Anal Chem* 2004; **76**: 1560–1570.

24. Zhang Z, Bast Jr RC, Yu Y *et al.* Three biomarkers identified from serum proteomic analysis for the detection of early stage ovarian cancer. *Cancer Res* 2004; **64**: 5882–5890.

25. Ye B, Cramer DW, Skates SJ *et al.* Haptoglobin-alpha subunit as potential serum biomarker in ovarian cancer: identification and characterization using proteomic profiling and mass spectrometry. *Clin Cancer Res* 2003; **9**: 2904–2911.

26. Yanagisawa K, Shyr Y, Xu BJ *et al.* Proteomic patterns of tumour subsets in non-small-cell lung cancer. *Lancet* 2003; **362**: 433–439.

27. Campbell S, Bhan V, Royston P, Whitehead MI, Collins WP. Transabdominal ultrasound screening for ovarian cancer. *BMJ* 1989; **299**: 1363–1367.

28. DePriest PD, Shenson D, Fried A *et al*. A morphology index based on sonographic findings in ovarian cancer. *Gynecol Oncol* 1993; **51**: 7–11.

29. Modesitt SC, Pavlik EJ, Ueland FR, DePriest PD, Kryscio RJ, van Nagell Jr JR. Risk of malignancy in unilocular ovarian cystic tumors less than 10 centimeters in diameter. *Obstet Gynecol* 2003; **102**: 594–599.

30. Kurjak A, Schulman H, Sosic A, Zalud I, Shalan H. Transvaginal ultrasound, color flow, and Doppler waveform of the postmenopausal adnexal mass. *Obstet Gynecol* 1992; **80**: 917–921.

31. Einhorn N, Sjovall K, Knapp RC *et al*. Prospective evaluation of serum CA 125 levels for early detection of ovarian cancer. *Obstet Gynecol* 1992; **80**: 14–18.

32. Menon U, Skates SJ, Lewis S *et al*. A prospective study using the risk of ovarian cancer algorithm to screen for ovarian cancer. *J Clin Oncol* 2005; **23**: In Press.

33. Jacobs IJ, Skates S, Davies AP *et al*. Risk of diagnosis of ovarian cancer after raised serum CA 125 concentration: a prospective cohort study. *BMJ* 1996; **313**: 1355–1358.

34. Adonakis GL, Paraskevaidis E, Tsiga S, Seferiadis K, Lolis DE. A combined approach for the early detection of ovarian cancer in asymptomatic women. *Eur J Obstet Gynecol Reprod Biol* 1996; **65**: 221–225.

35. Grover S, Quinn MA, Weidman P *et al*. Screening for ovarian cancer using serum CA125 and vaginal examination: report on 2550 females. *Int J Gynecol Cancer* 1995; **5**: 291–295.

36. van Nagell Jr JR, DePriest PD, Reedy MB *et al*. The efficacy of transvaginal sonographic screening in asymptomatic women at risk for ovarian cancer. *Gynecol Oncol* 2000; **77**: 350–356.

37. Sato S, Yokoyama Y, Sakamoto T, Futagami M, Saito Y. Usefulness of mass screening for ovarian carcinoma using transvaginal ultrasonography. *Cancer* 2000; **89**: 582–588.

38. Hayashi H, Yaginuma Y, Kitamura S *et al*. Bilateral oophorectomy in asymptomatic women over 50 years old selected by ovarian cancer screening. *Gynecol Obstet Invest* 1999; **47**: 58–64.

39. Tabor A, Jensen FR, Bock JE, Hogdall CK. Feasibility study of a randomised trial of ovarian cancer screening. *J Med Screen* 1994; **1**: 215–219.

40. Millo R, Facca MC, Alberico S. Sonographic evaluation of ovarian volume in postmenopausal women: a screening test for ovarian cancer? *Clin Exp Obstet Gynecol* 1989; **16**: 72–78.

41. Goswamy RK, Campbell S, Whitehead MI. Screening for ovarian cancer. *Clin Obstet Gynaecol* 1983; **10**: 621–643.

42. Kurjak A, Kupesic S. Transvaginal color Doppler and pelvic tumor vascularity: lessons learned and future challenges. *Ultrasound Obstet Gynecol* 1995; **6**: 145–159.

43. Vuento MH, Pirhonen JP, Makinen JI, Laippala PJ, Gronroos M, Salmi TA. Evaluation of ovarian findings in asymptomatic postmenopausal women with color Doppler ultrasound. *Cancer* 1995; **76**: 1214–1218.

44. Parkes CA, Smith D, Wald NJ, Bourne TH. Feasibility study of a randomised trial of ovarian cancer screening among the general population. *J Med Screen* 1994; **1**: 209–214.

45. Pavlik EJ, van Nagell Jr JR, DePriest PD *et al*. Participation in transvaginal ovarian cancer screening: compliance, correlation factors, and costs. *Gynecol Oncol* 1995; **57**: 395–400.

46. Beral V, Fraser P, Chilvers C. Does pregnancy protect against ovarian cancer? *Lancet* 1978; **1**: 1083–1087.

47. Schwartz M, Lerman C, Daly M, Audrain J, Masny A, Griffith K. Utilization of ovarian cancer screening by women at increased risk. *Cancer Epidemiol Biomarkers Prev* 1995; **4**: 269–273.

48. Wolfe CD, Raju KS. The attitudes of women and feasibility of screening for ovarian and endometrial cancers in inner city practices. *Eur J Obstet Gynecol Reprod Biol* 1994; **56**: 117–120.

49. Kew FM, Ashton VJ, Cruickshank DJ. Tolerability of transvaginal ultrasonography as an ovarian cancer screening test. *J Med Screen* 2004; **11**: 45–47.

50. Drescher CW, Nelson J, Peacock S, Andersen MR, McIntosh MW, Urban N. Compliance of average- and intermediate-risk women to semiannual ovarian cancer screening. *Cancer Epidemiol Biomarkers Prev* 2004; **13**: 600–606.

51. Hogg R, Friedlander M. Biology of epithelial ovarian cancer: implications for screening women at high genetic risk. *J Clin Oncol* 2004; **22**: 1315–1327.

52. Weiner Z, Beck D, Shteiner M *et al*. Screening for ovarian cancer in women with breast cancer with transvaginal sonography and color flow imaging. *J Ultrasound Med* 1993; **12**: 387–393.

53. Muto MG, Cramer DW, Brown DL *et al*. Screening for ovarian cancer: the preliminary experience of a familial ovarian cancer center. *Gynecol Oncol* 1993; **51**: 12–20.

54. Belinson JL, Okin C, Casey G *et al*. The familial ovarian cancer registry: progress report. *Cleveland Clin J Med* 1995; **62**: 129–134.

55. Menkiszak J. Jakubowska A. Gronwald J. Rzepka-Gorska I. Lubinski J. [Hereditary ovarian cancer: summary of 5 years of experience: in Polish] *Ginekol Pol* 1998; **69**: 283–287.

56. Karlan BY, Raffel LJ, Crvenkovic G *et al*. A multidisciplinary approach to the early detection of ovarian carcinoma: rationale, protocol design, and early results. *Am J Obstet Gynecol* 1993; **169**: 494–501.

57. Karlan BY, Baldwin RL, Lopez-Luevanos E *et al*. Peritoneal serous papillary carcinoma, a phenotypic variant of familial ovarian cancer: implications for ovarian cancer screening. *Am J Obstet Gynecol* 1999; **180**: 917–928.

58. Dorum A, Kristensen GB, Abeler VM, Trope CG, Moller P. Early detection of familial ovarian cancer. *Eur J Cancer* 1996; **32A**: 1645–1651.

59. Dorum A, Heimdal K, Lovolett K *et al*. Prospectively detected cancer in familial breast/ovarian cancer screening. *Acta Obstet Gynecol Scand* 1999; **78**: 906–911.

60. Taylor KJ, Schwartz PE. Cancer screening in a high risk population: a clinical trial. *Ultrasound Med Biol* 2001; **27**: 461–466.

61. Scheuer L, Kauff N, Robson M *et al*. Outcome of preventive surgery and screening for breast and ovarian cancer in BRCA mutation carriers. *J Clin Oncol* 2002; **20**: 1260–1268.

62. Laframboise S, Nedelcu R, Murphy J, Cole DE, Rosen B. Use of CA-125 and ultrasound in high-risk women. *Int J Gynecol Cancer* 2002; **12**: 86–91.

63. Tailor A, Bourne TH, Campbell S, Okokon E, Dew T, Collins WP. Results from an ultrasound-based familial ovarian cancer screening clinic: a 10-year observational study. *Ultrasound Obstet Gynecol* 2003; **21**: 378–385.

64. Fries MH, Hailey BJ, Flanagan J, Licklider D. Outcome of five years of accelerated surveillance in patients at high risk for inherited breast/ovarian cancer: report of a phase II trial. *Mil Med* 2004; **169**: 411–416

65. Urban N, Drescher C, Etzioni R, Colby C. Use of a stochastic simulation model to identify an efficient protocol for ovarian cancer screening. *Control Clin Trials* 1997; **18**: 251–270.

Index

Page numbers in *italics* refer to tables and figures.

Abused women *see* Domestic violence
α-fetoprotein (AFP), 1
Amnion, 27
Amniotic fluid embolism, 107
Amniotomy, 46
Anaphylaxis, penicillin, 73
Anterior colporrhaphy, 139
Antibiotics
  intrapartum prophylaxis, 70–1, *71–2*
    adverse effects, 73–4
  in pPROM management, 33
  resistance to, 73–4
Aortic aneurysm/dissection, 107, *108*
Appraisal of staff, 130
Artificial urinary sphincters (AUS), 142
Audit of practice, 130

Bacterial infection and pPROM, 29, 31
Bacterial vaginosis and preterm labour, 18, *19*,
  20, 30, 31
Barium enema in endometriosis diagnosis,
  189–90
Bladder neck buttress, 139
Bladder neck slings *see* Sling procedures
Breast cancer risk and PCOS, 153
Building a Safer NHS for Patients (DoH, 2002),
  119

CA125, 246–8, *249*
Caesarean section
  bowel perforation, 107
  rates and indications, 40
Calcium in myometrial cell contraction, 49

Cancers
  incidence and mortality, *243*
  see also specific cancers
Carbon dioxide (CO_2) laser surgery for
  endometriosis, 196–7
Cardiac causes of maternal death, *104*, 107–8
Cardiovascular disease risk with PCOS, 150,
  151, 152
Central obesity in PCOS, 150
Cephalopelvic disproportion, 40
  see also Labour, dysfunctional
Cerebral haemorrhage, 106
Cervical adenocarcinoma
  adenocarcinoma *in situ* (AIS; high-grade
    CGIN), 219, 220
    see also Cervical glandular intra-epithelial
      neoplasia (CGIN)
  and HPV infection, 222
  incidence, 219
  mean age at diagnosis, 222
  micro-invasive, 219, 221
Cervical cancer
  FIGO staging, 232–3
  imaging, 233
  management principles, 234
  natural history, 231–2
  nodal status assessment, 233
  screening programme modifications, 231
  see also Cervical adenocarcinoma
Cervical cancer, surgical management, 233–40
  fertility-sparing, 237
  Figo stages, *235*
    IA1, 234–5
    IA2, 235
    IB1–IIA, 236
    IIB and beyond, 236

III and beyond, 237
historical aspects, 233–4
intra-operative radiotherapy, 239
key points, 240
nerve-sparing, 238
recurrent disease, 238–9
Cervical cerclage, *19*, 20
Cervical damage and pPROM risk, 30
Cervical glandular intra-epithelial neoplasia (CGIN)
diagnosis, 222
key points, 227
low- and high-grade, 220
management
conservative, 222–5
during pregnancy, 226
follow-up, 226–7
hysterectomy, 225–6
pathogenesis, 221–2
pathology, 220–1
Cervical length measurement, 18, *19*, *20*, 21
Cervicovaginal fetal fibronectin test, 18, *19*, 20, 32
CGIN *see* Cervical glandular intra-epithelial neoplasia
Chemoradiation therapy for cervical cancer, 236, 237
Cholesterol, 151
Chorion, 27
Choroid plexus cysts, 9–10
Clindamycin resistance, 73
Clomiphene citrate, 154, 155
Cold-knife conisation (CKC), 223
Collagen in fetal membranes, 28
Colposuspension, 136, 138–9
Computed tomography (CT)
cervical cancer assessment, 233
endometriosis diagnosis, 190
Confidential Enquiries, 101–18
Confidential Enquiry into Maternal and Child Health (CEMACH)
future challenges, 116
maternal death case ascertainment, 103
origins, 101
perinatal death classification, 111
perinatal death enquiries, 109–10
remit, 101, 116
Confidential Enquiry into Maternal Deaths (CEMD)
cases reported by cause, *104*
death rate calculation, 105
history, 101–2
international role, 109
system, 102
see also Maternal deaths
Confidential Enquiry into Stillbirths and Deaths in Infancy (CESDI)
babies born at 27-28 weeks, 114–15
cases reported by cause, *112*
enquiry topics undertaken, *113*

history, 109–10
intrapartum deaths, 111, 113
one-in-ten sample of deaths, 114
perinatal death classification, 111
sudden unexpected deaths in infancy, 115
Continuity of care in obstetrics, 86–7
Copper-bearing intra-uterine devices, 210
Cornual pregnancies, 106
Corticosteroids in pPROM management, 33
Cot death, 115
Cyproterone acetate, 156

Dermoid ovarian cysts, 185
Detrusor overactivity and urinary incontinence surgery, 136–7
Diabetes mellitus and PCOS, 149, 150–1
Domestic violence, 53–63
defined, 53
epidemiology, 53–4
extent during pregnancy, 54
factors affecting women's disclosure of, 58
health professionals' responses
abused women's views on, 58–9
general approach, 56–7
research on maternity-based interventions, 59
routine enquiries, 57–8
summary of good practice, *60*
key points, 61
maternal and fetal health implications, 55–6
risk factors and indicators, 54–5
Domestic Violence Resource Manual (DoH, 2000), 57
Down's syndrome antenatal screening, 1–14
comparison of tests, *6*
development of tests, 1–2
first trimester, 2–5
arguments for, 3
biochemical markers, 4
nuchal translucency measurement, 3–4, 5
future developments
fetal ductus venosus waveform assessment, 11
fetal nasal bone assessment, 10–11
improvement strategies
benchmark timeframes, 7
integrated tests, 5–6
patient information, 7–8
key points, 11–12
National screening programme development, 8–9
second trimester, 2
soft markers, 9–10
Drosperinone, 156
Duloxetine, 135
Dysfunctional labour *see* Labour, dysfunctional
Dyslipidaemia in PCOS, 151
Dystocia *see* Labour, dysfunctional

Ehlers–Danlos syndrome, 30
Electrosurgery for endometriosis, 196–7
Emergency contraception, 209–17
  defined, 209
  key points, 215
  methods, 210
  potential users, 210
  research approaches, 209–10
  women's knowledge
    industrialised countries, 211–13
    non-industrialised countries, 213–14
Endometrial ablation procedures, 159–68
  discontinued, 164–5
  first generation
    audit of, 161
    endometrial resection, 159–60
    neodymium YAG laser, 159
    rollerball ablation, 160–1
    Versapoint, 161
  key points, 167
  new, 165
    Her Option, 165
    Hydro ThermAblator, 165–6
    NovaSure, 166–7
    Thermablate, 166
  second generation, 161–2
    audit of, 162
    microwave ablation, 163–4
    uterine thermal balloon, 162–3
Endometrial cancer/hyperplasia and PCOS,
  152–3
Endometrial laser interstitial thermal therapy
  (ELITT), 164
Endometriosis
  deep
    diagnosis, 201–3
    types, 200–1
  forms of, 194
  imaging, 183–91
    barium enema, 189–99
    CT, 190
    intravenous urography, 190
    key points, 191
    MRI, 185–9, 202, 203
    ultrasound, 183–5, 203
  ovarian endometrioma physiopathology,
    197–8
  postpartum, 68
  theories of, 193
Endometriosis, surgery for advanced disease,
  195–207
  deep endometriosis, 196
    complications, 205
    procedures, 203–5
    results, 205
  history of techniques, 195–6
  key points, 206
  laser and electrosurgery, 196–7

ovarian endometriomas
  cyst size, 198
  procedures, 198–9
  results, 199–200
  summarised, 199
Error management
  audit of practice, 130
  error analysis
    active failures, 124–5
    latent failures, 125–6
    person approach, 122–3
    Swiss cheese model of accident causation,
     123–4
    system approach, 123
  error reporting, 120–1
    National Patient Safety Agency, 121–2
  key points, 131
  lessons from high-reliability organisations,
    127
  process of error production, 129
  risk reduction, 128–30
  root-cause analysis, 127–8
Erythromycin resistance, 73–4
Ethinyl oestradiol, 156
Ethnicity and PCOS, 149
Exenterative surgery, 238–9

Fatty liver, 104, 107
Fertility prognosis with endometrial pathology
  and PCOS, 152–3
Fertility-sparing surgery
  cervical cancer, 237
  high-grade CGIN, 222–5
Fetal breathing movement test, 20–1
Fetal ductus venosus, 11
Fetal fibronectin test, 18, 19, 20, 32
Fetal health and domestic violence, 56
Fetal heart recording, 113
Fetal infection with GBS, 66
Fetal membranes, 27
Fetal nasal bones, 10–11
Fetoprotein, α-, (AFP), 1
FIGO staging of cervical cancer, 232–3
First and Second Trimester Evaluation of Risk
  (FASTER) trial, 5
Fistulas, 41

Gonadotrophin therapy, 155
Group B streptococcus (GBS) in pregnancy,
  65–76
  diagnosis, 70
  epidemiology
    incidence of neonatal sepsis, 67–8
    mother-to-child transmission, 66–7
    neonatal colonisation risk, 67
    prevalence of colonisation in pregnancy,
     66
  maternal infection, 66, 68

neonatal sepsis
 incidence, 67–8
 presentation and management, 69
 prognosis, 69–70
neonatal sepsis prevention
 efficacy of screening, 72–3
 impact of screening adoption in UK, 74
 intrapartum antibiotic prophylaxis, 70–1,
  71–2, 73–4
 management of high risk infants, 72
 screening strategies, 71
 UK practice and guidelines, 74–5
 Strep. agalactiae serotypes, 65–6
 vaccination, 75

Haemorrhage, *104*, 106
Haemorrhagic ovarian cysts, 185
Her Option, 165
Herald of Free Enterprise, 125–6
High-density lipoproteins (HDLs), 151
Hirsutism, 156
Home vs. hospital births *see* Place of birth
Human chorionic gonadotrophin (hCG), 1, 4
Human papillomavirus (HPV) infections, 222,
 231
Hydro ThermAblator (HTA), 165–6
Hyperandrogenism, 150, 156
Hyperinsulinaemia in PCOS, 148, 150
Hysterectomy
 high-grade CGIN treatment, 225–6
 Rutledge classification, 234
Hysterectomy, radical
 history, 233–4
 nerve-sparing technique, 238
Hysterectomy, total and subtotal, 169–81
 comparison of outcomes
  bowel function, 177
  cervical stump problems, 172–3
  hospital stay length, 173, *174*
  lower urinary tract symptoms, 175
  operation time, 173, *174*
  pelvic pain, 178
  peri-/postoperative complications, 175,
   176
  peri-operative blood loss, 173, *174*
  prolapse, 177
  quality of life, 175–7
  sexual life, 178, *179*
  urinary incontinence, 171–2
 factors in method choice, 169–70
 incidence rates, 170
 key points, 180

Infant deaths, 110–11, 115
Infection and pPROM, 29
Inhibin, 2
Insulin metabolism disturbances and PCOS,
 147, 148, 149, 150–1
Insulin sensitising agents, 155–6

Intra-operative radiotherapy (IORT), 239
Intrauterine growth restriction (IUGR), 111
Intravenous urography, 90
Intrinsic sphincter deficiency (ISD), 137

Labour
 advantages of shorter duration, 40–1
 phases of first stage, *42*, 43
 stencils, 43
 see also Place of birth
Labour, dysfunctional, 39–51
 active management technique, 45–6
  amniotomy, 46
  outcomes, 47–8
  oxytocin infusion, 46–7
 defined, 39
 diagnosis, 42
  partography, 42–4
 failure to progress, 40, 41–2
 importance, 40–1
 key points, 50
 pathophysiological research, 48–50
 primagravidae and multigravidae, 41
 terminology, 39–40
Labour, preterm, 15–25
 cause distribution, *16*
 child morbidity and mortality, 15
 prediction and treatment
  asymptomatic pregnant women, 18–20,
   22
  clinical context, 16–17
  key points, 23
  literature searches, 17
  statistical measures, 17–18
  symptomatic pregnant women, 20–2
 as risk factor for pPROM, 28–9
 see also Preterm prelabour rupture of the
  membranes
Laparoscopic colposuspension, 138–9
Laparoscopic ovarian diathermy, 155
Large loop excision of the transformation zone
 (LLETZ), 30, 223–4
Laser depilation, 156
Levonorgestrel emergency contraception, 210
Likelihood ratios (LRs), 17–18
Loop electrosurgical excision procedure (LEEP)
 and pPROM risk, 30

Magnetic resonance imaging (MRI)
 cervical cancer, 233
 endometriosis
  ovarian endometriomas, *186–7*, 187–8
  other sites of deposits, 188, *202*, 203
  sensitivity and specificity, 188–9
  technical aspects, 185, 187
MALDI-TOF mass spectrometry, 248
Marfan's syndrome, 107
Marshall Marchetti Krantz (MMK) procedure,
 139

Maternal anthropometry in preterm labour prediction, 18, *19*
Maternal deaths
    case identification by CEMACH, 103
    cases reported by cause, *104*
    coincidental, *104*, 108–9
    defined, 102–3
    direct, *104*, 105–7
    global picture, 109
    historical trends, 102
    indirect, *104*, 107–8
    late, 103, *104*
    rate calculation, 105
    subgroups, 103
Maternity Home Help Organization (Netherlands), 86
Matrix metalloproteinases, 28
Matrix-assisted laser desorption ionisation time of flight (MALDI-TOF) mass spectrometry, 248
Medical error management *see* Error management
Menorrhagia treatment *see* Endometrial ablation
Menstrual irregularity management in PCOS, 153, 154–5
Mental health impact of domestic violence, 56
Metformin, 155–6
Microwave endometrial ablation (MEA), 163–4
Mid-urethral tape procedures, 139–40
Midwives, 84
Mifepristone (RU486), 210, 212
Mistakes, 124, 125
    see also Error management
MISTLETOE project, 161
Model of Best Practice (DoH, 2003), 6–7
Myocardial infarction, 107, *108*
Myometrial physiology and dysfunctional labour, 48–50

National Patient Safety Agency (NPSA), 121–2
National Sentinel Caesarean Section Audit, 40
Needle excision of the transformation zone (NETZ), 224–5
Needle suspension procedures, 141
Neodymium YAG laser, 159
Neonatal sepsis, 65
    see also Group B streptococcus (GBS) in pregnancy
Neutrophil elastase, 28
NovaSure system, 166–7
Nuchal translucency (NT) measurement, 3–4, 5
Number needed to treat (NNT), 18

Obesity and PCOS, 150, 154
Obstetric Manual (2003), 79, 91–100
    codes for care providers, *91*
    decision tree, *92*
    indications list, 91–2

conditions developing during pregnancy, 96–9
    conditions occurring during birth, 99–100
    conditions occurring during the puerperium, 100
    obstetrical medical history, 95–6
    pre-existing gynaecological disorders, 94–5
    pre-existing non-gynaecological disorders, 92–4
Odds ratio (OR), 18
Oestriol, 1
Oestrogen emergency contraception, 210
Office for National Statistics (ONS), 103
Omissions, 129–30
ORACLE trial, 33
Oral contraceptive pill, 154
Organisation with a Memory, An (DoH, 2000), 119
Ovarian cancer
    management, 245
    presentation, 244
    survival rates, *244*
Ovarian cancer screening, 243–59
    acceptability of tests, 250–1
    cost-effectiveness, 255
    current randomised controlled trials, 250, *251*
    frequency, 255
    general population, *247*, 252, 254–5
    high-risk population, 252, *253*
    issue of 'latent phase', 245, 251–2
    key points, 256
    modalities
        tumour markers, 246–9, *253*
        ultrasound, 249
        vaginal examination, 246
        others, 249
    multimodal screening, *247*, 249–50
    prospective studies
        general population, *247*
        high-risk population, *253*
    specificity requirement, 245–6
Ovarian diathermy, 155
Ovulation induction, 153–4, 155
Oxytocin infusion, 46–7

PAPP-A, 4
Partogram Action Line Study, 44
Partography, 42–4
Patient safety, 119
    see also Risk management in obstetrics
Patient safety incidents (PSIs), 121
PCOS *see* Polycystic ovary syndrome
Pelvic exenteration, 238–9
Pelvic floor exercises, 134
Penicillin, 71, 73
Peri-urethral injections, 141
Perinatal deaths

cases reported by cause, *112*
CESDI/CEMACH classification of causes, 111
confidential enquiry programme
    babies born at 27-28 weeks, 114–15
    future for, 116
    intrapartum deaths, 111, 113
    one-in-ten sample, 114
    topics undertaken by CESDI, *113*
and place of birth, 83–6
reporting of, 111
trends, 110
Peripartum cardiomyopathy, 107
Photodynamic endometrial ablation, 164–5
Place of birth, 77–91
    caregivers' views, 86–7
    conditions to be met for home births, 89
    obstetric interventions and, 82–3
    perinatal mortality/morbidity and, 83–6
    pregnant women's attitudes, 87–8
    referral to secondary care during labour, 80–1
    risk selection of pregnancies, 78–9
    see also Obstetric Manual (2003)
Polycystic ovary syndrome (PCOS), 147–58
    breast cancer risk, 153
    cardiovascular disease risk
        central obesity, 150
        dyslipidaemia, 151
        impaired glucose tolerance/diabetes, 150–1
        in younger women, 151–2
    defined, 147–8, 149
    diagnosis, 148–9
    endometrial cancer/hyperplasia risk, 152–3
    key points, 157
    management, 153–4
        hyperandrogenism and hirsutism, 156
        infertility, 155
        with insulin sensitising agents, 155–6
        menstrual irregularity, 153, 154–5
        obesity, 154
    national/racial differences, 149
    prevalence, 148, 149
Positron emission tomography (PET), cervical cancer assessment, 233
Postcoital contraception *see* Emergency contraception
Postpartum endometriosis, 68
pPROM *see* Preterm prelabour rupture of the membranes
Pregnancy, CGIN management, 226
Pregnancy-induced hypertension, *104*, 106
Pregnancy-related deaths, defined, 103
Preterm labour *see* Labour, preterm
Preterm prelabour rupture of the membranes (pPROM), 27–38
    clinical risk factors, 28–30

complications, 32
defined, 27
diagnosis, 31–2
genetics, 30
key points, 35
management, 33–4
mechanism, 27–8
natural history, 32
prediction, 31
prevention, 31
previable, 34
Project 27/28, 114–15
Prolapse, 177
Proteome analysis in ovarian cancer screening, 248–9
Psychiatric causes of maternal death, *104*, 108
Puerperal psychosis, 108
Puerperal sepsis, *104*, 107
Pulmonary hypertension, 108
Pyoglitazone, 156

Quality of life after hysterectomy, 175–7

Radiofrequency induced endometrial ablation, 164
Radiotherapy for cervical cancer, 234, *235*, 236, 237
    intra-operative, 239
Relative risk (RR), 18
Renal pelvic dilation, 9, 10
Risk management in obstetrics, 119–32
    audit of practice, 130
    error analysis
        active failures, 124–5
        latent failures, 125–6
        person approach, 122–3
        Swiss cheese model of accident causation, 123–4
        system approach, 123
    errors within the NHS, *120*
    event reporting, 120–1
        National Patient Safety Agency, 121–2
        types of incidents, 122
    key points, 131
    lessons from high-reliability organisations, 127
    process of error production, *129*
    risk reduction, 128–30
    root-cause analysis, 127–8
Risk matrices, 128, *129*
Risk of ovarian cancer (ROC) algorithm, 248, 249, 250
Risk scoring, preterm labour, 18, *19*
Rollerball endometrial ablation, 160–1
Root-cause analysis, 127–8
Rosiglitazone, 156
RU486 (mifepristone), 210, 212
Rutledge classification of hysterectomies, 234

Sampson's theory of endometriosis, 193
SELDI-TOF mass spectrometry, 248
Sentinal lymph node identification, cervical cancer, 233
SENTRY programme, 73
Sepsis, puerperal, *104*, 107
Serum, Urine and Ultrasound Screening Study (SURUSS), 4
Sexual function
    after cervical cancer treatment, 232
    after hysterectomy, 178, *179*
Sling procedures
    efficacy, 140–1
    intrinsic sphincter deficiency treatment, 137
    recurrent stress incontinence treatment, 136
Small for gestational age (SGA) infants, 111
Smoking as pPROM risk factor, 28
Socio-economic group and domestic violence, 54–5
Spironolactone, 156
Staff appraisal, 130
Stillbirths, 110, 111, *112*, 114
Streptococcal infections *see* Group B streptococcus (GBS) in pregnancy
Stress incontinence
    after hysterectomy, *171*, 172
    duloxetine treatment, 135
    physiotherapy, 134
    symptomatic and urodynamic evaluation, 135
Stress incontinence surgery, 133–45
    concepts underlying methods, 133–4
    efficacy, 137–8
        anterior colporrhaphy, 139
        artificial urinary sphincter, 142
        bladder neck buttress, 139
        laparoscopic colposuspension, 138–9
        Marshall Marchetti Krantz procedure, 139
        mid-urethral tape procedures, 139–40
        needle suspensions, 141
        open colposuspension, 138
        peri-urethral injections, 141
        slings, 140–1
    factors influencing choice
        detrusor overactivity, 136–7
        intrinsic sphincter deficiency, 137
        previous surgery, 135–6
    key points, 142–3
Sudden infant death syndrome (SIDS), 115
Sudden unexpected deaths in infancy (SUDI), 115
Suicide, pregnancy-associated, 108
Surface-enhanced laser desorption ionisation time of flight (SELDI-TOF) mass spectrometry, 248

Tension-free vaginal tape (TVT), 136, 139–40
Thermablate system, 166
Thiazolinediones, 156
Thrombin, 29
Thrombosis/thromboembolism, *104*, 105
TNF-2 and preterm birth, 30
Tocolysis, *21*, 22, 33
Trachelectomy, radical, 237
Transcervical resection of the endometrium (TCRE), 160
Transobturator tape procedure, 140
Troglitazone, 155–6
Tumour markers for ovarian cancer, 246–9, *253*

UK Collaborative Trial of Ovarian Cancer Screening (UKCTOCS), 250, *251*
UK Familial Ovarian Cancer Screening Study (UKFOCSS), 252, *254*
Ultrasonography
    availability of dating scans, 8–9
    cervical length measurement, 18, *19*, *20*, 21
    Down's syndrome antenatal screening
        fetal ductus venosus waveform assessment, 11
        fetal nasal bone assessment, 10–11
        nuchal translucency measurement, 3–4, 5
        soft markers, 9–10
    endometrial thickness, 153, 154
    endometriosis, 183–5, 203
    fetal breathing movement, *20*, 21
    ovarian cancer screening, 249
    polycystic ovaries, 148
Urinary incontinence
    after hysterectomy, 171–2
    see also Stress incontinence; Stress incontinence surgery
US NIH Prostate, Lung, Colorectal and Ovarian (PLCO) Cancer Screening Trial, 250
Uterine rupture, 107
Uterine thermal balloons, 162–3

Vaccination against GBS, 75
Vaginal bleeding and pPROM, 29
Vaginal examination for ovarian cancer, 246
Venous thromboembolism, *104*, 105
Versapoint, 161
VestaBlate, 164
Vitamin C deficiency and pPROM, 29

Weight and PCOS, 148, 150, 154

Yuzpe regimen, 210